T0191717

Using Event-B for Critical Device Software Systems

Neeraj Kumar Singh

Using Event-B
for Critical
Device Software
Systems

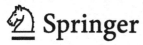 Springer

Neeraj Kumar Singh
Department of Computing and Software
McMaster University
Hamilton, Ontario
Canada

ISBN 978-1-4471-5790-8   ISBN 978-1-4471-5260-6 (eBook)
DOI 10.1007/978-1-4471-5260-6
Springer London Heidelberg New York Dordrecht

© Springer-Verlag London 2013
Softcover re-print of the Hardcover 1st edition 2013
This work is subject to copyright. All rights are reserved by the Publisher, whether the whole or part of
the material is concerned, specifically the rights of translation, reprinting, reuse of illustrations, recitation,
broadcasting, reproduction on microfilms or in any other physical way, and transmission or information
storage and retrieval, electronic adaptation, computer software, or by similar or dissimilar methodology
now known or hereafter developed. Exempted from this legal reservation are brief excerpts in connection
with reviews or scholarly analysis or material supplied specifically for the purpose of being entered
and executed on a computer system, for exclusive use by the purchaser of the work. Duplication of
this publication or parts thereof is permitted only under the provisions of the Copyright Law of the
Publisher's location, in its current version, and permission for use must always be obtained from Springer.
Permissions for use may be obtained through RightsLink at the Copyright Clearance Center. Violations
are liable to prosecution under the respective Copyright Law.
The use of general descriptive names, registered names, trademarks, service marks, etc. in this publication
does not imply, even in the absence of a specific statement, that such names are exempt from the relevant
protective laws and regulations and therefore free for general use.
While the advice and information in this book are believed to be true and accurate at the date of publication, neither the authors nor the editors nor the publisher can accept any legal responsibility for any
errors or omissions that may be made. The publisher makes no warranty, express or implied, with respect
to the material contained herein.

Printed on acid-free paper

Springer is part of Springer Science+Business Media (www.springer.com)

*Dedicated to Lord Krishna, and
My Loving Parents*

Preface

Software systems are pervasive in all walks of life and have become an essential part of our daily life. Information technology is one major area which provides powerful and adaptable opportunities for innovation, and it seems boundless. However, systems developed using computer-based logic have produced disappointing results. According to stakeholders, they are unreliable, at times dangerous, and fail to provide the desired outcomes. Most significant reasons of system failures are the poor development practices for system designs. This is due to the complex nature of modern software and lack of adequate and proper understanding. Software development provides a framework for simplifying a complex system to get a better understanding and to develop the higher fidelity quality systems at lower cost. Highly embedded critical systems, in areas such as automation, medical surveillance, avionics, etc., are susceptible to errors, which can lead to grave consequences in case of failures.

Formal methods have emerged as an alternative approach to ensuring the quality and correctness of the high confidence critical systems, overcoming limitations of the traditional validation techniques such as simulation and testing. The purpose of this book is to provide the use of formal techniques for the development of computing systems with high integrity. Specifically, it addresses the issue that formal methods are not well integrated into established critical systems development processes by defining a new development life-cycle, and a set of associated techniques and tools to develop highly critical systems using formal techniques from requirements analysis to automatic source code generation using several intermediate layers with a rigorous safety assessment approach. The verification and validation tasks are carried out in intermediate layers for providing a correct formal model with desired system behaviour according to stakeholder needs. This methodology combines the refinement approach with various tools including verification tool, model checker tool, real-time animator and finally, produces the source code into multiple languages using automatic code generation tool. The approach has been realised using Event-B formalism. This book presents a set of tools that helps to verify desired properties, which are undiscovered during the system development. Moreover, this approach helps to identify the potential problems at an early stage of the system development. This book also critically evaluates the proposed life-cycle methodology, and associated techniques and tools through a case study in the medical domain, the cardiac pacemaker.

In addition, the book addresses the formal representation of medical protocols, which is useful for improving the existing medical protocols. We formalise a real-world medical protocol (ECG interpretation) to analyse whether the formalisation complies with certain medically relevant protocol properties. The formal verification process discovers several anomalies in the existing protocols, and provides a hierarchical structure for efficient ECG interpretation that helps to find a set of conditions that can help to diagnose particular diseases at an early stage. The main objective of the developed formalism is to test correctness and consistency of the medical protocol.

Outline

This book proposes an advanced development technique for modelling the critical medical systems using stepwise refinement and introduces the rigorous techniques to analyse the complex behaviour. It covers basic and advanced notions of critical systems, real-time animator to find hidden requirements with the help of domain experts, refinement chart to analyse the refinement structure, automatic code generation, heart-model to provide the biological environment for closed-loop modelling and application scenarios for medical systems verification. Moreover, this book presents advanced notion of critical system development from requirement analysis to implementation. The chapters of this book are organised in a coherent way that will help the reader to understand the development of complex medical systems. The book is structured in 11 chapters. Chapters 2 to 7 cover methodology, and techniques and tools for developing any complex critical system related to medical, automotive or avionic domains. The rest of the chapters have particular emphasis in the medical domain. Chapter 2 presents a basic background and development life-cycle related to the safety critical systems. Chapter 3 describes modelling techniques using the Event-B modelling language. In Chap. 4, we propose a development life-cycle methodology for developing the highly critical software systems using formal methods from requirements analysis to code implementation using rigorous safety assessments. In Chap. 5, we propose a novel architecture to validate the formal model with real-time data set in the early stage of development without generating the source code. This architecture can be used for requirement traceability. In Chap. 6, the refinement chart is proposed to handle the complexity and for designing the critical systems. In Chap. 7, we present a tool that automatically generates efficient target programming language code (C, C++, Java and C#) from Event-B formal specification related to the analysis of complex problems. In this chapter, the basic functionality as well as the design-flow is described, stressing the advantages when designing this automatic code generation tool; EB2ALL. In Chap. 8, we present a methodology to model a biological system, like the heart.

The heart model is mainly based on electrocardiography analysis, which models the heart system at the cellular level. The main objective of this methodology is to model the heart system and integrate it with the medical device model like the cardiac pacemaker to specify a closed-loop system. Chapter 9 shows a complete formal development of a cardiac pacemaker using proposed techniques and tools from requirements analysis to automatic code generation. The methodology and techniques are presented in previous chapters. All the essential properties are proven according to the domain experts. In Chap. 10, we present a new application of formal methods to evaluate real-life medical protocols for quality improvement. In this study, we consider a real-life reference protocol (ECG Interpretation) which covers a wide variety of protocol characteristics related to several heart diseases. Chapter 11 summarises this book. The formal development of industrial size case studies, illustrations, and formalisation throughout the text will help the reader to understand the complexity of medical systems and master the intricacies of the more subtle aspects in critical systems analysis.

Acknowledgement

This book is based on my Ph.D. thesis and would not have been possible without the support of a number of people. I would like to express my deep and sincere gratitude to my supervisor Prof. Dominique Méry for his inspiring discussions, enduring supervision and encouragement. His wide knowledge and his logical way of thinking have been of great value for me. His extensive discussions, critical suggestions and interesting explorations around my work have been very helpful for this study. He has also been a kind and effective advisor, allowing me a great amount of freedom while being actively involved in my research and nudging me in the right directions. I thank to the French Ministry of University and Research for grant funding for my Ph.D. study.

I would like to thank the external referees of my Ph.D. thesis, Prof. John Fitzgerald from the University of Newcastle and Prof. Yamine Ait-Ameur from the LISI/ENSMA. It is an honour for me that they were willing to invest their valuable time and effort in the careful reviewing of my thesis. In fact, I am thankful to all members of my Ph.D. committee, Prof. Catherine Dubois, Dr. Yann Guermeur, Dr. Isabelle Perseil, Prof. Olivier Roux and Prof. Dr. Etienne Aliot for fruitful discussions and for the highest support they offered for my work. I am also very thankful to Dr. Isabelle Perseil and Prof. Dominique Méry, who encourage me to publish a book based on my thesis work. I thank Mr. Ben Bishop and Mrs. Beverley Ford from Springer for helping to facilitate the publication of this book.

My sincere thanks also goes to Dr. S. Ramesh, and Dr. Manorajan Satpathi, for offering me the summer internship opportunities in their group (India Science Lab, General Motor, Bangalore, India) and leading me working on diverse exciting projects. I would like to thank Amel Amblard (Clinical Research Manager, Sorin Group-ELA Medicals) and research team of Sorin Group, Paris to demonstrate current challenging problems and to show the development process of a cardiac pacemaker. Furthermore, I thank Prof. Dr. Etienne Alliot, Head of the Cardiology Department of CHU Nancy, and all his colleagues MD doctors, who share their experiences for implanting a cardiac pacemaker and give me an opportunity to learn about the heart system through their fruitful discussions. Furthermore, I am grateful to cardiologist experts Prof. Yves Juillière (MD, Cardiology) and Dr. Frédérique Claudot and biomedical experts Dr. Didier Fass from the INRIA/LORIA, who shared their experiences to discuss and to verify the correctness of the heart model.

I would like to extend my gratitude to Prof. Tom Maibaum and Assoc. Prof. Alan Wassyng from the McMaster University for their advices in the area of certification and pacemaker challenges. Furthermore, I want to acknowledge to Prof. Dominique Cansell, Dr. Stephan Merz, Dr. Pascal Fontaine and Dr. Denis Roegel from the INRIA/LORIA for their advice and time. I also thank Prof. P.K. Kalra from IIT Rajasthan, Prof. Prabhat Munshi from IIT Kanpur and Asst. Prof. M.H. Khan from IET Lucknow for their inspiration.

I thank colleagues, friends, and family members for their support, encouragement, patience, and ideas throughout my studies, including: Late Mr. Kamleshwar Singh, Mr. Jitendra Singh, Mr. Rajkumar Singh, Mr. Shankar Singh, Late Mr. Ratneshwar Singh, Mr. Ravindra Singh, Mr. Surendra Singh, Mr. Sikander Singh, Mr. Updesh Singh, Mr. Manoj Singh, Dr. Pramod, Dinesh, Anurag, and Yogendra.

Especially, I thank my parents, Mrs. Lalita Devi and Mr. Ram Babu Singh, my brothers, Er. Sanjay Singh and Mr. Ranjay Singh, for their continuous support and encouragement, and I thank my wife, Arti, for her valuable support.

Further Sources

This book is based on several sources, particularly chronicles three years of working towards the author's Ph.D. thesis [10]. Chapter 4 covers some material from an article in the Innovations in Systems and Software Engineering [3] and also covers some material from previous work at SoICT [6]. Chapter 5 is an extended version of a previous paper at CSDM [1] and ISoLA [2]. Chapter 6 is a derived version of an article in the ACM Transactions on Embedded Computing Systems [9]. Chapter 7 is a substantially extended version of a previous paper at SoICT [4] that presents the basic framework and development of plug-ins for automatic code generation. In Chap. 8, we extend a previous paper at FHIES [7]. Chapter 9 is a significantly improved and detailed case study on the cardiac pacemaker in the International Journal of Discrete Event Control Systems [5]. Chapter 10 is also detailed version of an article at FHIES [8].

References

1. Méry, D., & Singh, N. K. (2010). Real-time animation for formal specification. In M. Aiguier, F. Bretaudeau, & D. Krob (Eds.), *Complex systems design & management* (pp. 49–60). Berlin: Springer.

2. Méry, D., & Singh, N. K. (2010). Trustable formal specification for software certification. In T. Margaria & B. Steffen (Eds.), *Lecture notes in computer science: Vol. 6416. Leveraging applications of formal methods, verification, and validation* (pp. 312–326). Berlin: Springer.

3. Méry, D., & Singh, N. (2011). A generic framework: From modeling to code. In *Innovations in systems and software engineering* (pp. 1–9).

4. Méry, D., & Singh, N. K. (2011). Automatic code generation from Event-B models. In *Proceedings of the second symposium on information and communication technology*, SoICT'11 (pp. 179–188). New York: ACM.

5. Méry, D., & Singh, N. K. (2011). Functional behavior of a cardiac pacing system. *International Journal of Discrete Event Control Systems, 1*(2), 129–149.

6. Méry, D., & Singh, N. K. (2012). Critical systems development methodology using formal techniques. In *Proceedings of the third symposium on information and communication technology*, SoICT'12 (pp. 3–12). New York: ACM.

7. Méry, D., & Singh, N. K. (2012). Formalization of heart models based on the conduction of electrical impulses and cellular automata. In Z. Liu & A. Wassyng (Eds.), *Lecture notes in computer science: Vol. 7151. Foundations of health informatics engineering and systems* (pp. 140–159). Berlin: Springer.

8. Méry, D., & Singh, N. K. (2012). Medical protocol diagnosis using formal methods. In Z. Liu & A. Wassyng (Eds.), *Lecture notes in computer science: Vol. 7151. Foundations of health informatics engineering and systems* (pp. 1–20). Berlin: Springer.

9. Méry, D., & Singh, N. K. (2013). Formal specification of medical systems by proof-based refinement. *ACM Transactions on Embedded Computing Systems, 12*(1), 15:1–15:25.

10. Singh, N. K. (2011). *Reliability and safety of critical device software systems*. PhD thesis, Department of Computing Science, Université Henri Poincaré-Nancy 1.

York, UK   Neeraj Kumar Singh
April 2013

Contents

Chapter 1
Introduction

Abstract The primary goal of this book is to advance the use of formal techniques for the development of computing systems with high integrity. Specifically, the book makes an analysis of critical system software that the formal methods are not well integrated into established critical systems development processes. This book presents formalism for a new development life-cycle, and a set of associated techniques and tools to develop the highly critical systems using formal techniques from requirements analysis to automatic source code generation using several intermediate layers with rigorous safety assessment approach. The approach has been verified using the Event-B formalism. The efficacy of formalism has been evaluated through a "Grand Challenge" case study, relative to the development of a cardiac pacemaker.

In this chapter, we present the motivation of this work and main concepts of our proposed approach for developing a new methodology for system development, and associated techniques and tools.

1.1 Motivation

Nowadays, software systems have penetrated into our daily life in many ways. Information technology is one major area, which provides powerful, and adaptable opportunities for innovation. However, sometimes computer-based developed systems are producing disappointed results and fail to produce the desired results according to work requirements and stakeholder needs. They are unreliable, and eventually dangerous. As a cause of system failure, poor developments practices [10, 16, 32, 38, 39] are one of the most significant. This is due to the complex nature of modern software and lack of understanding. Software development provides a framework for simplifying a complex system to get a better understanding and to develop the higher-fidelity system at a lower cost. Highly embedded critical systems, such as automotive, medical, and avionic, are susceptible to errors, which are not sustainable in case of failure. Any failure in these systems may be two types of consequences: *direct consequences* and *indirect consequences*. Direct consequences lead to finance, property losses, and personal injuries, while indirect consequences lead to income lost, medical expenses, time to retain another person, and decrease employee moral, etc. Additionally, and most significantly potential loss is customer trust for a product failure. In this context, a high degree of safety

N.K. Singh, *Using Event-B for Critical Device Software Systems*,
DOI 10.1007/978-1-4471-5260-6_1, © Springer-Verlag London 2013

and security is required to make amenable to the critical systems. A system is considered to accomplish the current task safely in case of a system failure. A formal rigorous reasoning about algorithms and mechanisms beneath such a system is required to precisely understand the behaviour of systems at the design level. However, to develop a reliable system is a significantly complicated task, which affects the reliability of a system.

Formal methods-based development [9, 14, 37] is a standard and popular approach to deal with the increasing complexity of a system with assurance of correctness in the modern software engineering practices. Formal methods-based techniques increasingly control safety-critical functionality in the development of the highly critical systems. These techniques are also considered as a way to meet the requirements of the standard certificates [6, 8, 12, 13] to evaluate a critical system before use in practice. Furthermore, critical systems can be effectively analysed at early stages of the development, which allows to explore conceptual errors, ambiguities, requirements correctness, and design flaws before implementation of an actual system. This approach helps to correct errors more easily and with less cost. We formulate the following objectives related to a critical system development:

- Establishing a unified theory for the critical systems development.
- Building a comprehensive and integrated suite of tools for the critical systems that can support verification activities, including formal specification, model validation, real-time animation and automatic code generation.
- Environment modelling for the development of a closed-loop system for verification purposes.
- Refinement-based formal development to achieve less error-prone models, easier specification for the critical systems and reuse of such specification for further designs.
- Model-based development and component-based design frameworks.
- System integration of critical infrastructure. Possibility of annotating models for different purposes, (e.g., directing the synthesis or hooking to verification tools).
- Evidence-based certification through animation.
- Requirements and metrics for certifiable assurance and safety.

The enumerated objectives are covered in this book through developing a new development life-cycle methodology and a set of associated techniques and tools for developing the critical systems. The development life-cycle methodology is a development process for the systems to capture the essential features precisely in an intuitive manner. A development methodology including a set of techniques and tools is developed for handling the stakeholders requirements, refinement-based system specification, verification, model animation using real-time data set through a real-time animator, and finally automatic source code generation from the verified formal specification to implement a system.

The formal verification and model validation offers to meet the challenge of complying with FDA's QSR, ISO, IEEE, CC [6, 8, 12, 13] quality system directives. According to the FDA QSR, validation is the "confirmation by examination and provision of objective evidence that the particular requirements for a specific

intended use can be consistently fulfilled". Verification is "confirmation by examination and provision of objective evidence that specified requirements have been
fulfilled" [11, 21]. All the proposed approaches may also help to obtain the certification standards [6, 8, 12, 13] in the area of critical system development.

1.2 Approach

In this book, we present a development life-cycle methodology, a framework for
real-time animator [19], refinement chart [31], a set of automatic code generation tools [7, 18, 22] and formal logic based heart model for closed-loop modelling [25, 29]. The development methodology and associated tools are used for
developing a critical system from requirements analysis to code implementation,
where verification and validation tasks are used as intermediate layers for providing a correct formal model with desired system behaviour at the concrete level. Our
approach of specification and verification is based on the techniques of abstraction
and refinement. Introducing a new set of tools helps to verify the desired properties, which are hidden at the early stage of the system development. For example,
a real-time animator provides a new way to discover hidden requirements according to the stakeholders. It is an efficient technique to use the real-time data set, in
a formal model without generating the source code in any target programming language [19], which also provides a way for domain experts (i.e. medical experts) to
participate in the system development process (medical device development). A basic description about development methodology and all associated techniques and
tools are provided in the following paragraphs:

We propose a new methodology, which is an extension of the waterfall model [3,
5, 34, 35] and utilises rigorous approaches based on formal techniques to produce a
reliable critical system. This methodology combines the refinement approach with
a verification tool, model checker tool, real-time animator and finally generates the
source code using automatic code generation tools. The system development process
is concurrently assessed by the safety assessment approaches [15, 33, 36] to comply
with certification standards [6, 8, 12, 13]. This life-cycle methodology consists of
seven main phases: first, informal requirements, resulting in a structured version of
the requirements, where each fragment is classified according to a fixed taxonomy.
In the second phase, informal requirements are formalised using a formal modelling
language, with a precise semantics, and enriched with invariants and temporal constraints. The third phase consists of refinement-based formal verification to test the
internal consistency and correctness of the specifications. The fourth phase is the
process of determining the degree to which a formal model is an accurate representation of the real world from the perspective of the intended uses of the model using
a model-checker. The fifth phase is used to animate the formal model with real-time
data set instead of *toy-data*, and offers a simple way for specifiers to build a domain-
specific visualisation that can be used by domain experts to check whether a formal
specification corresponds to their expectations. The six phase generates the source

code from the verified system specifications and final phase is used for acceptance testing of the developed system. This approach is useful to verify complex properties of a system and to discover the potential problems like deadlock and liveness at an early stage of the system development.

According to the development life cycle of a critical system, we emphasise the requirements traceability using a real-time animator [19]. Formal modelling of requirements is a challenging task, which is used to reasoning in earlier phases of the system development to make sure completeness, consistency, and automated verification of the requirements. The real-time animation of a formal model has been recognised to be a promising approach to support the process of validation of requirement's specification. The principle is to simulate the desired behaviours of a given system using formal models in the real-time environment and to visualise the simulation in some form which appeals to stakeholders. The real-time environment assists in the construction, clarification, validation and visualisation of a formal specification. Such an approach is also useful for evidence-based certification.

Refinement techniques [1, 2, 4] serve a key role for modelling a complex system in an incremental way. A refinement chart is a graphical representation of a complex system using a layering approach, where functional blocks are divided into multiple simpler blocks in a new refinement level, without changing the original behaviour of the system. The final goal of using this refinement chart is to obtain a specification that is detailed enough to be effectively implemented, but also to correctly describe the system behaviours. The purpose of the refinement chart is to provide an easily manageable representation for different refinements of the systems. The refinement chart offers a clear view of assistance in "system" integration. This approach also gives a clear view about the system assembly based on operating modes and different kinds of features. This is an important issue not only for being able to derive system-level performance and correctness guarantees, but also for being able to assemble components in a cost-effective manner.

Another important step in the software-development life cycle is the code implementation. In this context, we have developed an automatic code generation tool [7, 18, 22, 23] for generating an efficient target programming language code (C, C++, Java and C#) from Event-B formal specifications related to the analysis of complex problems. This tool is a collection of plug-ins, which are used for translating Event-B formal specifications into different kinds of programming languages. The translation tool is rigorously developed with safety properties preservation. We present an architecture of the translation process, to generate a target language code from Event-B models using Event-B grammar through syntax-directed translation, code scheduling architecture, and verification of an automatic generated code.

A closed-loop model of a system is considered as a *de facto* standard for critical systems in the medical, avionic, and automotive domains for validating the system model at the early stages of system development, which is an open problem in the area of modelling. The cardiac pacemaker and implantable cardioverter-defibrillators (ICDs) are key critical medical devices, which require closed-loop modelling (integration of system and environment modelling) for verification purpose to obtain a certificate from the certification bodies. In this context, we propose a methodology to model a biological system related to the heart system, which provides a biological environment for building the close loop system for the cardiac pacemaker [27]. The heart model is mainly based on electrocardiography analysis, which models the heart system at the cellular level. The main objective of this methodology is to model the heart system and integrate with a medical device model like the cardiac pacemaker to specify a closed-loop model. Industries have been striving for such a kind of approach for a long time in order to validate a system model under the virtual biological environment [27].

Assessment of the proposed framework, and techniques and tools are scrutinised through the development of a cardiac pacemaker. The cardiac pacemaker is a pilot project of the international "Grand Challenge". This book covers a complete development process of a cardiac pacemaker using the proposed life-cycle framework and developed tools [17, 20, 24] from requirements analysis to code implementation.

Formal techniques are useful not only for critical-systems, but it can be used to verify required safety properties in other domains, for example, in the clinical domain to verify the correctness of protocols and guidelines [26, 27, 30]. Clinical guidelines systematically assist practitioners with providing appropriate health care for specific clinical circumstances. Today, a significant number of guidelines and protocols are lacking in quality. Indeed, ambiguity, and incompleteness are common anomalies in the medical practices. Our main objective is to find anomalies and to improve the quality of medical protocols using well-known mathematical formal techniques, such as Event-B. In this study, we use the Event-B modelling language to capture guidelines for their validation for improving the protocols. An appropriateness of the formalism is given through a case study, relative to a real-life reference protocol (ECG Interpretation) that covers a wide variety of protocol characteristics related to several heart diseases.

1.2.1 Outline

The book is structured in 11 chapters. Chapter 2 presents a basic background and development life-cycle related to the safety critical systems. Chapter 3 describes modelling techniques using the Event-B modelling language. In Chap. 4, we propose a development life-cycle methodology for developing the highly critical software systems using formal methods from requirements analysis to code implementation using rigorous safety assessments. In Chap. 5, we propose a novel architecture to validate the formal model with real-time data set in the early stage of development without generating the source code [19]. This architecture can be used for requirement traceability. In Chap. 6, the refinement chart is proposed to handle the complexity and for designing the critical systems. In Chap. 7, we present a tool that automatically generates efficient target programming language code (C, C++, Java and C#) from Event-B formal specification related to the analysis of complex problems. In this chapter, the basic functionality as well as the design-flow is described, stressing the advantages when designing this automatic code generation tool; EB2ALL [7, 18, 22, 23, 28]. In Chap. 8, we present a methodology to model a biological system, like the heart. The heart model is mainly based on electrocardiography analysis, which models the heart system at the cellular level. The main objective of this methodology is to model the heart system and integrate it with the medical device model like the cardiac pacemaker to specify a closed-loop system. Chapter 9 presents a complete formal development of a cardiac pacemaker using proposed techniques and tools from requirements analysis to automatic code generation. In Chap. 10, we present a new application of formal methods to evaluate real-life medical protocols for quality improvement. An assessment of the proposed approach is given through a case study, relative to a real-life reference protocol (ECG Interpretation) which covers a wide variety of protocol characteristics related to several heart diseases. We formalise the given reference protocol, verify a set of interesting properties of the protocol and finally determine anomalies. Chapter 11 summarises this book.

References

1. Abrial, J.-R. (1996). *The B-book: Assigning programs to meanings*. New York: Cambridge University Press.
2. Abrial, J.-R. (2010). *Modeling in Event-B: System and software engineering* (1st ed.). New York: Cambridge University Press.
3. Acuña, S. T., & Juristo, N. (2005). *International series in software engineering. Software process modeling*. New York: Springer.
4. Back, R. J. R. (1981). On correct refinement of programs. *Journal of Computer and System Sciences*, *23*(1), 49–68.
5. Bell, R., & Reinert, D. (1993). Risk and system integrity concepts for safety-related control systems. *Microprocessors and Microsystems*, *17*, 3–15.
6. CC. Common criteria. http://www.commoncriteriaportal.org/.
7. EB2ALL (2011). Automatic code generation from Event-B to many programming languages. http://eb2all.loria.fr/.
8. FDA. Food and Drug Administration. http://www.fda.gov/.
9. Gaudel, M.-C., & Woodcock, J. (Eds.) (1996). *Lecture notes in computer science: Vol. 1051. Proceedings, FME'96: Industrial benefit and advances in formal methods*. Third international symposium of formal methods Europe, co-sponsored by IFIP WG 14.3, Oxford, March 18–22, 1996. Berlin: Springer.
10. Gibbs, W. W. (1994). Software's chronic crisis. *Scientific American*, September.
11. High Confidence Software and Systems Coordinating Group (2009). *High-confidence medical devices: Cyber-physical systems for 21st century health care* (Technical report). NITRD. http://www.nitrd.gov/About/MedDevice-FINAL1-web.pdf.
12. IEEE-SA. IEEE Standards Association. http://standards.ieee.org/.
13. ISO. International Organization for Standardization. http://www.iso.org/.
14. Jetley, R., Purushothaman Iyer, S., & Jones, P. (2006). A formal methods approach to medical device review. *Computer*, *39*(4), 61–67.
15. Leveson, N. G. (1991). Software safety in embedded computer systems. *Communications of the ACM*, *34*, 34–46.
16. Leveson, N. G., & Turner, C. S. (1993). An investigation of the Therac-25 accidents. *Computer*, *26*, 18–41.
17. Méry, D., & Singh, N. K. (2009). *Pacemaker's functional behaviors in Event-B* (Research report). MOSEL-LORIA-INRIA-CNRS: UMR7503-Université Henri Poincaré-

Nancy I-Université Nancy II-Institut National Polytechnique de Lorraine. http://hal.inria.fr/inria-00419973/en/.

18. Méry, D., & Singh, N. K. (2010). *EB2C: A tool for Event-B to C conversion support*. Poster and tool demo submission, published in a CNR technical report in SEFM.

19. Méry, D., & Singh, N. K. (2010). Real-time animation for formal specification. In M. Aiguier, F. Bretaudeau, & D. Krob (Eds.), *Complex systems design & management* (pp. 49–60). Berlin: Springer.

20. Méry, D., & Singh, N. K. (2010). Technical report on formal development of two-electrode cardiac pacing system. MOSEL-LORIA-INRIA-CNRS: UMR7503-Université Henri Poincaré-Nancy I-Université Nancy II-Institut National Polytechnique de Lorraine. http://hal.archives-ouvertes.fr/inria-00465061/en/.

21. Méry, D., & Singh, N. K. (2010). Trustable formal specification for software certification. In T. Margaria & B. Steffen (Eds.), *Lecture notes in computer science: Vol. 6416. Leveraging applications of formal methods, verification, and validation* (pp. 312–326). Berlin: Springer.

22. Méry, D., & Singh, N. K. (2011). Automatic code generation from Event-B models. In *Proceedings of the second symposium on information and communication technology*, SoICT'11 (pp. 179–188). New York: ACM.

23. Méry, D., & Singh, N. K. (2011). *EB2J: Code generation from Event-B to Java*. Short paper presented at the 14th Brazilian symposium on formal methods, SBMF'11.

24. Méry, D., & Singh, N. K. (2011). Functional behavior of a cardiac pacing system. *International Journal of Discrete Event Control Systems, 1*(2), 129–149.

25. Méry, D., & Singh, N. K. (2011). Technical report on formalisation of the heart using analysis of conduction time and velocity of the electrocardiography and cellular-automata. MOSEL-LORIA-INRIA-CNRS: UMR7503-Université Henri Poincaré-Nancy I-Université Nancy II-Institut National Polytechnique de Lorraine. http://hal.inria.fr/inria-00600339/en/.

26. Méry, D., & Singh, N. K. (2011). Technical report on interpretation of the electrocardiogram (ECG) signal using formal methods. MOSEL-LORIA-INRIA-CNRS: UMR7503-Université Henri Poincaré-Nancy I-Université Nancy II-Institut National Polytechnique de Lorraine. http://hal.inria.fr/inria-00584177/en/.

27. Méry, D., & Singh, N. K. (2012). Closed-loop modeling of cardiac pacemaker and heart. In *Foundations of health informatics engineering and systems*.

28. Méry, D., & Singh, N. K. (2012). *Formal development and automatic code generation: Cardiac pacemaker*. New York: ASME Press.

29. Méry, D., & Singh, N. K. (2012). Formalization of heart models based on the conduction of electrical impulses and cellular automata. In Z. Liu & A. Wassyng (Eds.), *Lecture notes in computer science: Vol. 7151. Foundations of health informatics engineering and systems* (pp. 140–159). Berlin: Springer.

30. Méry, D., & Singh, N. K. (2012). Medical protocol diagnosis using formal methods. In Z. Liu & A. Wassyng (Eds.), *Lecture notes in computer science: Vol. 7151. Foundations of health informatics engineering and systems* (pp. 1–20). Berlin: Springer.

31. Méry, D., & Singh, N. K. (2013). Formal specification of medical systems by proof-based refinement. *ACM Transactions on Embedded Computing Systems, 12*(1), 15:1–15:25.

32. Price, D. (1995). Pentium FDIV flaw-lessons learned. *IEEE MICRO, 15*(2), 86–88.

33. Redmill, M. C. F., & Catmur, J. (1999). *System safety: HAZOP and software HAZOP* (1st ed.). Chichester: Wiley.

34. Schumann, J. M. (2001). *Automated theorem proving in software engineering*. New York: Springer.

35. Wichmann, B. A., & British Computer Society (1992). *Software in safety-related systems* (Special report). BCS.

36. Wilkinson, P. J., & Kelly, T. P. (1998). Functional hazard analysis for highly integrated aerospace systems. In *Certification of ground/air systems seminar* (pp. 4–146). New York: IEEE. Ref. No. 1998/255.

37. Woodcock, J., & Banach, R. (2007). The verification grand challenge. *Journal of Universal Computer Science, 13*(5), 661–668.

38. Yeo, K. T. (2002). Critical failure factors in information system projects. *International Journal of Project Management, 20*(3), 241–246.
39. Zhang, Y., Jones, P. L., & Jetley, R. (2010). A hazard analysis for a generic insulin infusion pump. *Journal of Diabetes Science and Technology, 4*(2), 263–283.

Chapter 2
Background

Abstract Formal methods based system development is considered as a promising approach to develop the safe critical systems. This chapter discusses the standard safety life-cycle, traditional safety analysis techniques, traditional system engineering approach, standard design methodologies and safety standards that are used for developing the critical systems. Furthermore, we have given a list of successful industrial case studies based on formal techniques. Moreover, we discuss the role of medical device regulations. Finally, this chapter shows the usability of formal techniques for developing the critical systems and to motivate for developing a new methodology, and associated techniques and tool in the context of medical device development, which are covered in the remaining chapters.

2.1 Introduction

Critical systems are tremendously grown in functionality in both software and hardware, and due to increasingly the complexity of critical systems it is very hard to predict the absence of failure. Moreover, some of these failures may cause catastrophic financial loss, time or even human life. One of the main objectives of software engineering is to provide a framework to develop a critical system that operates reliably despite this complexity. It has been shown in [97, 113] that the promising results are achievable only through the use of formal methods in the development process. More than a decade, several formal methods based techniques and tools are used by industries and academic research projects [62, 111]. The backbone of formal methods is considered to be mathematics, which often supports related techniques and tools based on logico-mathematical theory for specifying and verifying the complex systems. The techniques and tools based on formal methods provide a certain level of reliability under some constraints. Formal verification is considered as a benchmark technique, particularly in the area of safety critical systems, where important safety properties are required to prove rigorously before implementing a system. However, the use of formal methods helps to speculate the hidden peculiarity of a system like inconsistencies, ambiguities, and incompleteness.

In the past, formal methods based technique was not into practice in the software development life-cycle due to the use of complex mathematical notations; inadequate tools support and too hard to apply. Special training was required to use

N.K. Singh, *Using Event-B for Critical Device Software Systems*,
DOI 10.1007/978-1-4471-5260-6_2, © Springer-Verlag London 2013

formal methods to apply in the system development process. Increasingly, number of successful development of techniques and tools related to the formal methods, the industries have started to adopt it for verifying the safety properties of complex systems [13, 14, 23, 97]. For verifying a critical system, industries prefer to use formal methods-based techniques such as model checking or theorem proving in place of the traditional simulation techniques. In both areas related to the model checking and theorem proving, the researchers and practitioners are performing more and more industrial-sized case studies [9, 11, 13, 24, 38, 61, 62, 78], and thereby gaining the benefits of using formal methods.

This chapter briefly discusses safety critical systems, examines the use of formal techniques to provide safety and reliability, analysis the use of traditional safety techniques for software, surveys on regulations for medical devices, and gives a list of successful industrial case studies based on formal techniques. Reliability and safety are the most important attributes of critical systems. The main objective of this chapter is to provide information about current safety issues in medical domain particularly for the safety critical software systems. It should be noted that the formal methods are the most important techniques that are applicable for a safety related software development for medical devices using several classical safety analysis techniques.

2.1.1 Structure of This Chapter

This chapter contains a concise survey that reviews the existing literatures relating to the development and analysis of a software for safety critical systems, which identifies current valuable approaches for developing the safety critical software, and reviews the methods and analysis techniques available to the system developers. Section 2.2 gives an overview about reliability and safety. Section 2.3 presents a role of a software in safety-critical systems and Sect. 2.4 describes safety life-cycle for critical systems. Section 2.5 presents traditional safety analysis techniques. Section 2.6 explores the traditional system engineering approach, and Sect. 2.7 gives a list of standard design methodologies for the system development process. Section 2.8 depicts about safety standards, and Sect. 2.9 presents medical device standards and discusses the current issues of regulations. Section 2.10 presents a list of industrial projects related to the formal methods, and finally, Sect. 2.11 discusses the use of formal methods for the safety critical software systems.

2.2 Reliability and Safety

2.2.1 Reliability

Reliability is a fundamental attribute for the safe operation of any critical system. According to the Institute of Electrical and Electronic Engineers (IEEE), "*Reliability is the ability of a system or component to perform its required functions under stated conditions for a specified period of time*" [54]. Reliability can be used for prediction, analysing, preventing and mitigating failure over time of a complex critical system. In the context of safety, there are several elements of reliability. These elements are operational reliability and performance reliability. Operational reliability can estimate the probability of failure of a system, while performance reliability measures the adequacy of features to successfully perform under the specific conditions. Reliability analysis aims to protect a system from failures of its components, software and hardware [67].

A fundamental challenge in reliability analysis is the uncertainty for failure occurrences and consequences. To protect a system, a quantitative approach has been pushed forward for the design, regulation and management of the safety of hazardous systems. The reliability assurance is a process that is considered by manufacturers during product development according to the regulating standards [18, 22, 33, 54, 58]. The reliability is quantified in terms of probability. Reliability has a time oriented characteristic that can be expressed as the Mean Time Between Failures (MTBF) [95]. When we use probability or characteristics of the underlying life distribution to measure reliability, it must be emphasised that reliability is a relative measure of the performance of a system. It is relative to the user requirements, system failures, expected lifetime of the device, operating environment conditions, system functionality and behaviour of the system changes with time.

Reliability engineering is a function to calculate the expected reliability of a system, process and behaviour in advance. The main objective of reliability engineering is to deliver reliable product in order to satisfy behaviour requirements, safe operation, lower cost, and to maintain company reputation [95]. Nowadays, reliability engineering is a well established discipline that can provide an integration of formal methods to investigate the system requirements, correctness of the system by addressing the following questions: (1) why a system fails? (2) how to develop a reliable system? (3) how to measure the reliability of design, process and operation of a system? and (4) how to maintain system reliability during system operation through fault diagnosis and prediction [17, 116].

2.2.2 Safety

Safety can be defined as "*freedom from those conditions that can cause death, injury, occupational illness, or damage to or loss of equipment or property, or damage to the environment*" [83]. Safety can provide some standards to ensure quality and functionality of a system. The safety standards eliminate all potential risks that can cause loss of life, injuries or property damage. Critical systems that meet certification standards, are safe to use in practice. It provides confidence to the user to use for their purpose in daily life.

Safety is like reliability that concentrate on the designing phase of a system. A system must be designed for safety. System safety is an engineering and management discipline that encapsulates human, machine, environment, designing, testing, operating and maintaining system to achieve acceptable risk within the timing and cost constraints in the system life-cycle [56]. Hazard analysis can improve the safety that defines real or potential conditions that can cause injuries, illness, loss of system, property or damage environment.

2.2.3 Safety vs. Reliability

As a conventional approach, it is assumed that a reliable system is safer and vice versa. However, it is not always true and it can lead to a lot of confusion to analysis a system failure. Actually, it is often true that the safer system can be less reliable. For example, an inoperative elevator can provide maximum level of safety. The inoperative elevator cannot do any functionality like opening or closing the door, moving up or down, after pressing any button. To use the elevator, in this state is always safe, but the reliability of the elevator is zero. The inoperative elevator has not any functionality, it is absolutely unreliable and ineffective to use for moving up or down to different floors. To improve the safety of a reliable system, system designer introduces some elements to add the functionalities. Such as, designers can introduce elements and controls for moving up or down of the elevator. These new elements can reduce the reliability of the elevator. Such that, a sensor can provide a proper opening or closing door operation. If the sensor is out-of-order, then the elevator will not move. Here, the sensor behaviour reduces the reliability and increases the safety of the system.[1]

Reliability and safety are the main attributes to determine effectiveness of a system, where effectiveness is influenced by the life-cycle activities related to the design, manufacturing, use and disposal of the product [22]. IEC 60513 [50], fundamental aspects of safety standards for medical electrical equipment, provides a safety standard for developing the medical systems that assures the basic safety and essential performance. IEC 60601 [52] address reliability stating that "*reliability of functioning is regarded as a safety issue (for life-supporting equipment) and where interruption of an examination or treatment is considered as a hazard for the patient.*"

According to the FDA [33] regulation safety is defined as: "There is a reasonable assurance that a device is safe when it can be determined, based upon valid scientific evidence, that the probable benefits to health from the use of the device for its intended use and conditions of use, when accompanied by adequate directions and warnings against unsafe use, outweigh any probable risks." Effectiveness is defined thus: "There is a reasonable assurance that a device is effective when it can be determined, based upon valid scientific evidence, that is a significant portion of the target population, the use of the device for its intended uses and conditions of use, when accompanied by adequate directions to use and warnings against unsafe use, will provide clinically significant results" [94].

---

[1]http://www.aldservice.com/en/safety/what-is-safety.html.

2.3 Software in Safety-Critical Systems

Software is a vital part of any system, especially in embedded systems, where it is used to control the whole functionality of the systems. The embedded systems have major role to control the behaviour of the safety critical systems. When we use these systems, we consider that their risk has been minimised and uses of the systems are effectively safe. The system is not only safe, but we also expect other attributes like reliable and cost effective. Main safety-critical systems are commercial aircraft, medical care, train signalling systems, air traffic control, nuclear power, and weapons, where any kind of failure can quickly lead to human life in danger, loss of equipment, and so on. The industries are responsible for designing and delivering the safety-critical systems according to the standards authorities [18, 33, 54, 58], which satisfy the requirements.

To address the problem of system's failure related to the software errors for example, overdoses from Therac-25 for treating cancer through radiation [74], the overshooting of the runway at Warsaw airport by an Airbus A320 [79], Intel Pentium floating point divide [91], 5000 adverse events for Insulin Infusion Pump (IIP) reported by FDA [114, 115] and Ariane 5 flight 501 going off [76]. All these problems and many more are considered as a part of the "software crisis". The term "software crisis" has been introduced in late 1960s to describe the failures of the systems in which software-development problems cause the entire system [36]. In 1968, a meeting is organised by NATO related to the software crisis. This crisis had as its root cause the problem of complexity brought about in many cases by sheer length of programs combined with a poor control over how each line of code affects the overall system. Almost three decades later, this problem still remains as indicated in [36].

Software crisis is a well-known problem for other engineering disciplines, and over the years of experience has been accumulated to provide effective solutions: the technology has been available, and it has been shown to work with a very high degree of confidence. Software are using frequently in the system development, which is also classified as an engineering discipline, so it would seem natural that one can apply the insights and quickly surmount any hurdles. However, it is true that the engineering insights are applicable to modern the critical-system development to come over the traditional approaches of the system development.

2.3.1 Software Safety and Reliability

Increasing size and complexity of software in critical systems, the software has a primary threat for the reliability. Most of the reliability engineering techniques address failures in hardware components. Software architecture analysis methods concentrate to analyse the quality and behaviour of a system at the early stage of the system development. Several useful reliability engineering techniques are available in literature to analyse and design a reliable system. A comprehensive survey of these techniques is given in [70, 77]. Software quality has been promoted in the software architecture analysis domain. The software architecture is an important process that helps to predict important qualities of a system and to identify the potential risks [29]. To provide an early reliability analysis that covers software components, it is advantageous to utilise both results from software architecture analysis and conventional reliability analysis approaches [101].

According to the IEEE, software safety can be defined as *"freedom from software hazard,"* where *software hazard is defined as "a software condition that is a prerequisite to an accident,"* and an *accident is defined as "an unplanned event or series of events that results in death, injury, illness, environmental damage, or damage to or loss of equipment or property"* [54]. The use of formal methods in software development process provides safety assurance that the software does not show any failure cases. There are several techniques that are used to identify the software bugs at the early stage of the system development. Each phase of the software development is verified and validated using several techniques from requirements analysis to code generation [54, 55].

International regulatory standards provide guidelines for designing, operating and maintaining the critical systems [48]. To analyse the reliability, the hardware and software barriers must take into account. However, hardware barriers are more reliable than the software barriers according to the past history of the system functionality in terms of performance, proof-checking, and regress testing of the hardware components [32]. In a complex system, self-test are not sufficient to identify potential failures. Therefore, proof-checks are used to perform at regular intervals to cope with undetected hardware failures.

The hardware systems are subject to ageing and wear. Ageing and wear characteristics of the hardware systems provide a way to calculate the reliability using MTBF. However, the software systems are not applicable to use statistical technique like MTBF for reliability calculation, because software systems are not subject to ageing and wear. Tools and techniques related to the software failures are not similar to the hardware failures due to different characteristics of both software and hardware systems. The software systems do not follow the physical laws of degradation or failure as per the hardware systems [116].

The software reliability is an important challenge in the area of safety critical systems, where software may be used to control the hardware components. The software failures can be identified using software-centric approach and system-centric viewpoint. The software-centric approach looks for failure modes and to evaluate their probabilities, and the system-centric viewpoint is based on practical observation related to the specifications and requirements, which encapsulate software design failures.

The fault injection method is a technique for quantitative analysis of the software failure that deliberately inject faults in the software and count the number of times that the software maintains its function in spite of the injected fault [1, 46, 105]. However, this approach is not effective to discover all hidden failures. Hence, another feasible approach to building the reliable software is to use the systematic software development process. The main objective is to evaluate different fault tolerant approaches throughout the software development process [116].

Fig. 2.1 Safety life-cycle
(adapted from [53])

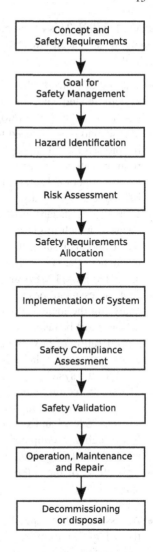

2.4 The Safety Life-Cycle for Critical Systems

Safety is a most important system property, that should be methodically analysed along the system life-cycle. A number of standards and recommended practices define the processes and the objectives of the safety life-cycle, such as IEC 61598 [53], MODEF [30]. Figure 2.1 depicts a stepwise implementation of the system development safety life-cycle. The main objective of this development cycle is to guide system designers and developers in what they need to do in order to claim that their systems are acceptably safe for their intended uses. The purpose of the overall safety life-cycle is to force safety to be addressed independently of functional issues, thus overcoming the assumption that functional reliability will automatically produce safety [53, 92]. This development cycle is accepted by all industry sectors in developing the advanced safe critical systems. The life-cycle phases are briefly described as follows:

- The initial concept phase is used to identify the functional requirements of the system, related environment where the system will be operated, and possible design approaches for developing the system.
- The second phase is used to set the goal for management and technical activities to consider the safety implications of the developing system through assessing the required safety level to ensure that the system achieves and maintains the required level of functional safety. The goal should be produced at the beginning of system life-cycle and it must be reviewed at regular interval.
- In Phase 3, hazard identification process is applied to identify the possible hazards, which might arise during construction, installation, operation, maintenance and disposal of the system. This hazard identification process is applicable throughout the system life-cycle. The main formal techniques for hazard analysis are FHA, FTA, FMEA and HAZOP.
- Risk assessment process is used to identify a set of possible risks through analysing the identified hazards, and check against tolerability criteria. A set of actions must be taken to reduce the overall risks. The action can be decided under consideration of possible consequences of hazards to a tolerable level. The risk assessment process helps to discover possible requirements for the safety integrity level for the system.
- The safety requirements are separately assessed for different parts of the system and the whole system is reviewed to ensure that the risk will be reduced to an acceptable level and system is safe in use. Any critical system is too complex in functionality. To implement the safety functions, a simple technology should be used to avoid the overall complexity of the system.
- This phase of the safety life-cycle is related to system implementation, where safety related parts or components are implemented to satisfy the safety requirements.
- Assessment of the specific components or parts of the system must comply with the safety requirements to ensure that the component of the system meets the given safety requirements. The assessment process is based on analysis and auditing techniques.
- Safety validation phase is used to verify the system against the claimed safety properties. This process assures that the system have been achieved a set of goals and system is safe to use in practice. Moreover, during the verification process arising problems are also resolved.
- This phase of safety life-cycle related to the system operation and maintenance, which ensures that the system will be safe during the maintenance process. Various safety related system problems arise due to a poor maintenance process. Thus the system must be designed for maintainability. The use of the system in different environment should also be analysed to evaluate the system behaviour and must ensure the safety of the system.

- Finally, safety considerations that may apply during decommissioning should also be taken into account. Thus an assessment of the impact of the decommissioning should be made on both the components and the process of the system. This process will use hazard and risk assessment approaches to determine the level of safety-related work. The safety related work must be satisfied during the decommissioning activity of the critical system.

2.5   Traditional Safety Analysis Techniques

Safety provides protection from hazard to human life, the environment or property. There are not such a magical thing that can guarantee for absolute safety. However, a system can be enough safe that can accept any risk related to the life, environment or property. The risk can be measured through probability and the complex calculations of a system, while a system can be failed due to use of any harmful substances in the process. However, software is not a harmful substance. Software can be used to control the system behaviour using a set of processes. Moreover, the software can contribute to safety, e.g. through control over hazardous physical processes [72]. Software hazard and safety analysis refer to the process of assessing and to make contribution to design a safety software. According to [81], four safety-relevant elements of a system development process are defined as follows:

1. Identifying hazards and associated safety requirements.
2. Designing the system to meet its safety requirements.
3. Analysing the system to show that it meets its safety requirements.
4. Demonstrating the safety of the system by producing a safety case.

2.5.1   Hazard Analysis

Software development life-cycle and engineering techniques are used to design and develop a system to meet all the functional requirements. These techniques place a little effort to examine failure cases of a system. However, a highly critical system like aviation, medical or automotive needs to consider all possible failure scenarios to avoid from any hazard. Different kinds of techniques may be employed for safety assessment from hazard analysis. When a system has many components, then take a modular approach for analysing a system using System Hazard Analysis (SHA) and Subsystem Hazard Analysis (SSHA). The SHA discovers all associated hazards of a system, while the SSHA discovers how an operation of a particular component affects on the whole system.

The SHA and SSHA analyses are performed by several techniques, which are provided by the standard authorities. Traditional safety analysis techniques such as Hazard and Operability study (HAZOP) [92], Functional Hazard Assessment (FHA) [109], Fault Tree Analysis (FTA) [73], and Failure Mode Effects Analysis

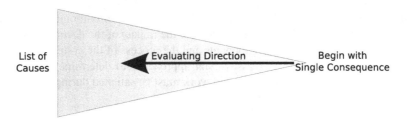

List of
Causes

Evaluating Direction

Begin with
Single Consequence

Fig. 2.2 FTA—Evaluating back from consequence to cause

(FMEA) [31] are standards to apply for hardware intensive systems that are also applicable for the software systems. Traditional safety analysis therefore begins by defining the hazards associated with a system, determines their severity, and then attempts to identify the factors that can initiate the hazards. These safety analysis techniques provide a rigorous way to examine the causes and their consequences of the identified hazards.

Functional Hazard Assessment (FHA)

Hazard are unfavourable conditions that a system should avoid to occur or must be identified in advance. Once the hazards are known that it becomes possible to trace backwards from the hazards to the particular events that can cause them. Functional Hazard Assessment (FHA) is used to identify such type of hazards that can be occurred because of functional failure. The safety analysis techniques concentrate on defining the required functionality and analysing the consequences of failures. The FHA is an informal process that is used to document hazards and determine their severity. The FHA produces a list hazards in tabular form with different degree of severity [109].

Fault Tree Analysis (FTA)

Where a system is self-contained, having its boundaries well defined, one focuses on the hazards that are internal to the system, which may be termed faults. Thus, a fault is always a hazard, but not conversely. At this level, we have another technique to analyse the systems using Fault Tree Analysis (FTA) [73]. The FTA is a safety analysis technique that is deductive and top-down method of analysing system design and performance to identify all the possible failures or errors. It is based on a feedback process that can start with a system level hazard and try to discover backward for identifying all the possible causes of hazards (see Fig. 2.2). The FTA shows a list of hazards according to the hazard level. Although, the FTA has limited use for identifying the faults of a system using a visual technique that can trace higher level events down to their contributing events in form of failures, errors or faults. The FTA is represented in a tree structure that shows various factors to contribute a high

Fig. 2.3 FTA tree

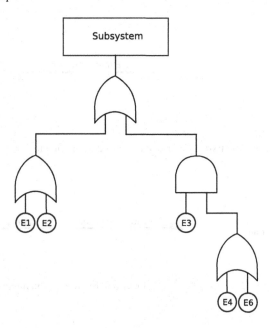

level event. The fault trees can also be used in a confirmatory role where they are
particularly useful in showing that a probability requirement for a hazardous failure mode has been met by the system. Figure 2.3 depicts a basic architecture of the
FTA. In this figure, highest level event (hazard) is traced backward to identify the
source of errors or faults. Events and gates in fault tree analysis are represented by
symbols. The source of errors or faults are known as the base events (errors) [73].

Failure Mode Effects Analysis (FMEA)

Failure modes and effects analysis (FMEA) is a step-by-step approach [31] to identify the possible hazards in a complex system that facilitates the identification of
potential problems in the design or process by examining the effects of lower level
failures. The FTA safety analysis technique is based on top-down approach, while
the FMEA is used a bottom-up approach. In this bottom-up analysis, the technique
determines possible failures of a system and produces a list of probable failures according to the degree of severity. The feed-forward technique of the FMEA is used
to discover possible failures or errors through forward tracing (see Fig. 2.4). FMEA
is useful for evaluating a new process prior to implementation, and for assessing the
impact of proposed changes on the existing processes. The output of FMEA presents
in a tabular form that describes the failure modes, in which something might fail,
and the consequences of those failures.

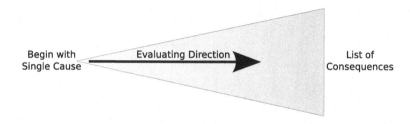

Fig. 2.4 FMEA—Evaluating forward from cause to consequences

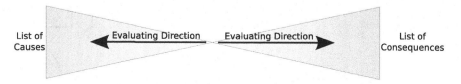

Fig. 2.5 HAZOP—Evaluating from the fault in both directions for causes and consequences

Hazard and Operability Analysis (HAZOP)

Hazard and operability studies (HAZOP) are more commonly used at the broadest level for analysing process plants like chemical and nuclear industries [57]. The HAZOP supports the chemical process industry, takes a representation of a system and analyses how its operation may lead to an unsafe deviation from the intent of the system [57] with special attention to the environment of operation. This technique is very popular in industries because it aims to predict possible failures, and identify their impact.

HAZOP [92] is a most prominent formal technique for identification of the hazards. This technique examines all the essential components and their interconnections of a system to explore the possible causes of errors and their consequences. Particularly, HAZOP is a powerful technique for exploring the interaction between parts of a system. HAZOP is based on a theory that assumes risk events are caused by deviations from design or operating intentions. Identification of such deviations is assessment and generally facilitated by using a set of "guide words" as a systematic list that includes process, and deviation perspectives. HAZOP starts to analyse in both directions, backwards to explore its possible causes, and forwards to examine its consequences (see Fig. 2.5).

A set of safety analysis techniques like FHA, FTA, FMEA, and HAZOP, is used to identify a list of base events that can contribute to hazardous conditions. A list of events gives the general categories of safety properties required to the requirement model of a system. A more detailed discussion of the system hazard analyses (SHA) with the software perspective is provided in [57, 72].

2.5.2 Risk Assessment and Safety Integrity

A risk assessment is simply a careful examination of the past data related to the hazard's analysis for the similar systems; from the reliability assessments of components of the system being developed; and other sources. The outcome of the risk assessment presents some kind of gradation and may be expressed in terms of what constitutes a tolerable and intolerable risk. This outcome results help for regulating industrial risk, and to determine whether a risk is unacceptable, acceptable or somewhere in between. Lots of factors are used for determining the risk based on quantitative and qualitative analyses [8]. Using a risk classification of accidents according to the frequency and severity usefully serves as a relatively simple basis for its determination.

Assessment of a risk can decide a necessary level of safety that can be achieved from various functions of a system. This is an issue of safety integrity, which is defined as, *"Safety integrity is the likelihood of a safety-related system achieving the required safety functions under all the stated conditions within a stated period of time"* [108]. The system activities are contributing to the integrity may be characterised by two kinds of requirements:

1. Generation of the new safety requirements of a system is resulting from the design and development.
2. Ensuring that what is being built meets the requirements that have already been specified.

Here, the first requirement is related to the requirement analysis and hazard analyses of a system. The second requirement is related to the reliability engineering techniques, whose consideration may have to be sustained throughout the development as the design evolves with modification to interfaces, rearrangement of components or other kinds of changes. To apply the several techniques like FHA, HAZOP, FMEA and FTA for the fault prediction, fault removal, fault avoidance and fault tolerance, and to achieve the system integrity require together with methods and design of the system, are the main resources for measuring the system reliability [103].

A safety of a system may be simply characterised by a process of reducing risks to appropriate effect. The main objective of a qualitative or quantitative risk assessment is to establish the level of tolerability for any identified risk. If a risk falls in between the states of 'intolerable' and 'acceptable' then any risk must be reduced to 'as low as reasonably practicable'. This is known as the ALARP principle as illustrated in Fig. 2.6. The width of the triangle is proportionate to the level of risk and thus also to the amount of resources that can be justified to reduce it. A comprehensive survey of risks and safety integrity is provided in [8].

2.5.3 Safety Integrity and Assurance

Finally, there is always a question in the development of critical system, "What is the assurance level according to the certain level of integrity of the system?". In

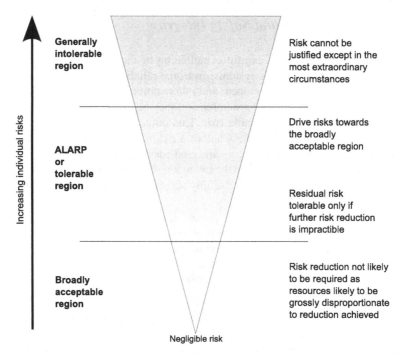

Increasing individual risks

Generally intolerable region — Risk cannot be justified except in the most extraordinary circumstances

ALARP or tolerable region — Drive risks towards the broadly acceptable region

Residual risk tolerable only if further risk reduction is impractible

Broadly acceptable region — Risk reduction not likely to be required as resources likely to be grossly disproportionate to reduction achieved

Negligible risk

Fig. 2.6 ALARP model of risk level

order to safety assurance of the developed system may be certified as safe, there must be a set of documents, which provides detail justification of the safety. This document contains a list of all hazard's cases with log details and various arguments for indicating that how the system has reached at the required safety levels. The safety case brings in all the aforementioned risk analyses, risk reductions and other integrity and reliability measures, often presenting various statistical evidence. It is a considerable huge amount of a task involves lots of documentation. A software SAM (Safety Arguments Manager) is recognised to support this process and allows to manage all the developing safety cases [82].

2.6 Traditional System Engineering Approach

A critical system uses a standard life-cycle to achieve a certificate from the standard authorities [18, 33, 54, 58]. A system can be considered safe if all the hazards have been eliminated, or the risk associated hazards have been reduced to an acceptable level. Software is a part of a system, which is used within the system to operate the system safely. The integrated software within a system does not show any kind of misbehaviour. However, if the same software is used by multiple systems then the software must have similar behaviour in each system. However, sometimes it is not true. It is believed that each system is different, with different requirements, different risk level with different hazard's characteristics, it is impossible to know if software is safe without considering the behaviour of the software as a part of the system which it is controlling. Therefore, when considering the process for developing a safe software, it is crucial that the whole system of which the software is a part is considered, as well as the software itself [12].

2.6.1   The Software Safety Life-Cycle

In the past several years, different types of software development life-cycle have been identified. All of them have their own merits and limitations according to the problem complexity, size and type of the system. This book will not enter into a discussion about different life-cycle process models. A detailed description about each life-cycle process model is available in [4, 80, 90, 99]. Here, we only discuss about life-cycle process model related to the safety critical software system.

In recognition of the distinctive nature of safety-related systems, there is a standard development process known as V-model, which is widely accepted by large companies and defence. It is an extension of the standard Waterfall model [4, 8, 98, 108]. The V-model represents a software-development process, where the process steps are bent upwards after the coding phase to form the typical V shape. The V-model presents the relationships between each phase of the development life-cycle and its associated phase of testing. V-model is also called verification and validation model (V & V). This process uses a very intensive testing for removing bugs or errors, which may appear during any stage of the system development.

The typical process of developing a safety-critical software system is generally time-consuming. Most of the development processes are based on the V-model, which is illustrated diagrammatically in Fig. 2.7. This model identifies the major elements of the development process and indicates the structured, and typically sequential, nature of the development process. The sequential nature of development is generally considered essential for reasons of managing communication and scale, for scheduling different phases and disciplines, for managing traceability (which is mandated by relevant safety standards) and for the certification purposes.

In order to produce a safety-related software according to this framework, various techniques are recommended. These include the application of structured analysis techniques to generate a visible modular construction (the principles of modularity are expounded in [89]), and diversity in design, implementation and maintenance to avoid faults due to common mode failures. Many such techniques are very widely applicable, and although they are usefully brought into the safety-critical context, there is not so much literature devoted solely to their use in this specific area. Nevertheless, material is available: for instance, there have been reviews such as [28, 103] to help designers and managers as to the suitability of mainstream programming languages for the safety-critical systems.

Safety requires a lot of integrity, and this is recognised in the safety life-cycle model which separates the specification of safety requirements into purely func-

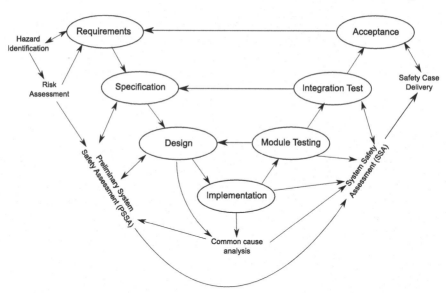

Fig. 2.7 The V model of safety-critical system development

tional requirements and safety-integrity requirements. The safety integrity requirements are calculated individually for each of the functions previously identified.
Having done this, one may concentrate on providing the high levels of assurance
on the safety-critical aspects. We intend using the safety life-cycle model as a basis,
with a view to ascertaining its suitability to support the production of formal models with high integrity. Our contention is that we treat carefully the non-functional
requirements and to put forward a selection of viewpoints and methods highlighting
further the safety concepts, which are often subtle, then the life-cycle model can
be effective [103]. A safe system can be characterised as one in which risks from
hazards have been minimised throughout a system life. The process of providing
hazard analyses and risk assessments are thus crucial activities to ensure the safety
of a system.

In Fig. 2.7, Preliminary System Safety Analysis (PSSA) and System Safety Analysis (SSA) are the collection of various techniques like FTA, HAZOP, FMEA, etc.
The aim of all these techniques is to identify failures and derive the safety requirements, which prevent from the occurrence of the hazard. FTA focuses on the different components of a system, while HAZOP focus on the flow between components. There are also a number of other techniques, which are used in the PSSA for
analysing failures, an overview can be found in [87].

2.7 Standard Design Methodologies

A design is a meaningful engineering representation of a higher-level interpretation
of a system, which is actually a part of an implementation in a source code. Design

process is traceable using reverse engineering technique to the actual stakeholders requirements. The quality of a system can be assessed through predefined criteria for a good design. Analysis and design methods for software have been evolving over the years, each with its approach for modelling needs a world-view into software [86]. The following methodologies are common, which are used in current practices.

- Structured Analysis and Structured Design (SA/SD)
- Object Oriented Analysis and Object Oriented Design (OOA/OOD)
- Formal Methods (FM) and Model-based Development

SA/SD techniques provide means to create and evaluate a good design of the systems. This technique covers functional decomposition, data flow and information modelling. OOA/OOD considers the whole system into abstract entities called objects, which can contain information (data) and have associated behaviour. It is in practice from last 30 years, which is used in several big projects. It contains Object-Oriented Analysis and Design (OOA/OOD) method, Object modelling Technique (OMT) Object-Oriented Analysis and Design with Applications (OOADA), Object-Oriented Software Engineering (OOSE) and UML. Formal Methods (FM) and Model-based development are a set of techniques and tools based on mathematical modelling and formal logic that are used to specify and verify requirements and designs for the systems and software [86]. Formal method is also a process that allows the logical properties of a computer system to be predicted from a mathematical model of a system by means of a logical calculation. Formal methods can be used for formal specification, formal verification and software models (with automatic code generation) [86].

2.7.1 Design for Reliability

Reliability is an attribute of a system that is derived from research, concept and design through analysing the capacity and performance under the working environment. The reliability level can be established during design phase of the system development. However, a subsequent testing and production cannot improve the reliability without any modification in the basic design. Design reliability techniques integrating with the development process for assuring the safety of a system. Reliability becomes a difficult design parameter due to the increasing complexity and limited knowledge of the system requirements. If reliability is an important attribute of a system then it is quantified during specification of the design requirements.

Reliability is essential for a healthcare and medical devices, which need to be safe and effective. Medical device manufacturers and regulating bodies like the Food and Drug Administration (FDA) [33] and Center for Devices and Radiological Health (CDRH) [22] have a responsibility for assuring the safety and effectiveness of medical devices. The CDRH has standards to analyse system specification, design requirements, and usability of a system. The CDRH [22] requires a complete and accurate requirements of any medical system for designing and manufacturing a safe system. The CDRH allows premarket review to identify relevant information for processing, manufacturing, assembly handling, maintenance and disposal of the system. Moreover, the CDRH also seeks to determine if the manufacturer has captured the important aspects of the development life-cycle for producing a product [59, 66]. However, the CDRH is also concerned with potential users like patient or clinician, who will use the device. FDA requires product performance to be verified [59, 60, 66] and validated [59, 66]. The FDA supports the performance and safety assessment of a system through providing the evidence that the system is adequate to use in practice. The FDA regulatory oversight of the manufacturing process through the Quality System Regulation [59, 66].

Increasing complexity and safety recalls in the medical systems advocate a new approach for a good design for reliability (DFR) in the medical industries [42]. DFR describes the tools and techniques that can support product and process design to ensure the system reliability. The DFR is a process that spans the entire product development cycle from concept to release of a product. The DFR [42] indicates the following paradigms that are essential to design a complex medical system:

1. Spend significant effort on requirement analysis
2. Critical failure is not an option for medical devices
3. Measure reliability in terms of total Life-cycle cost
4. Don't just design for reliability, design for durability
5. Design for prognostics to minimise surprise failures

2.8 Safety Standards

It is perhaps best to start by considering the various standards that exist for industries, which develop the safety critical systems. Standards are documented agreements containing technical specifications, which produce precise criteria, consistent rules, procedures to ensure reliability, software processes, methods, products, services and use of products, are fit for their purpose in this world. Standards include a set of issues corresponding to the product functionality and compatibility, facilitate interoperability including designing, developing, enhancing, and maintaining. A set of protocols and guidelines, which are produced by the standards, are consistent and universally acceptable for the product development. The standards allow to understand the quality of different products for competing with them, and provide a way to verify the credibility of a new product [22, 54, 58].

Verification and validation (V & V) are part of the certification process for any critical system. There are several reasons, why certification is required for any critical system. For example, medical device like a cardiac pacemaker must obtain a certificate before to use in practices. Certification of the product not only assures about the safety, but also helps to a customer to gain confidence to buy and to use the product, which is also important for commercial reasons like having a sales advantage to industry. Certifications are usually carried out by some national and international authorities. Certification can be applicable to an organisation, tools or methods, or systems or products. The main objective of the certification bodies is to provide assurance that an organisation can achieve a certain level of proficiency, and that they agree to the certain standards or criteria. In the case of product certification, there are always issues for the certification, whether a methodology or development process is certified or not.

There are many international standards bodies. More than 300 software standards and 50 organisations are developing software standards [34]. Standards come in many different flavours, for example, de-facto standards, local, national and international standards. Some of the standards are more specific related to the defence, financial, medical, nuclear, transportation, etc. (see the Appendix).

There are number of standards addressing safety and security of a system related to the software development. For example, avionics RTCA-Do-178B [96] or the IEC 61508 [35, 53] as the fundamental standard for the functional safety of E/E/EP systems [35, 53]. The IEC 62304 [51] standard is for the software life-cycles of medical device development that addresses to achieve more specific goals through standard process activity, and helps to design the safe systems. All the necessary requirements for each life-cycle process are provided by the IEC 62304. The process standard IEC 62304 [51] is a collection of two other standards ISO 14791 and ISO 13485, where the ISO 14791 standard is for quality, and the ISO 13485 is for risk management.

Institute of Electrical and Electronics Engineers (IEEE) standards [54] provides a safety assurance level for industries, including: power and energy, biomedical and health care, information technology, transportation, nanotechnology, telecommunication, information assurance, and many more. The IEEE standard is approved by authority and considers the users recommendations before apply into the development process. All these standards are reviewed at least every five years to qualify the new amendments in the systems.

Food and Drug Administration (FDA) [68] is established by US Department of Health and Human Services (HHS) in 1930 for regulating the various kinds of product like food, cosmetics, medical devices, etc. The FDA is now using standards in the regulatory review process to provide a safety to the public before using any product. The FDA provides some guidelines on the recognition to use of and consensus standards. The FDA is interested in the standards because they can help to serve as a common yardstick to assist with mutual recognition, based on the signed Mutual Recognition Agreement between the European Union and United States. The FDA standard classifies the medical devices based on risk and the use of medical devices. The FDA provides some standard guidelines for the medical devices, and the medical devices require to meet these standards. Time to time lots of amendments have been done in the FDA standards [33, 68] according to the use of medical devices to provide a safety.

Common Criteria (CC) [18] is an international standard that allows an evaluation of security for the IT products and technology. The CC is an international standard (ISO/IEC 15408) [58] for computer security certification. CC is a collection of existing criteria: European (Information Technology Security Evaluation Criteria

(ITSEC)), US (Trusted Computer Security Evaluation Criteria (TCSEC)) and Canadian (Canadian Trusted Computer Product Evaluation Criteria (CTCPEC)) [19–21]. The CC enables an objective evaluation to validate that a particular product or system satisfies a defined set of security requirements. The CC provides a framework for the computer users, vendors and testing organisations for fulfil their requirements and assures that the process of specification, implementation and testing of a product has been conducted in a rigorous and standard manner.

There are several ways to tackle the complexity issues of software, which major the software at industrial scales and usability of the software. The Software Engineering Institute, funded by the military, has produced a Capability Maturity Model (CMM) [90] by which may be assessed the quality of management in a software engineering team. The CMM broadly refers to a process improvement approach that is based on a process model. A process model is a structured collection of practices that describe the characteristics of effective processes; the practices included are those proven by experience to be effective. The CMM can be used to assess an organisation against a scale of five process maturity levels. Each level ranks the organisation according to its standardisation of processes in the subject area being assessed.

2.9 Regulations for Medical Devices

All kinds of medical products have to comply with national or international regulatory bodies that can provide safety assurance to use the medical products. The pathway from product design to the final product is often unclear and number of challenges and questions increase as medical device become more complex. The regulating bodies cover the essential requirements to regulate the standards of safety and performance of the medical devices. Medical device manufacturers agree to follow medical device development standards to provide the life-saving technologies to patient without compromising in safety with low cost.

The past decades shows several recalls related to the safety issues in the medical devices [63]. Everyday lots of defects are reported by consumers that are a serious consequence due to medical device failures. Faults in medical devices, such as pacemakers, defibrillators, artificial hip, and stents, have caused severe patient injuries and deaths. In 2006, FDA reported 116,086 device related injuries, 96,485 malfunctions, and 2,830 deaths; a more recent independent analysis claims there were 4,556 device-related deaths in 2009 [45, 63]. These recalls have raised many questions related to the device development process, designing and testing tools, and resources are adequate to ensure that the developed device are safe and secure to use in practice. However, the adoption of medical regulations has increased the rates of infant mortality, life expectancy, and premature and preventable deaths all over the world.

2.9.1 Device Classification

The Food and Drug Administration (FDA) has classified all the medical devices into three classes based-on the safety and effectiveness level [93]. The safety and effectiveness levels are categorised in the low, medium and high risks, respectively. Device classification determines different types of regulatory requirements that must be followed by the medical device manufacturers.

Class I

Class I devices are sufficient to provide reasonable assurance of the safety and effectiveness of the device with minimal potential for harm. The devices of this class are simpler than the Class II and Class III. These devices are subject to only general controls. Manufacturer registration with the FDA, good manufacturing techniques, branding and marking of the products are the main issues that are covered under the general controls [93]. These general controls are sufficient to provide safety and effectiveness of the devices. Class I devices are exempt from the premarket notification and the FDA determines low risk of illness or injuries to patient [93]. Class I devices include tongue depressors, bedpans, elastic bandages, examination gloves, and hand held surgical instruments and other similar types of common equipment.

Class II

Class II devices more complex than Class I devices, and the general controls of the Class II are insufficient to assure safety and effectiveness. To provide such assurances, additional methods are required [93]. Class II devices are also subject to special control in addition to the general controls of Class I. Special controls may include standard performance, labelling requirements and premarket review to reduce or mitigate risk. Class II assures that the used devices will not because of injuries or harm to patients. X-ray machines, powered wheelchairs, infusion pump, surgical drapes, surgical needles, suture material and acupuncture needles are the main devices of this class.

Class III

Class III devices have insufficient information to assure safety and effectiveness solely through the general and special controls that are sufficient for Class I and Class II devices [93]. In addition of the general controls of Class I, premarket approval and a scientific review are needed to ensure the safety and effectiveness of the Class III devices. Class III devices are described as those for which "insufficient information exists to determine that general controls are sufficient to provide reasonable assurance of its safety and effectiveness or that application of special controls that can provide such assurance and if, in addition, the device is life-supporting or life-sustaining, or for the use of substantial importance for preventing impairment of human health, or if the device presents a potential unreasonable risk of illness or injury" [93]. Class III includes devices which are life-supporting or life-sustaining, and devices which present a high or potentially unreasonable risk of illness or injury to a patient. Class III includes complex devices like heart valve, breast implants, implanted cerebral stimulator and cardiac pacemaker.

2.9.2 Regulation Issues

Development in the area of medical devices is rapidly changing. Over the last 25 years, medical devices have evolved from analog to digital systems. In the current development, microprocessor, software, smart sensor and actuator are the main components of medical systems. Most of the medical devices are based-on embedded real-time system. The functionality of these complex systems is mainly based on software to provide robustness, safety and effectiveness. An embedded system may be used for special-purpose computer system to perform any particular task due to resource limitation. The life of medical devices has decreased due to more rapid innovation in enabling technology and demand for the more robust systems. Increasing complexity of the medical systems has raised many recalls. Regulating bodies are used to control the quality of medical devices and to provide safety in use. The current development techniques and existing tools are not sufficient to provide assurance to use any medical device. Due to failure cases and constraints in exiting approach, the regulating bodies have offered several research challenges in the area of medical device development. The following challenges provide a framework for thinking about the main issues of current medical regulations [22, 33, 110]:

- A new platform and implementation technologies is required to support science- and engineering-based design, development, and certification to analysis the quality of advanced medical devices and new emerging technologies.
- Software based on medical devices must be validated according to the state of the art taking into account the principles of development life-cycle, risk management, validation and verification.
- Simulation based closed-loop modelling is required to evaluate the medical devices.
- Use quantitative analysis to evaluate a risk and to identify the safety issues of medical devices.
- Preventing from a malicious malfunction of software of the medical devices, and handling the emerging issues for information security and privacy.
- To provide a protection against emerging infectious diseases and terrorism.
- To use a formal methods-based design techniques to develop the medical devices.
- Developing a new approach to use clinical data in evaluating medical devices.
- Development of the robust, safe and sustainable medical devices with low manufacturing cost with increasing quality and performances.

2.10   Industrial Application of Formal Methods

This section surveys previous works related to the critical system development. A common theme in much of this work is to use formal methods. Formal methods provide numerous tools and techniques for solving the different kinds of problems. Mainly formal methods are applicable for verification and validation of a system. Formal methods are used to verifying the specification of a system. Although the safety-critical systems have got the confidence in the development due to use of formal methods, such techniques are applicable in a wide variety of application areas in industry. Formal methods have been used to improve the quality of the system as well as verifying the correctness of a system at an early stage of the system development. A set of examples that pioneered the application of formal methods, to more recent examples that illustrate the current state of the art. Here, we have given a list of industrial applications, where formal methods have been used in the projects. A detail survey of all these projects is presented in [13, 14, 23, 97].

2.10.1   IBM's Customer Information Control System

A successful application of formal methods was the verification of the Customer Information Control System (CICS) in 1980, which was collaborated between Oxford University and IBM Hursley Laboratories [49]. The overall system contains more than 750,000 lines of code. Some part of the code was produced from Z specifications, or partially specified in Z, and the resulting specifications were verified using a rigorous approach. Some tools, related to the type checking and parsing were developed during the project, which were used to assist the specifier and code inspector. More than 2000 pages of formal specifications were developed for verifying the system. Measurements taken by IBM throughout the development process indicated an overall improvement in the quality of the product, a reduction in the number of errors discovered, and earlier detection of errors found in the process [23]. Furthermore, it was estimated that the use of formal methods reduced 9 % of the development cost for the new release of the software.

2.10.2   The Central Control Function Display Information System (CDIS)

The Center Control Function Display (CDIS) System was delivered from Praxis to the UK Civil Aviation Authority in 1992 for London's airspace as a new air traffic management system [39]. The CDIS system consists of fault tolerant architecture of a distributed network, where more than 100 computers are linked together. Formal methods were used at various levels of the system development. The requirements analysis phase was represented by formal descriptions using structured notations.

The VDM [10] tool was used for specifying the whole system, which specified concurrent system behaviours. At the product design level, the VDM code was refined into more concrete specifications, and a lower level code was formally specified and developed using CCS [85]. The productivity of the system was better than the traditional system development and the quality of the system was improved through finding some faults.

2.10.3 The Paris Métro Signalling System (SACEM)

The SACEM system [44] was developed by several industrial partners GEC Alsthom, MATRA Transport and CSEE (Compagnie des Signaux et d'Entreprises Électriques) in 1989. The system was responsible for controlling the RER commuter train system Paris. The existing system was made of embedded software and hardware, where software had 21000 lines of code. Some parts of the SACEM software were formally specified in the B modelling language [2] for the proving purpose. The SACEM project is an example of "reverse engineering" process, where formal specification and verification were conducted after developing the code. Finally, the system was certified by the French railway authority.

ClearSy has developed the screen door controllers for Paris metro line using B formal methods [71]. The models are developed using correct by construction approach and to prove the absence of failure in the system behaviour. A constructive process was used during system specification and design leads to a high-quality system.

2.10.4 The Traffic Collision Avoidance System (TCAS)

Formal specification of the Traffic Collision Avoidance System (TCAS) [15] is another interesting example of the application of formal methods in the air-traffic transport domain. The TCAS system is used by all commercial aircraft for reducing the chance of a mid-air collision. In early 1990s, a safety critical system research group at the University of California, produced a formal requirements specification for the TCAS due to occurring some flaws in the original TCAS specification. The formal specification was developed into Requirements State Machine Language (RSML) [75], which is based on a variant of Statecharts [40]. The original specification was not supported by existing formal methods tools, but nevertheless, it was very useful for the project reviewers, in the sense of improving the original specification. Heimdahl et al. [43] successfully checked the consistency and completeness of the TCAS specification and provably-correct code generated from the RSML specification.

2.10.5 The Rockwell AAMP5 Microprocessor

The microcode of AAMP5 microprocessor was formally specified and verified, which was produced by Rockwell [84]. This project was undertaken by Collins Commercial Avionics (CCA) and SRI. The AAMP5 microprocessor has a complex architecture, designed for Ada language and implements floating-point arithmetic in the microcode. PVS theorem prover [26] was used for specifying and verifying the microcode of the AAMP5 instructions.

2.10.6 The VIPER Microprocessor

VIPER microprocessor was developed with a simple architecture, specifically for the safety critical applications [27]. Formal methods were used throughout the development cycle of VIPER, at the different level using different techniques. This work was conducted by the Royal Signals and Radar Establishment (RSRE). Some parts of the system were specified by the HOL theorem prover and LCF-LSM language [37]. Mainly top level specification and abstract level view for register transfer level were carried out in the HOL. There was not any significant result through this formal verification except finding some minor flaws in the system, which had no concerns for the fabricators of the chip.

2.10.7 INMOS Transputer

In 1985, a microprocessor manufacturing company INMOS starts to use the formal program specification, transformation and proof techniques for designing a microprocessor. Formal methods based techniques were used for designing or developing the components of the INMOS Transputer. Different types of formal techniques like, Z, Occam and CSP were the main tools for specifying system requirements. For example, the Z specification language was used to specify the IEEE Floating Point Standard, and the combined approach of Z and Occam was used to design the scheduler, for the microprocessor. Later, the CSP with other formal techniques were used in design and verification of new features on the third generation Transputer (T9000), Virtual Channel Processor (VCP). The VCP is a device that allows several logical connections between two processors that was implemented by a single physical connection. This successful application of formal methods offers to apply into a hardware engineering environment [25].

2.10.8 The Mondex Electronic Purse

In this section, we have mentioned the Mondex Electronic Purse as a significant example of the use of formal methods in an industrial-scale application. The Mondex

Electronic Purse [16, 100, 112] is an electronic system for e-commerce, based on smart card, produced by NatWest Development Team. Electronic purse must ensure the security of each transaction. Formal methods were used by a several group of researchers for verifying the protocol of money transfer over an insecure and lossy medium. The whole formal specification of the Mondex system was developed and proved from an abstract model to concrete model using refinement approach. The abstract model was focused specially on the safety properties of the system.

2.10.9 Darlington: Trip Computer Software

This case study describes the computerised shutdown system of Darlington Nuclear Generating Station (DNGS). The shutdown application contains two independent systems, Shutdown System One (SDS1) and Shutdown System Two (SDS2). The SDS1 is operated by dropping neutron-absorbing rods into the core; the SDS2 is operated by liquid poison injection into the moderator [25, 107]. The Trip computers are connected with plant sensor to shutdown the system, whenever shutdown is required. This Trip computers are used alone to concern the safety issues. The shutdown systems were required a high level of confidence to obtain the certification standard. The regulatory bodies were not sure to check the validity of the software. Thus, the formal techniques were used to identify the discrepancies in the shutdown systems. The verification process was conducted on the complete system. The entire process is reported in [5]. The final system was redesigned or modified according to the regulators and concludes that the new develop system is safe for use.

2.10.10 The BOS Control System

The BOS Software is an automatic system, which is used to protect the harbour of Rotterdam from flooding, while concurrently also controls the ship traffic [104]. BOS controls a movable barrier, taking decisions of when and how the barrier has to move, based on chaotic behaviour of water level, tidal info, and weather preconditions. BOS is a highly critical system, which is characterised by IEC 61508 [53]. The design and implementation of the BOS were undertaken by CMG Den Haag B.V., in collaboration with a formal methods team at University of Twente. Different kinds of methodologies were applied during development of the system. Mainly formal methods were used to specify the crucial part of the system for validating the system specification. The control part of the system was formally specified in PROMELA and the data part into Z specification language. The formal validation of the design focused on the communication protocol between BOS and an environment. The final implementation of the system was done in C++ which was generated from Z specification. At the initial level of the system development, formal methods helped to uncover several issues in the existing system. Overall use of the formal methods improves the quality of the system.

2.10.11 NIST Token-Based Access Control System (TBACS)

Token-Based Access Control System (TBACS) is a smart card access control system that is based on cryptographic technique. This system was developed by US National Institute for Standard and Technology (NIST) [25], where they used formal techniques in order to verify all the essential safety properties. A set of permitted and prohibited actions were the main safety properties that were mainly focused on information access and transmission. These safety properties were formally expressed in mathematical logic using a set of invariants. In this development process, a theorem prover tool FDM was used for verification purpose. The FDM tool was very useful to identify a significant flaw related to the smart token that was easily removed without any excessive cost of the system development. The TBACS experiment provides a proper guidelines to satisfy related standards.

2.10.12 The Intel® Core™ i7 Processor Execution Cluster

Intel Core i7 processor [65] is used to verify using formal methods. The Intel Core i7 processor is a multi-core processor, where formal methods were used for pre-silicon validation of the execution cluster EXE, a component that is responsible for carrying out data computations for all microinstructions. The EXE cluster implements more than 2,700 microinstructions and supports multi-threading. The formal methods were used here to verify the data-path, control logic, and the state of the components. Formal methods based on symbolic simulation, and inductive invariants were used in the validation process of the processor. The significant contribution was of this project that the formal verification completely replaced traditional coverage driven testing and proved that the formal verification was a viable alternative approach for traditional testing techniques in terms of time and costs with respect to quality of the system.

Here, we have presented a list of projects related the critical system development using formal methods. All these projects have used different kinds of formal techniques for discovering the bugs at the early stage of the system development and have shown that formal methods could be a significant approach for verifying the systems. Formal method techniques are very expensive and hard to apply in the system development process due to complexity of mathematics and the limitations of existing tools [26, 64, 88]. Main limitations are, each tool based on formal method can be used for only specific purpose, and a formal model developer requires good experience to use formal methods and knowledge of related mathematics. To know the significant use of formal methods [13, 14, 23, 97] as well as handling its complexity, in this book, we propose a new development life-cycle methodology, where each step is based on formal techniques. In this context, we develop a chain of techniques and tools for supporting the system development life-cycle using formal techniques from requirement analysis to code generation.

2.11 Formal Methods for Safety-Critical Systems

This section presents the use of formal methods in the critical device system software development through providing some informal definitions of the main concepts.

2.11.1 Why Formal Methods?

Providing a high integrity system with the embedded software requires a careful argument for its justification. Demonstrating the requirements through sufficient statistical evidence based on testing, and other general reliability measures has been shown to be doubtful. Thus, some other kinds of arguments have to be written, which must be precise—in language that is well-defined, whose meaning is clear, and with the ability to prove statements without doubt. Since natural language is unable to fulfil such demands, the only possible solution is to use a mathematical approach—formal methods [103].

A formal approach is an ideal for verification, the activity guaranteeing correctness, that we are building the system right and particularly, that successive refinements of a specification are consistent with each other. More than that, the discipline which they encourage often leads to a more careful analysis of the most basic assumptions and definitions in the design, a benefit which is often understated [103]. In particular, they may point to ambiguities in the requirements' definition. Formal methods are thus effective for validation—making sure that we are building the right system [13, 47, 102].

The main objective of formal methods is to help developers to build the reliable systems. Formal methods is a cutting-edge technology for developing the critical systems, where high safety and security are required. Mathematics is a basic foundation for formal logic that provides some ways to discover potential errors at the early stage of the development. Figure 2.8 presents modified V-model after introducing formal methods in a development process. This figure shows that module testing and integration testing are not required due to formally verified system at the specification and design level. Formal methods help to reduce the burden of exhaustive testing, which are used by the traditional development. Formal techniques verify the whole system at the early stage of the system development during specification and design, and to prove the correctness of the system. We cannot say that formal method is a silver bullet, but it is more reliable than the other traditional development approaches. Now formal methods' techniques are feasible to apply for any larger and complex problems.

2.11.2 Motivation for Their Use

The use of formal methods is very limited in current industrial practice. It is mainly used for verification and validation of any specific part of the system. Specifically,

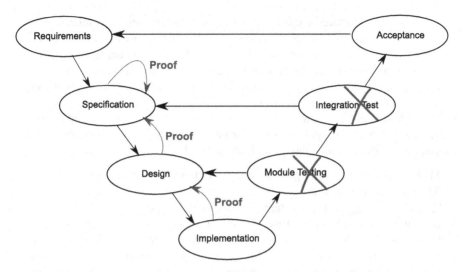

Fig. 2.8 The V-model of safety-critical system development using formal methods

it addresses that the formal methods are not well integrated into established critical system development processes. There are a number of reasons for this. First, the application of formal methods requires high abstraction and mathematical skills to write specifications and conduct proofs, and to read and understand formal specifications and proofs, especially when they are very complex. Second, existing formal methods do not offer usable and effective methods to use in the well-established industrial software process. There are lots of effective tools are available, which are crucial for formal methods application, but existing tools are not able to support a complete formal software-development process, although tools supporting the use of formal methods in limited areas are available in [26, 64, 88]. To make formal methods more practical and acceptable in industry, some substantial changes must be made.

This book proposes a development life-cycle and a set of associated techniques and tools to develop the highly critical systems using formal techniques from requirements analysis to automatic source code generation. In this context, we have developed a set of techniques and tools related to the Event-B modelling language [3]. Event-B modelling language is only used for verifying the part of a system. There is not a set of supporting tools, which can be used for the formal software development. The proposed techniques and tools have filled all missing tools and provide a rigorous framework for the system development process. The proposed approach is evaluated through a "Grand Challenge" case study, relative to the development of the cardiac pacemaker. This case study is related to the medical domain. Our main objective is to use this case study to show the effectiveness of our proposed approach and give the evidence that developed techniques and tools are applicable for any critical systems.

In this book, we have provided some possible solutions for the emerging problems in the area of software engineering related to the development of the critical systems. We have captured some missing things in the existing tools related to the formal methods that are essentially required for developing any highly critical system. We have proposed a set of new techniques and tools to model the critical systems, which cover some set of weakness in the existing approach. No one method or tool can serve all purposes. From the experience, we have learnt what kinds of techniques can have the most impact. To be attractive to the practitioners, methods and tools should satisfy the following criteria, where we realise that some of these criteria are ideals, but it is still good to strive for them and some of the basic criteria [23] are required in the development of methods and tools:

1. Methods and tools should provide significant benefits for developing a system, when starting to use them.
2. Helps for writing clear, consistent and unambiguous specifications.
3. It should be possible to amortise the cost of a method or tool over many uses. For example, it should be possible to derive benefits from a single specification at several points in a programme life-cycle: in design analysis, code optimisation, test case generation, and regression testing. Moreover existing developed specification can be reused for other development processes.
4. Methods and tools should work in conjunction with each other and with common programming languages and techniques. Developers should not have to "buy into" a new methodology completely to begin receiving benefits. The use of tools for formal methods should be integrated with that of tools for traditional software development, for example, compilers and simulators.
5. Notations and tools should provide a starting point for writing formal specifications for developers who would not otherwise write them. The knowledge of formal specifications needed to start realising benefits should be minimal.
6. Methods and tools should support evolutionary system development by allowing partial specification and analysis of selected aspects of a system.

A new method or tool should have precise strengths and weakness, limitations, modelling assumptions and to support for ease integration with other technique's, etc. Clear selection criteria helps the potential users to decide what method or tool is most appropriate for the particular problem. Given that no formal methods technique is likely to be suitable for describing and analysing every aspect of a complex system, a practical approach is to use different methods in combination. Based on the results of the survey performed in this chapter it is possible to identify the contribution that this book makes. We have given our motivation for developing new techniques and tools as follows:

- *Development life-cycle methodology*: This is the heart of the book, which presents a methodology for the critical system development from requirement analysis to automatic code generation with standard safety assessment approach. It is an extension of the waterfall model [8, 108] with some rigorous approaches to produce a reliable critical system. This methodology combines the refinement approach with a verification tool, model checker tool, real-time animator and finally generates the source code using automatic code generation tools. This kind of approach is very useful to develop the whole system using formal techniques and to verify the complex properties of a system and to discover the potential problems.

- *Environment modelling*: The most challenging problem is an environment modelling, for instance, to validate and verify the correct behaviour of a system model, requires an interactive formal model (an environment formal model). For example, a cardiac pacemaker or cardioverter-defibrillators (ICDs) formal models require a heart model to verify the correctness of the developed system. No any tools and techniques are available to provide an environment modelling to verify the developed system model. The main objective is to use formal approach for modelling the medical device and biological environment to verify the correctness of the medical systems.

  To model a biological environment (the heart) for a cardiac pacemaker or cardioverter-defibrillators (ICDs), we propose a method for modelling a mathematical heart model based on logico-mathematical theory. The heart model is based on electrocardiography analysis [7, 41, 69], which models the heart system at cellular level [106]. The main key feature of this heart model is the representation of all the possible morphological states of the electrocardiogram (ECG) [6, 7]. The morphological states represent the normal and abnormal states of the electrocardiogram (ECG). The morphological representation generates any kind of heart model (patients model or normal heart model using ECG). This model can observe a failure of impulse generation and failure of impulse propagation.

- *Refinement chart*: There are several ways to handle the design complexity of a system. Refinement technique is the most common approach, which facilitates to build a system gradually. We have discovered a very simple way to present the whole system based on operational behavioural using a refinement chart. The refinement chart is a graphical representation of a complex system using layering approach, where functional blocks are divided into multiple simpler blocks in a new refinement level, without changing the original behaviour of the system. The final goal to use this refinement chart is to obtain a specification that is detailed enough to be effectively implemented, but also to correctly describe the requirements of a system. The purpose of the refinement chart is to provide an easily manageable representation for different refinements of a system. The refinement chart offers a clear view of assistance in "system" integration. This approach also gives a clear view about the system assembling based on the operating modes and different kinds of features. For example, if a developer does not want to provide any particular feature in any system, then using the refinement chart, it is possible to find that removable feature easily and not to include in the final development system. However, it can also provide the information that, which other parts will be affect-able, when we remove the particular operating modes.

- *Real-time animator*: Lots of formal methods based animator are available for different formal languages. But all kinds of animator use only *toy-data* sets. No any tool is available for real-time data testing without generating the source code of the system. We have provided an architecture to use a set of real-time data for animation using formal specification. Here, we have discovered that the medical experts are unable to understand the complex formal specifications, so that we have proposed a new technique to apply a real-time data set to animate the formal specification and a domain expert can anticipate in the system development. Another objective is to develop this technique also for requirement traceability according to the domain experts. For example, through the animation of the formal model using real-time data set, domain experts can help to find the missing behaviour of a system.

- *Automatic source code generation form formal models*: Different kinds of code generation tools are available, and can generate source code into any programming languages but the main constraint is that all those tools are not applicable to generating the codes from Event-B modelling language. The main objective is to develop a set of code generation tools, which can support automatic code generation into several programming languages from Event-B modelling language and supports in the development life-cycle of a critical system from requirement analysis to code generation.
- *Integration of different approaches*: We proposed a new framework to compose different kinds of formal techniques to model a critical system to overcome the existing problems. An integration of formal techniques in the development process of a critical system provides the modelling concepts with formal semantics that captures at a high-level of abstraction. Modelling concepts should not be restricted due to apply the verification techniques for checking the correctness of a system. However, the system specifier should have the freedom to use the intuitive modelling concepts neglecting the complexity they impose on verification. The integration framework should bridge the gap between modelling concepts and input that is required for verification tools. For instance, integration of theorem prover and model checker can be used for verifying the essential properties. The compositional reasoning strategies using theorem prover and model checking can reduce the verification effort and to verify the required safety properties. The model checker helps to discover lots of errors and strengthening the safety properties through careful cross analysis of the model animation. System specifications are verified by both the model checker and theorem prover tools to prove the absence of any error.

References

1. Abdelmoez, W., Nassar, D. M., Shereshevsky, M., Gradetsky, N., Gunnalan, R., Ammar, H. H., et al. (2004). Error propagation in software architectures. In *Proceedings, 10th international symposium on software metrics* (pp. 384–393).
2. Abrial, J.-R. (1996). *The B-book: Assigning programs to meanings*. New York: Cambridge University Press.
3. Abrial, J.-R. (2010). *Modeling in Event-B: System and software engineering* (1st ed.). New York: Cambridge University Press.
4. Acuña, S. T., & Juristo, N. (2005). *International series in software engineering. Software process modeling*. Berlin: Springer.

5. Archinoff, G. H., Hohendorf, R. J., Wassyng, A., Quigley, B., & Borsch, M. R. (1990). *Verification of the shutdown system software at the Darlington nuclear generating station.* Presented at the international conference on control instrumentation and nuclear installations, Glasgow.

6. Artigou, J. Y., & Monsuez, J. J. (2007). *Cardiologie et maladies vasculaires.* Paris: Elsevier Masson.

7. Bayes, B. V. N., de Luna, A., & Malik, M. (2006). The morphology of the electrocardiogram. In *The ESC textbook of cardiovascular medicine* (pp. 1–36). Oxford: Blackwell.

8. Bell, R., & Reinert, D. (1993). Risk and system integrity concepts for safety-related control systems. *Microprocessors and Microsystems, 17,* 3–15.

9. Berry, G., Bouali, A., Fornari, X., Ledinot, E., Nassor, E., & de Simone, R. (2000). ESTEREL: A formal method applied to avionic software development. *Science of Computer Programming, 36*(1), 5–25.

10. Bjørner, D., & Jones, C. B. (Eds.) (1978). *The Vienna development method: The metalanguage.* London: Springer.

11. Blanc, L., & Dissoubray, S. (2000). Esterel methodology for complex system design. *Microelectronic Engineering, 54*(1–2), 163–170.

12. Blanchard, B. S., & Fabrycky, W. J. (2006). *Prentice Hall international series in industrial and systems engineering. Systems engineering and analysis.* Upper Saddle River: Pearson Prentice Hall.

13. Bowen, J., & Stavridou, V. (1993). Safety-critical systems, formal methods and standards. *Software Engineering Journal, 8*(4), 189–209.

14. Bozzano, M., & Villafiorita, A. (2010). *Design and safety assessment of critical systems* (1st ed.). Boston: Auerbach.

15. Britt, J. J. (1994). Case study: Applying formal methods to the traffic alert and collision avoidance system (TCAS) II. In *Ninth annual conference on computer assurance,* COMPASS'94 (pp. 39–51).

16. Butler, M., & Yadav, D. (2007). An incremental development of the Mondex system in Event-B. *Formal Aspects of Computing, 20*(1), 61–77.

17. Cai, K.-Y. (1996). *Introduction to fuzzy reliability.* Norwell: Kluwer Academic.

18. CC. Common criteria. http://www.commoncriteriaportal.org/.

19. CC (2009). Common criteria for information technology security evaluation, part 1: Introduction and general model. http://www.iec.ch/.

20. CC (2009). Common criteria for information technology security evaluation, part 2: Security functional requirements. http://www.iec.ch/.

21. CC (2009). Common criteria for information technology security evaluation, part 3: Security assurance components. http://www.iec.ch/.

22. CDRH (2006). Safety of marketed medical devices. Center for Devices and Radiological Health, US FDA.

23. Clarke, E. M., & Wing, J. M. (1996). Formal methods: State of the art and future directions. *ACM Computing Surveys, 28,* 626–643.

24. Cousot, P., Cousot, R., Feret, J., Mauborgne, L., Miné, A., Monniaux, D., et al. (2007). Combination of abstractions in the Astrée static analyzer. In *Lecture notes in computer science. Proceedings of the 11th Asian computing science conference on advances in computer science: Secure software and related issues* (pp. 272–300). Berlin: Springer.

25. Craigen, D., Gerhart, S., & Ralston, T. (1993). An international survey of industrial applications of formal methods. In J. P. Bowen & J. E. Nicholls (Eds.), *Workshops in computing. Z user workshop,* London, 1992 (pp. 1–5). London: Springer. ISBN 978-3-540-19818-5.

26. Crow, J., Owre, S., Rushby, J., Shankar, N., & Srivas, A. (1995). *A tutorial introduction to PVS.* Computer Science Laboratory, SRI International.

27. Cullyer, W. J. (1989). Implementing high integrity systems: The viper microprocessor. *IEEE Aerospace and Electronic Systems Magazine, 4*(6), 5–13.

28. Cullyer, W. J., Goodenough, S. J., & Wichmann, B. A. (1991). The choice of computer languages for use in safety critical systems. *Software Engineering Journal, 6,* 51–58.

29. Dobrica, L., & Niemelä, E. (2002). A survey on software architecture analysis methods. *IEEE Transactions on Software Engineering, 28*(7), 638–653.
30. Draft defence standard 00-56 (1996). Safety management requirements for defence systems containing programmable electronics. Ministry of Defence, UK.
31. Eubanks, C. F., Kmenta, S., & Ishii, K. (1996). System behavior modeling as a basis for advanced failure modes and effects analysis. In *Proceedings of the ASME design engineering technical conference*. London: UCL Press.
32. Fankhauser, H. (2001). Safety functions versus control functions. In U. Voges (Ed.), *Lecture notes in computer science: Vol. 2187. Computer safety, reliability and security* (pp. 66–74). Berlin: Springer.
33. FDA. Food and Drug Administration. http://www.fda.gov/.
34. Fries, R. C. (2011). *Handbook of medical device design*. New York: Dekker.
35. Gall, H. (2008). Functional safety IEC 61508/IEC 61511 the impact to certification and the user. In *Proceedings of the 2008 IEEE/ACS international conference on computer systems and applications*, AICCSA'08 (pp. 1027–1031). Washington: IEEE Comput. Soc.
36. Gibbs, W. W. (1994). Software's chronic crisis. *Scientific American*, September.
37. Gordon, M. J. C. (1983). *LCF-LSM: A system for specifying and verifying hardware*. University of Cambridge Computer Laboratory.
38. Halbwachs, N., Caspi, P., Raymond, P., & Pilaud, D. (1991). The synchronous dataflow programming language Lustre. In *Proceedings of the IEEE* (pp. 1305–1320).
39. Hall, A. (1996). Using formal methods to develop an ATC information system. *IEEE Software, 13*(2), 66–76.
40. Harel, D. (1987). *Algorithmics: The spirit of computing*. Boston: Addison-Wesley Longman.
41. Harrild, D. M., & Henriquez, C. S. (2000). A computer model of normal conduction in the human atria. *Circulation Research, 87*, 25–36.
42. Hegde, V., & Raheja, D. (2010). Design for reliability in medical devices. In *Reliability and maintainability symposium (RAMS), 2010 proceedings—annual* (pp. 1–6).
43. Heimdahl, M. P. E., & Leveson, N. G. (1996). Completeness and consistency in hierarchical state-based requirements. *IEEE Transactions on Software Engineering, 22*, 363–377.
44. Hennebert, C., & Guiho, G. (1993). SACEM: A fault tolerant system for train speed control. In *The twenty-third international symposium on fault-tolerant computing*, FTCS-23 (pp. 624–628). Digest of papers.
45. High Confidence Software and Systems Coordinating Group (2009). *High-confidence medical devices: Cyber-physical systems for 21st century health care* (Technical report). NITRD. http://www.nitrd.gov/About/MedDevice-FINAL1-web.pdf.
46. Hiller, M., Jhumka, A., & Suri, N. (2001). An approach for analysing the propagation of data errors in software. In *Proceedings of the 2001 international conference on dependable systems and networks (formerly: FTCS)*, DSN'01 (pp. 161–172). Washington: IEEE Comput. Soc.
47. Hinchey, M. G., & Bowen, J. P. (1995). *Prentice Hall international series in computer science. Applications of formal methods*. London: Prentice Hall.
48. Hokstad, P., & Corneliussen, K. (2004). Loss of safety assessment and the IEC 61508 standard. *Reliability Engineering & Systems Safety, 83*(1), 111–120.
49. Houston, I., & King, S. (1991). CICS project report experiences and results from the use of Z in IBM. In S. Prehn & W. Toetenel (Eds.), *Lecture notes in computer science: Vol. 551. VDM'91 formal software development methods* (pp. 588–596). Berlin: Springer.
50. IEC60513 (1994). International Electrotechnical Commission: Fundamental aspects of safety standards for medical electrical equipment. http://www.iec.ch/.
51. IEC62304 (2006). International Electrotechnical Commission: Medical device software—software life-cycle processes. http://www.iec.ch/.
52. IEC60513 (2007). International Electrotechnical Commission: Medical electrical equipment. http://www.iec.ch/.
53. IEC61508 (2008). IEC functional safety and IEC 61508: Working draft on functional safety of electrical/electronic/programmable electronic safety-related systems. http://www.iec.ch/.

54. IEEE-SA. IEEE Standards Association. http://standards.ieee.org/.
55. IEEE Std. 1012-1998. IEEE standard for software verification and validation. http://standards.ieee.org/.
56. IEEE Std. 1074-1997. IEEE standard for developing software life cycle processes. http://standards.ieee.org/.
57. Imperial Chemical Industries Ltd., Chemical Industries Association, & Chemical Industry Safety and Health Council (1977). *A guide to hazard and operability studies*. London: Chemical Industry Safety and Health Council of the Chemical Industries Association.
58. ISO. International Organization for Standardization. http://www.iso.org/.
59. ISO 13485. International Organization for Standardization: Medical devices—quality management systems—requirements for regulatory purposes. http://www.iso.org/.
60. ISO 14971. International Organization for Standardization: Medical devices—application of risk management to medical devices. http://www.iso.org/.
61. Jetley, R. P., Carlos, C., & Purushothaman Iyer, S. (2004). A case study on applying formal methods to medical devices: Computer-aided resuscitation algorithm. *International Journal on Software Tools for Technology Transfer, 5*(4), 320–330.
62. Jetley, R., Purushothaman Iyer, S., & Jones, P. (2006). A formal methods approach to medical device review. *Computer, 39*(4), 61–67.
63. Johnson, J. A. (2012). FDA regulation of medical devices. http://www.fas.org/sgp/crs/misc/R42130.pdf.
64. Jones, C. B. (1990). *Systematic software development using VDM* (2nd ed.). Upper Saddle River: Prentice Hall.
65. Kaivola, R., Ghughal, R., Narasimhan, N., Telfer, A., Whittemore, J., Pandav, S., et al. (2009). Replacing testing with formal verification in Intel Core^{tm} i7 processor execution engine validation. In *Proceedings of the 21st international conference on computer aided verification*, CAV'09 (pp. 414–429). Berlin: Springer.
66. Kanholm, J. (2003). *ISO 13485:2003 & FDA QSR, 21 CFR 820, quality manual: 34 procedures and forms*. Los Angeles: AQA Press.
67. Kapur, K. C. (2007). *Reliability and maintainability* (pp. 1921–1955). New York: Wiley.
68. Keatley, K. L. (1999). A review of the FDA draft guidance document for software validation: Guidance for industry. *Quality Assurance, 7*(1), 49–55.
69. Khan, M. G. (2008). *Rapid ECG interpretation*. Clifton: Humana Press.
70. Laprie, J. C. C., Avizienis, A., & Kopetz, H. (Eds.) (1992). *Dependability: Basic concepts and terminology*. Secaucus: Springer.
71. Lecomte, T., Servat, T., & Pouzancre, G. (2007). Formal methods in safety-critical railway systems. In *10th Brazilian symposium on formal methods*, Ouro Preto (pp. 29–31).
72. Leveson, N. G. (1991). Software safety in embedded computer systems. *Communications of the ACM, 34*, 34–46.
73. Leveson, N. G., & Harvey, P. R. (1983). Software fault tree analysis. *The Journal of Systems and Software, 3*(2), 173–181.
74. Leveson, N. G., & Turner, C. S. (1993). An investigation of the Therac-25 accidents. *Computer, 26*, 18–41.
75. Leveson, N. G., Heimdahl, M. P. E., Hildreth, H., & Reese, J. D. (1994). Requirements specification for process-control systems. *IEEE Transactions on Software Engineering, 20*(9), 684–707.
76. Lions, J. L. (Chairman) (1996). *Ariane 5 flight 501 failure: Report by the inquiry board* (Technical report). Paris: European Space Agency.
77. Lyu, M. R. (Ed.) (1996). *Handbook of software reliability engineering*. Hightstown: McGraw-Hill.
78. Macedo, H. D., Larsen, P. G., & Fitzgerald, J. (2008). Incremental development of a distributed real-time model of a cardiac pacing system using VDM. In *Lecture notes in computer science. Proceedings of the 15th international symposium on formal methods*, FM'08 (pp. 181–197). Berlin: Springer.

79. Main Commission (1994). *Report on the accident to Airbus A320-211 aircraft in Warsaw on 14 September 1993* (Technical report). Warsaw: Aircraft Accident Investigation.
80. Marciniak, J. J. (2002). *Encyclopedia of software engineering* (2nd ed.). New York: Wiley.
81. McDermid, J. A. (2002). Software hazard and safety analysis. In *Proceedings of the 7th international symposium on formal techniques in real-time and fault-tolerant systems*, FTRTFT'02 (pp. 23–36). London: Springer. Co-sponsored by IFIP WG 2.2.
82. McDermid, H. C., Forder, J., & Storrs, G. (1993). Sam—a tool to support the construction, review and evolution of safety arguments. In *Directions in safety-critical systems* (pp. 195–216). London: Springer.
83. MIL-STD-882C (1993). System safety program requirements. US DoD. http://www.system-safety.org/.
84. Miller, S. P., & Srivas, M. (1995). Formal verification of the AAMP5 microprocessor: A case study in the industrial use of formal methods. In *Proceedings, Workshop on industrial-strength formal specification techniques* (pp. 2–16).
85. Milner, R. (1982). *A calculus of communicating systems*. Secaucus: Springer.
86. NASA Technical Team (2004). *NASA software safety guidebook* (Technical report). NASA Technical Standard.
87. Neumann, P. (1995). Safeware: System safety and computers. *Software Engineering Notes*, *20*, 90–91.
88. Overture. Overture: Formal modelling in VDM. http://www.overturetool.org/.
89. Parnas, D. L. (1972). On the criteria to be used in decomposing systems into modules. *Communications of the ACM*, *15*, 1053–1058.
90. Paulk, M. C. (1995). *The SEI series in software engineering. The capability maturity model: Guidelines for improving the software process*. Reading: Addison-Wesley.
91. Price, D. (1995). Pentium FDIV flaw-lessons learned. *IEEE MICRO*, *15*(2), 86–88.
92. Redmill, M. C. F., & Catmur, J. (1999). *System safety: HAZOP and software HAZOP* (1st ed.). Chichester: Wiley.
93. Register, O. F. (1999). *Code of federal regulations. Guidance for industry and FDA: Regulation of medical devices: Background information for international officials*.
94. Register, O. F. (2011). *Code of federal regulations. Title 21, Food and drugs, Pt. 1-99* (p. 511). Revised as of April 1, 2011. US Independent Agencies and Commissions. ISBN 9780160883941.
95. Rouse, W. B., & Compton, W. D. (2009). Systems engineering and management. *Information, Knowledge, Systems Management*, *8*(1–4), 231–240.
96. RTCA (1992). Do-178B, software considerations in airborne systems and equipment certification. Committee: SC-167. http://www.rtca.org/.
97. Rushby, J. (1995). *Formal methods and their role in the certification of critical systems* (Technical report). Safety and reliability of software based systems (twelfth annual CSR workshop).
98. Schumann, J. M. (2001). *Automated theorem proving in software engineering*. New York: Springer.
99. Sommerville, I. (1995). *Software engineering* (5th ed.). Redwood City: Addison-Wesley Longman.
100. Stepney, S., Cooper, D., & Woodcock, J. (2000). *An electronic purse: Specification, refinement, and proof* (Technical monograph PRG-126). Oxford University Computing Laboratory Programming Research Group.
101. Tekinerdogan, B., Sozer, H., & Aksit, M. (2008). Software architecture reliability analysis using failure scenarios. *The Journal of Systems and Software*, *81*(4), 558–575.
102. Thomas, M. (1993). The industrial use of formal methods. *Microprocessors and Microsystems*, *17*, 31–36.
103. Trafford, P. J. (1997). *The use of formal methods for safety-critical system*. PhD thesis, Kingston University.

104. Tretmans, J., Wijbrans, K., & Chaudron, M. R. V. (2001). Software engineering with formal methods: The development of a storm surge barrier control system revisiting seven myths of formal methods. *Formal Methods in System Design, 19*(2), 195–215.

105. Voas, J. (1997). Error propagation analysis for cots systems. *Computing and Control Engineering Journal, 8*(6), 269–272.

106. von Neumann, J. (1966). *Theory of self-reproducing automata.* Chicago: University of Illinois Press. A. W. Burks (Ed.).

107. Wassyng, A., & Lawford, M. (2003). Lessons learned from a successful implementation of formal methods in an industrial project. In K. Araki, S. Gnesi, & D. Mandrioli (Eds.), *Lecture notes in computer science: Vol. 2805. FME 2003: Formal methods* (pp. 133–153). Berlin: Springer.

108. Wichmann, B. A., & British Computer Society (1992). *Software in safety-related systems* (Special report). BCS.

109. Wilkinson, P. J., & Kelly, T. P. (1998). Functional hazard analysis for highly integrated aerospace systems. In *Certification of ground/air systems seminar* (pp. 4–146). New York: IEEE. Ref. No. 1998/255.

110. Wizemann, T. (Ed.) (2010). *Public health effectiveness of the FDA 510(k) clearance process: Balancing patient safety and innovation: Workshop report.* Washington: National Academies Press.

111. Woodcock, J., & Banach, R. (2007). The verification grand challenge. *Journal of Universal Computer Science, 13*(5), 661–668.

112. Woodcock, J., Stepney, S., Cooper, D., Clark, J. A., & Jacob, J. (2008). The certification of the Mondex electronic purse to ITSEC level E6. *Formal Aspects of Computing, 20*(1), 5–19.

113. Woodcock, J., Larsen, P. G., Bicarregui, J., & Fitzgerald, J. (2009). Formal methods: Practice and experience. *ACM Computing Surveys, 41*, 19:1–19:36.

114. Xu, H., & Maibaum, T. (2012). An Event-B approach to timing issues applied to the generic insulin infusion pump. In Z. Liu & A. Wassyng (Eds.), *Lecture notes in computer science: Vol. 7151. Foundations of health informatics engineering and systems* (pp. 160–176). Berlin: Springer.

115. Zhang, Y., Jones, P. L., & Jetley, R. (2010). A hazard analysis for a generic insulin infusion pump. *Journal of Diabetes Science and Technology, 4*(2), 263–283.

116. Zio, E. (2009). Reliability engineering: Old problems and new challenges. *Reliability Engineering & Systems Safety, 94*(2), 125–141.

Chapter 3
The Modelling Framework: Event-B

Abstract This chapter presents an overview of the Event-B notations that are used to formalise the cardiac pacemaker case study. Event-B has evolved from the Classical B for specifying and reasoning about reactive systems. Main motivation to select Event-B is targeted at an incremental modelling style where a system is defined abstractly, and later interesting properties are introduced in an incremental fashion using a stepwise refinement. The use of refinement represents a system at different levels of abstraction and the use of mathematical proof verifies consistency between the refinement levels. Event-B is an event-based approach which is defined in terms of a few simple concepts describing a discrete event system and proof obligations that permit verification of properties of an event system. This chapter explains the fundamental concepts and formal notations of Event-B modelling language. Event-B is provided with tool support in the form of an open and extensible Eclipse-based IDE called Rodin, which is a platform for the Event-B specification and verification.

3.1 Introduction

3.1.1 Overview of B

Classical B is a state-based method developed by Abrial for specifying, designing and coding software systems. It is based on Zermelo-Fraenkel set theory with the axiom of choice. Sets are used for data modelling, *Generalised Substitutions* are used to describe state modifications, the refinement calculus is used to relate models at varying levels of abstraction, and there are a number of structuring mechanisms (machine, refinement, implementation), which are used in the organisation of a development. The first version of the B method is extensively described in The B-book [2]. It is supported by the Atelier B tool [21] and by the B Toolkit [10].

Central to the classical B approach is the idea of a software operation which will perform according to a given specification if called within a given pre-condition. Subsequent to the formulation of the classical approach, Abrial and others have developed a more general approach in which the notion of *event* is fundamental. An

N.K. Singh, *Using Event-B for Critical Device Software Systems*,
DOI 10.1007/978-1-4471-5260-6_3, © Springer-Verlag London 2013

event has a firing condition (a guard) as opposed to a pre-condition. It may fire when its guard is true. Event based models have proved useful in requirement analysis, modelling distributed systems and in the discovery/design of both distributed and sequential programming algorithms.

After an extensive experience with B, current work by Abrial is proposing the formulation of a second version of the method [3]. This distills experience gained with the event-based approach and provides a general framework for the development of *discrete systems*. Although this widens the scope of the method, the mathematical foundations of both versions of the method are the same.

3.1.2 Proof-Based Development

Proof-based development methods [2, 7, 34] integrate formal proof techniques in the development of software systems. The main idea is to start with a very abstract model of the system under development. Details are gradually added to this first model by building a sequence of more concrete ones. The relationship between two successive models in this sequence is that of *refinement* [2, 7, 9, 19]. The essence of the refinement relationship is that it preserves already proved *system properties* including safety properties and termination.

A development gives rise to a number of, so-called, *proof obligations*, which guarantee its correctness. Such proof obligations are discharged by the proof tool using automatic and interactive proof procedures supported by a proof engine [21, 22].

At the most abstract level it is obligatory to describe the static properties of a model's data by means of an *invariant* predicate. This gives rise to proof obligations relating to the consistency of the model. They are required to ensure that data properties which are claimed to be invariant are preserved by the events or operations of the model. Each refinement step is associated with a further invariant which relates the data of the more concrete model to that of the abstract model and states any additional invariant properties of the (possibly richer) concrete data model. These invariants, so-called *gluing invariants* are used in the formulation of the refinement proof obligations.

The goal of a B development is to obtain a *proved model*. Since the development process leads to numerous proof obligations, the mastering of proof complexity is a crucial issue. Even if a proof tool is available, its effective power is limited by classical results over logical theories and we must distribute the complexity of proofs over the components of the current development, e.g. by refinement. Refinement has the potential to decrease the complexity of the proof process whilst allowing for traceability of requirements.

B models rarely need to make assumptions about the *size* of a system being modelled, e.g. the number of nodes in a network. This is in contrast to model checking approaches [20]. The price to pay is to face possibly complex mathematical theories and difficult proofs. The re-use of developed models and the structuring mechanisms available in B help in decreasing the complexity. Where B has been exercised on known difficult problems, the result has often been a simpler proof development than has been achieved by users of other more monolithic techniques [33].

3.1.3 Scope of the B Modelling

The scope of the B method concerns the complete process of software and system development. Initially, the B method was mainly restricted to the development of software systems [11, 26, 30] but a wider scope for the method has emerged with the incorporation of the event based approach [1, 3, 5, 14, 15] and is related to the systematic derivation of reactive distributed systems. Events are simply expressed in the rich syntax of the B language. Abrial and Mussat [5] introduce elements to handle liveness properties. The refinement of the event-based B method does not deal with fairness constraints but introduces explicit counters to ensure the happening of abstract events, while new events are introduced in a refined model. Among case studies developed in B, we can mention the METEOR project [11] for controlling train traffic, the PCI protocol [18], the IEEE 1394 Tree Identify Protocol [6]. Finally, B has been combined with CSP for handling communications systems [13, 14] and with action systems [15]. The proposal can be compared to the action systems [8], UNITY programs [19] and TLA$^+$ [28] specifications but there is no notion of abstract fairness like in TLA$^+$ or in UNITY.

3.1.4 Structure of This Chapter

This chapter presents basic information about Event-B modelling language. Section 3.2 explores the related techniques and Sect. 3.3 presents the Event-B modelling notation. Section 3.4 gives an idea about modelling actions over states, and Sect. 3.5 represents the proof obligations. Section 3.6 gives detail about model refinement, and finally, Sect. 3.7 discusses about the decomposition approach in modelling.

3.2 Related Techniques

The B method is a state-based method integrating set theory, predicate calculus and generalised substitution language. We briefly compare it to related notations.

Like Z [25, 37], B is based on the ZF set theory; both notations share the same roots, but we can point to a number of interesting differences. Z expresses state change by use of before and after predicates, whereas the predicate transformer semantics of B allows a notation which is closer to programming. Invariants in Z are incorporated into operation descriptions and alter their meaning, whereas the invariant in B is checked against the state changes described by operations and events to ensure consistency. Finally, B makes a careful distinction between the logical properties of pre-conditions and guards, which are not clearly distinguished in Z.

The refinement calculus used in B for defining the refinement between models in the event-based B approach is very close to Back's action systems, but tool support for action systems appears to be less mechanised than B.

TLA^+ [29, 32] can be compared to B, since it includes set theory with the ϵ operator of Hilbert. The semantics of TLA^+ temporal operator is expressed over traces of states whereas the semantics of B actions is expressed in the weakest precondition calculus. Both semantics are equivalent with respect to safety properties, but the trace semantics of TLA^+ allows an expression of fairness and eventuality properties that is not directly available in B.

VDM [23, 27] is a method with similar objectives to classical B. Like B it uses partial functions to model data, which can lead to meaningless terms and predicates, e.g. when a function is an applied outside its domain. VDM uses a special three valued logic to deal with indefiniteness. B retains classical two valued logic, which simplifies proof at the expense of requiring more care with indefiniteness. Recent approaches to this problem will be mentioned later. ASM [12, 24, 35] and B share common objectives related to the design and the analysis of (software/hardware) systems. Both methods bridge the gap between human understanding and formulation of real-world problems and the deployment of their computer-based solutions. Each has a simple scientific foundation: B is based on set theory, and ASM is based on the algebraic framework with an abstract state change mechanism. An Abstract State Machine is defined by a signature, an abstract state, a finite collection of rules and a specific rule; rules provide an operational style very useful for modelling specification and programming mechanisms. Like B, ASM includes a refinement relation for the incremental design of systems; the tool support of ASM is under development, but it allows one to verify and to analyse ASMs. In applications, B seems to be more mature than ASM, even if ASM has several real successes like the validation [38] of Java and the Java Virtual Machine.

3.3 The Event-B Modelling Notation

Event-B [4], unlike Classical B [2], does not have a fixed syntax. We summarise the concepts of the Event-B modelling language [4, 17] developed by Abrial and indicate the links with the tool called Rodin [36]. Here, we present the basic notation for Event-B using some syntax. We proceed like this to improve legibility and help the reader remembering the different constructs of Event-B. The syntax should be understood as a convention for presenting Event-B models in a textual form rather than defining a language.

Event-B [4] modelling language has mainly two main constructs *contexts* and *machines*, which are used to model a system. Contexts is used to formalise the static

Fig. 3.1 Relationship
between constructs: Machine
and Contexts

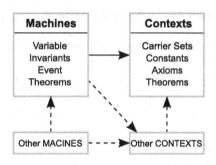

parts of the system, while Machines is used to specify dynamic behaviour of the
system. Context can be extended by other contexts and referenced by machines.
A dynamic part of the system, machines can be refined by machines. Figure 3.1
depicts basic constructs and their relationship.

3.3.1 Contexts

Contexts express the axiomatic static properties of the models. Contexts may contain carrier sets (s), constants (c), axioms, and theorems. The carrier sets are just
represented by their name. The different carrier sets of a context are completely independent, and that are supposed to be non-empty. The constants are defined using
a set of predicates. The predicates of a system require to satisfy properties $\mathcal{P}(s, c)$.
A set of axioms can describe properties of the carrier sets and the constants. Theorems are derived properties that can be proved from the axioms. Proof obligations
associated with contexts are straightforward: the stated theorems must be proved,
which follow from the predefined axioms and theorems. Additionally, a context may
be indirectly seen by machines. Namely, a context C can be seen by a machine M
indirectly if the machine M explicitly sees a context which is an extension of the
context C.

3.3.2 Machines

A machine is a known as a formal discrete model that expresses dynamic behavioural properties of a system. The machine model contains a set of state variables
(x), invariants $I(x)$, theorems, events (e), and variants. A variable x represents the
state of the machine. The variables, like constants, correspond to simple mathematical objects: sets, binary relations, functions, numbers, etc. They are constrained by
invariants $I(x)$. Invariants $I(x)$ are supposed to hold whenever the value of variables changes.

A machine is organising events modifying state variables, and it uses static informations defined in a context. These basic structure mechanisms are extended

Table 3.1 Set-theoretical notation

Name	Syntax	Definition
Binary relation	$s \leftrightarrow t$	$(\mathcal{P})(s \times t)$
Composition of relations	$r_1 ; r_2$	$\{x, y \mid x \in a \,\wedge\, y \in b \,\wedge\, \exists z.(z \in c \,\wedge\, x, z \in r_1 \,\wedge\, z, y \in r_2)\}$
Inverse relation	r^{-1}	$\{x, y \mid x \in \mathcal{P}(a) \,\wedge\, y \in \mathcal{D}(b) \,\wedge\, a \mapsto b \in r\}$
Domain	$dom(r)$	$\{a \mid a \in s \,\wedge\, \exists b.(b \in t \,\wedge\, a \mapsto b \in r)\}$
Range	$ran(r)$	$dom(r^{-1})$
Identity	$id(s)$	$\{x, y \mid x \in s \,\wedge\, y \in s \,\wedge\, x = y\}$
Restriction	$s \lhd r$	$id(s) ; r$
Co-restriction	$r \rhd s$	$r ; id(s)$
Anti-restriction	$s \lhd\!\!\!- r$	$(dom(r) - s) \lhd r$
Anti-co-restriction	$r \rhd\!\!\!- s$	$r \rhd (ran(r) - s)$
Image	$r[w]$	$ran(w \lhd r)$
Overriding	$q \lhd\!\!\!+ r$	$(dom(r) \lhd q) \cup r$
Partial function	$s \nrightarrow t$	$\{r \mid r \in s \leftrightarrow t \,\wedge\, (r^{-1} ; r) \subseteq id(t)\}$

by the refinement mechanism which provides a mechanism for relating an abstract model and a concrete model by adding new events or by adding new variables. This mechanism allows us to develop gradually Event-B models and to validate each decision step using the proof tools. The refinement relationship should be expressed as follows: a model M is refined by a model P, when P is simulating M. The final concrete model is close to the behaviour of the real system that is executing events using real source code. We give details now on the definition of events, refinement and guidelines for developing the complex system models.

3.4 Modelling Actions over States

The event-driven approach [4, 17] is based on the Classical B notation [2]. It extends the methodological scope of basic concepts to take into account the idea of *formal reactive models*. Briefly, a formal reactive model is characterised by a (finite) list x of *state variables* possibly modified by a (finite) list of *events*, where an invariant $I(x)$ states properties that must always be satisfied by the variables x and *maintained* by the activation of the events. Table 3.1 presents some set-theoretical notations of Event-B [4] and Classical B [2], which are used to formalise a system. We summarise the definitions and principles of formal models and explain how they can be managed by tools [36].

Each event is composed of a guard $G(t, x)$ and an action $R(t, x)$, where t are local variables the event may contain. The guard states the necessary condition under which an event may occur, and the action describes how the state variables evolve when the event occurs. The first general form for an event is as follows:

$$\boxed{\textbf{ANY } t \textbf{ WHERE } G(x, t) \textbf{ THEN } x : |R(x, x', t) \textbf{ END}}$$

Table 3.2 List of generalised substitutions

Type	Generalised substitution
Empty	*skip*
Deterministic	$x := E(x, t)$
Non-deterministic	$x :\in E(x, t)$
	$x : \mid P(x, x')$

Second form of an event (e), when event (e) has not any local variable (t), then an event is represented as follows:

$$\boxed{\textbf{WHEN } G(x) \textbf{ THEN } x : \mid R(x, x') \textbf{ END}}$$

Third form of an event (e), when event (e) has not any guard (G) and local variable (t), then an event is represented as follows:

$$\boxed{\textbf{BEGIN } x : \mid R(x, x') \textbf{ END}}$$

The first form for an event means that it is guarded by a guard that states the necessary condition for this event to occur. The guard is represented by $\exists t \cdot G(t, x)$. It defines a possibly non-deterministic event where t represents a vector of distinct local variables. It is also semantically equivalent to $\exists t \cdot (G(t, x) \wedge R(x, x', t))$. In the first, second and third forms, *before-after* predicate $BA(e)(x, x')$, associated with each event e, describes the event as a logical predicate expressing the relationship linking the values of the state variables just before (x) and just after (x') the *execution* of event e. The third form of the event (e) is used for initialisation.

Generalised substitutions (see Table 3.2) are also borrowed from the B notation [2]. They provide a means to express changes to state variable values. The action of an event is composed of mainly three kinds of assignments: *skip* (do nothing), deterministic assignment and non-deterministic assignment. Where x is a variable, E is an expression and P is a predicate. The value of x in each case depends on its corresponding expression/predicate. For example, $x :\in E(x, t)$, x will be assigned as an element of $E(x, t)$. In the case of $x : \mid P(x, x')$, x will be assigned as a value satisfying the predicate P. $x : \mid P(x, x')$ is a more general substitution form of an assignment predicate. This should be read as x *is modified in such a way that the value of x afterwards, denoted by x', satisfies the predicate* $P(x, x')$, where x' denotes the *new value* of the vector and x denotes its *old value*.

3.5 Proof Obligations

Proof obligations are generated by Rodin tool [36]. Different kinds of proof obligations are produced by Rodin tool that are as follows: WD (well-definedness), INV (Invariant Preservation), GRD (Guard Strengthening), SIM (Action Simulation), FIS (Feasibility), etc. The WD proof obligations are generated to ensure that formal predicates and expressions are well defined, which covers generally axioms, invariants, event guards/actions. The Rodin tool supports well-definedness to aid the activities of modelling and proving [2]. The INV proof obligations are generated to guarantee that the invariants are always preserved whenever the machine state changes. Proof obligations (INV 1 and INV 2) are produced by the Rodin tool [36] from events to state that an invariant condition $I(x)$ is preserved. Their general form follows immediately from the definition of the before-after predicate $BA(e)(x, x')$ of each event e and $grd(e)(x)$ is safety of the guard $G(t, x)$ of the event e:

> (INV1) $Init(x) \Rightarrow I(x)$
> (INV2) $I(x) \wedge BA(e)(x, x') \Rightarrow I(x')$

The generated GRD proof obligation ensures that the guard of a concrete event is a correct refinement of the corresponding guard of the abstract event. Finally, the generated SIM proof obligations aim to ensure that the abstract actions are refined correctly by the action of the corresponding concrete event as specified by any gluing invariants. Note that it follows from the two guarded forms of the events that this obligation is trivially discharged when the guard of an event is false. Whenever this is the case, the event is said to be *disabled*.

The proof obligation FIS expresses the feasibility of the event e with respect to the invariant I. By proving feasibility we achieve that $BA(e)(x, y)$ provides an after state whenever $grd(e)(x)$ holds. This means that the guard indeed represents the enabling condition of the event. The intention of specifying a guard of an event is that the event may always occur when the guard is true. There is, however, some interaction between guards and non-deterministic assignments, namely $x : |BA(e)(x, x')$. The predicate $BA(e)(x, x')$ of an action $x : |BA(e)(x, x')$ is not satisfiable or the set S of an action $v :\in S$ is empty. Both cases show violations of the event feasibility proof obligation.

> (FIS) $I(x) \wedge grd(e)(x) \Rightarrow \exists y . BA(e)(x, y)$

We say that an assignment is feasible if there is an after-state satisfying the corresponding before-after predicate. For each event its feasibility must be proved. Note, that for deterministic assignments, the proof of feasibility is trivial. Furthermore, note that feasibility of the initialisation of a machine yields the existence of an initial state of the machine. It is not necessary to require an extra initialisation.

It is sometimes useful to state that the model which has been defined is deadlock free, that it can run for ever. This is very simply done by stating that the disjunction of the event guards always hold under the properties of the constant and the invariant. This is shown as follows, where $G_1(e)(x), \ldots, G_n(e)(x)$ denotes the guards of events.

> (DKLF) $I(x) \Rightarrow G_1(e)(x) \vee G_2(e)(x), \ldots, G_n(e)(x)$

3.6 Model Refinement

The refinement of a formal model allows us to enrich the model via a *step-by-step* approach and is the foundation of our correct-by-construction approach [31]. Refinement provides a way to strengthen invariants and to add details to a model. It is also used to transform an abstract model to a more concrete version by modifying the state description. This is done by extending the list of state variables (possibly suppressing some of them), by refining each abstract event to a set of possible concrete version, and by adding new events. The abstract (x) and concrete (y) state variables are linked by means of a *gluing invariant* $J(x, y)$. A number of proof obligations ensures that,

- each abstract event is correctly refined by its corresponding concrete version;
- each new event refines *skip*;
- no new event takes control for ever;
- relative deadlock freedom is preserved.

Details of the formulation of these proofs follow. We suppose that an abstract model AM with variables x and invariant $I(x)$ is refined by a concrete model CM with variables y and gluing invariant $J(x, y)$. Event e is in abstract model AM and event f is in concrete model CM. Event f refines event e. $BA(e)(x, x')$ and $BA(f)(y, y')$ are predicates of events e and f, respectively. We have to prove the following statement, corresponding to proof obligation (1):

$$I(x) \wedge J(x, y) \wedge BA(f)(y, y') \Rightarrow \exists x' \cdot (BA(e)(x, x') \wedge J(x', y'))$$

A set of new introduced events in a refinement step can be viewed as hidden events not visible to the environment of a system and are thus outside the control of the environment. In Event-B, requiring a new event to refine *skip* means that the effect of the new event is not observable in the abstract model. Any number of executions of an internal action may occur in between each execution of a visible action. Now, proof obligation (2) states that $BA(f)(y, y')$ must refine *skip* $(x' = x)$, generating the following simple statement to prove (2):

$$I(x) \wedge J(x, y) \wedge BA(f)(y, y') \Rightarrow J(x, y')$$

The third kind of proof obligation is related to the progress of its execution, where a standard technique is to introduce a variant $V(y)$ that is decreased by each new event (to guarantee that an abstract step may occur). This leads to the following simple statement to prove (3):

$$I(x) \wedge J(x, y) \wedge BA(f)(y, y') \Rightarrow V(y') < V(y)$$

The relative deadlock freeness [16] is the property to prove that the concrete model does not introduce additional deadlocks. We give formalisms for reasoning about the guards of an event in the concrete and abstract models: $grds(AM)$ represents the disjunction of the guards of events of the abstract model, and $grds(CM)$ represents the disjunction of the guards of events of the concrete model. Relative deadlock freeness is now easily formalised as the following proof obligation (4):

$$I(x) \wedge J(x, y) \wedge grds(AM) \Rightarrow grds(CM)$$

In refining a model, an existing event can be refined by strengthening the guard and/or the before-after predicate (effectively reducing the degree of non-determinism), or a new event can be added to refine the skip event. The feasibility condition is crucial to avoiding possible states that have no successor, such as division by zero. Furthermore, this refinement guarantees that the set of traces of the refined model contains (up to stuttering) the traces of the resulting model. The refinement of an event e by an event f means that the event f simulates the event e.

The Event-B modelling language is supported by the Rodin platform [36] and has been introduced in publications [2, 4, 17], where there are many case studies and discussions about the language itself and the foundations of the Event-B approach. The language of *generalised substitutions* is very rich, enabling the expression of any relation between states in a set-theoretical context. The expressive power of the language leads to a requirement for help in writing relational specifications, which is why we should provide guidelines for assisting the development of Event-B models.

3.7 Decomposition

A large system needs several refinement steps to model the whole system from an abstract to the concrete level. Increasing refinement steps introduces many state variables to specify the desired behaviour of a system. Increasing number of state variables makes the system too complex that becomes impossible to manage. Decomposition is a process that can split the whole system into several independent subsystems. The decomposition process reduces the overall complexity of the system that helps to apply the refinement technique on each subsystem. All the independent subsystems are put together to form a single model that can guaranteed to be a refinement of the original one [4].

For developing a large complex model, it is necessary to decompose a model $\mathcal{M}$ into sub-models. Suppose the model $\mathcal{M}$ can be decomposed into two sub-models $\mathcal{P}$ and $\mathcal{Q}$. The decomposition process divides a set of events and variables of the model $\mathcal{M}$ into two groups related to the sub-models $\mathcal{P}$ and $\mathcal{Q}$. However, there are always some variables those are shared by both sub-models. The shared variables are known as *external variables*, and to handle these shared variables we need to introduce some *external events*.

Figure 3.2 presents the decomposition process of the model $\mathcal{M}$ into the sub-models $\mathcal{P}$ and $\mathcal{Q}$. A variable v_2 is an *external variable* and ex_3 and ex_2 are *external events* of the sub-models $\mathcal{P}$ and $\mathcal{Q}$, respectively. Other variables v_1 and v_3 are the *internal variables*, and e_1, e_2, e_3 and e_4 are internal events of the sub-models $\mathcal{P}$ and $\mathcal{Q}$.

Each subsystem can be refined independently after successful decomposition of the system. Such as, subsystems $\mathcal{P}$ and $\mathcal{Q}$ can be refined into $\mathcal{PR}$ and $\mathcal{QR}$ (see Fig. 3.2). The refined model $\mathcal{PR}$ contains the *internal variables* u_1 and *external variables* u_2. Similarly, the refined model $\mathcal{QR}$ contains *internal variables* u_2 and *external variables* u_3. The shared external variables v_2 are common in both decomposed models that must be refined in a same way. The desired properties must be

Fig. 3.2 Decomposition

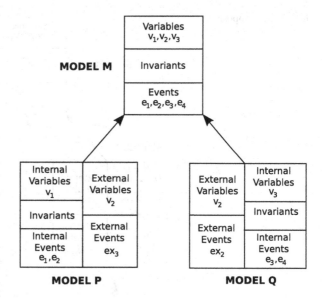

preserved at the concrete level using the gluing invariants $v_2 = h(u_2)$. The final system can be achieved through re-compositioning (see Fig. 3.3) of the refined sub-systems $\mathcal{PR}$ and $\mathcal{QR}$. It can be achieved through conjoining the invariants of both models and removing the external events. Finally, we need to prove that the final re-composed model $\mathcal{MR}$ is indeed a refinement of the original model $\mathcal{M}$. In order to prove that it is sufficient to prove the following:

> External events ex_3 in $\mathcal{P}$ and ex_2 in $\mathcal{Q}$ are refined to event e_3 and e_2 in $\mathcal{M}$

3.8 Tools Environments for Event-B

The Event-B modelling language is supported by the Atelier B [21] environment and by the Rodin platform [36]. Both environments provide facilities for editing machines, refinements, contexts and projects, for generating proof obligations corresponding to the given properties, for proving proof obligations in an automatic or/and interactive process and for animating models. The internal prover is shared by the two environments and there are hints generated by the prover interface for helping the interactive proofs. However, the refinement process of machines should be progressive when adding new elements to a given current model and the goal is to distribute the complexity of proofs through the proof-based refinement. These tools are based on logical and semantical concepts of Event-B models (machines, contexts, refinement) and our methodology for modelling the medical devices can be built from them.

Fig. 3.3 Re-composition

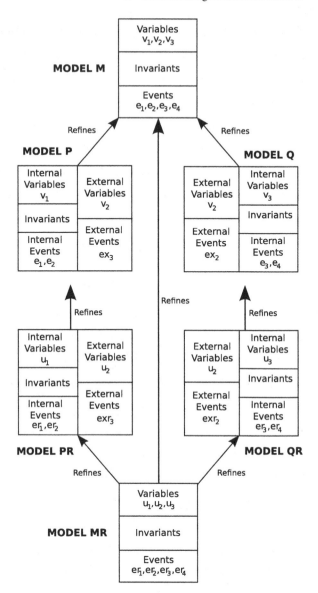

References

1. Abrial, J.-R. (1996). Extending B without changing it (for developing distributed systems). In H. Habrias (Ed.), *1st conference on the B method* (pp. 169–190).
2. Abrial, J.-R. (1996). *The B-book: Assigning programs to meanings*. New York: Cambridge University Press.
3. Abrial, J.-R. (2003). B#: Toward a synthesis between Z and B. In D. Bert, J. P. Bowen, S. King, & M. Waldén (Eds.), *Lecture notes in computer science: Vol. 2651. ZB 2003: Formal specification and development in Z and B* (pp. 168–177). Berlin: Springer.

4. Abrial, J.-R. (2010). *Modeling in Event-B: System and software engineering* (1st ed.). New York: Cambridge University Press.
5. Abrial, J.-R., & Mussat, L. (1998). Introducing dynamic constraints in B. In *Proceedings of the second international B conference on recent advances in the development and use of the B method*, B'98 (pp. 83–128). London: Springer.
6. Abrial, J.-R., Cansell, D., & Méry, D. (2003). A mechanically proved and incremental development of IEEE 1394 tree identify protocol. *Formal Aspects of Computing, 14*(3), 215–227.
7. Back, R. J. R. (1981). On correct refinement of programs. *Journal of Computer and System Sciences, 23*(1), 49–68.
8. Back, R. J. R. (1988). A calculus of refinements for program derivations. *Acta Informatica, 25*, 593–624.
9. Back, R.-J. J., Akademi, A., & Von Wright, J. (1998). *Refinement calculus: A systematic introduction* (1st ed.). New York: Springer.
10. B-Core Ltd. (1996). *B-toolkit user's manual, release 3.2.*
11. Behm, P., Benoit, P., Faivre, A., & Meynadier, J.-M. (1999). Météor: A successful application of B in a large project. In J. Wing, J. Woodcock, & J. Davies (Eds.), *Lecture notes in computer science: Vol. 1708. FM'99—formal methods* (pp. 369–387). Berlin: Springer.
12. Börger, E., & Stärk, R. (2003). *Abstract state machines: A method for high-level system design and analysis*. Berlin: Springer.
13. Butler, M. J. (1996). Stepwise refinement of communicating systems. *Science of Computer Programming, 27*(2), 139–173.
14. Butler, M. (2000). CSP2B: A practical approach to combining CSP and B. *Formal Aspects of Computing, 12*, 182–196.
15. Butler, M., & Waldén, M. (1999). Parallel programming with the B method. In E. Sekerinski & K. Sere (Eds.), *Formal approaches to computing and information technology (FACIT). Program development by refinement* (pp. 183–195). London: Springer.
16. Cansell, D., & Méry, D. (2007). Proved-patterns-based development for structured programs. In V. Diekert, M. Volkov, & A. Voronkov (Eds.), *Lecture notes in computer science: Vol. 4649. Computer science—theory and applications* (pp. 104–114). Berlin: Springer.
17. Cansell, D., & Méry, D. (2008). The Event-B modelling method: Concepts and case studies. In D. Bjørner & M. C. Henson (Eds.), *Monographs in theoretical computer science. Logics of specification languages* (pp. 47–152). Berlin: Springer.
18. Cansell, D., Gopalakrishnan, G., Jones, M., Méry, D., & Weinzoepflen, A. (2002). Incremental proof of the producer/consumer property for the PCI protocol. In *Proceedings of the 2nd international conference of B and Z users on formal specification and development in Z and B*, ZB'02 (pp. 22–41). London: Springer.
19. Chandy, K. M., & Misra, J. (1988). *Parallel program design: A foundation*. Reading: Addison-Wesley. ISBN 0-201-05866-9.
20. Clarke, E. M., Grumberg, O., & Peled, D. (2001). *Model checking*. Cambridge: MIT Press.
21. ClearSy. Atelier B. http://www.clearsy.com.
22. ClearSy, Aix-en-Provence (2004). B4FREE. http://www.b4free.com.
23. Fitzgerald, J. (2007). The typed logic of partial functions and the Vienna development method. In D. Bjørner & M. C. Henson (Eds.), *EATCS textbook in computer science. Logics of specification languages* (pp. 431–465). Berlin: Springer.
24. Gurevitch, Y. (1995). Evolving algebras 1993: Lipari guide. In *Specification and validation methods* (pp. 9–36). Oxford: Oxford University Press.
25. Henson, M. C., Deutsch, M., & Reeves, S. (2007). Z logic and its applications. In D. Bjørner & M. C. Henson (Eds.), *EATCS textbook in computer science. Logics of specification languages* (pp. 467–569). Berlin: Springer.
26. Hoare, J., Dick, J., Neilson, D., & Holm Sørensen, I. (1996). Applying the B technologies on CICS. In *FME 96* (pp. 74–84). Berlin: Springer.
27. Jones, C. B. (1990). *Systematic software development using VDM* (2nd ed.). Upper Saddle River: Prentice Hall.

28. Lamport, L. (1994). A temporal logic of actions. *ACM Transactions on Programming Languages and Systems, 16*(3), 872–923.
29. Lamport, L. (2002). *Specifying systems: The TLA$^+$ language and tools for hardware and software engineers*. Reading: Addison-Wesley.
30. Lano, K., Bicarregui, J., & Sanchez, A. (1999). Invariant-based synthesis and composition of control algorithms using B. In *FM'99—B users group meeting—Applying B in an industrial context: Tools, lessons and techniques* (pp. 69–86).
31. Leavens, G. T., Abrial, J.-R., Batory, D., Butler, M., Coglio, A., Fisler, K., et al. (2006). Roadmap for enhanced languages and methods to aid verification. In *Fifth international conference on generative programming and component engineering*, GPCE 2006 (pp. 221–235). New York: ACM.
32. Merz, S. (2007). The specification language TLA$^+$. In D. Bjørner & M. C. Henson (Eds.), *EATCS textbook in computer science. Logics of specification languages* (pp. 381–430). Berlin: Springer.
33. Moreau, L., & Duprat, J. (2001). A construction of distributed reference counting. *Acta Informatica, 37*, 563–595.
34. Morgan, C. (1990). *Prentice Hall international series in computer science. Programming from specifications*. Upper Saddle River: Prentice Hall.
35. Reisig, W. (2007). Abstract state machines for the classroom. In D. Bjørner & M. C. Henson (Eds.), *EATCS textbook in computer science. Logics of specification languages* (pp. 1–32). Berlin: Springer.
36. RODIN (2004). Rigorous open development environment for complex systems. http://rodin-b-sharp.sourceforge.net.
37. Spivey, J. M. (1987). *Understanding Z: A specification language and its formal semantics*.
38. Stärk, R., Schmid, J., & Börger, E. (2001). *Java and the Java virtual machine*. Berlin: Springer.

Chapter 4
Critical System Development Methodology

Abstract Formal methods have emerged as an alternative approach to ensuring the quality and correctness of the high confidence critical systems, overcoming limitations of the traditional validation techniques such as simulation and testing. This chapter presents a methodology for developing critical systems from requirement analysis to automatic code generation with standard safety assessment approach. This methodology combines the refinement approach with various tools including verification tool, model checker tool, real-time animator and finally, produces the source code into many languages using automatic code generation tools. This approach is intended to contribute to further the use of formal techniques for developing the critical systems with high integrity and to verify the complex properties, which help to discover potential problems.

4.1 Introduction

Software quality assurance for critical systems is an emerging market. New tools and techniques are developed to provide an assurance that systems will never show any failure. These tools and techniques are used for designing critical systems like avionics, medical devices and automotive. New developed tools and techniques are varied according to the diversity in critical systems. For example, in the medical domain, small systems like a pacemaker, requires different kinds of tools and

---

Sections of this chapter are adapted from the original publication: Méry, D., & Singh, N. K. (2012). Critical systems development methodology using formal techniques. In *Proceedings of the third symposium on information and communication technology*, SoICT'12, Ha Long (pp. 3–12). New York: ACM.

ACM COPYRIGHT NOTICE. Copyright © 2012 by the Association for Computing Machinery, Inc. Permission to make digital or hard copies of part or all of this work for personal or classroom use is granted without fee provided that copies are not made or distributed for profit or commercial advantage and that copies bear this notice and the full citation on the first page. Copyrights for components of this work owned by others than ACM must be honored. Abstracting with credit is permitted. To copy otherwise, to republish, to post on servers, or to redistribute to lists, requires prior specific permission and/or a fee. Request permissions from Publications Dept., ACM, Inc., fax +1 (212) 869-0481, or permissions@acm.org.

N.K. Singh, *Using Event-B for Critical Device Software Systems*,
DOI 10.1007/978-1-4471-5260-6_4, © Springer-Verlag London 2013

techniques than the other large systems like imaging for diagnostics or surgery navigation, patient monitoring system, etc.

Software is an essential part of any critical system, which realises system's functionality and software reliability for gaining confidence. From the last few years, the use of critical systems has been increased [69]. These devices may sometimes malfunction. Device-related problems are responsible for many accidents. A lot of deaths and injuries have been reported by the US Food and Drug Administration's (FDA) caused by failure of medical devices [51], which advocate safety and security issues for using it. Certification standards have found that many accidents due to system failure, are caused by product design and engineering flaws, which are considered as the firmware problems [16, 28].

Manufacturers have the freedom to tailor the process and to select appropriate methodology according to their specific needs. A lack of information about process and product qualities leads to uncertainness about the appropriateness of the methodology. Software development measures both processes in the quality management plan and associated safety cases related to the approval of the products. Formal methods are usually applied for analysing assumptions, relationships, and requirements of the system.

Software certification is performed by certification standards, like FDA, IEC/ISO, IEEE [35, 36, 43], which do not prove the correctness of a system. If a product receives certification, it simply means that it has met all the requirements needed for certification. It does not mean that the product is *bug-free*. Therefore, the manufacturer cannot use certification to avoid assuming its legal or moral obligations. Many standards consist of functional requirements on the particular medical products; there are also a number of standards, which address system safety and software development. For example, IEC-62304 [34] process standard for the quality and risk management of medical devices.

The scope of formal methods is limited in the current industrial practices, which address that the formal methods are not well integrated into established critical system development processes. Formal methods need high abstraction and mathematical skills to write specifications and conduct proofs, and to read and understand formal specifications and proofs, especially when they are complex, are the main reasons for not using in practices. Another important cause is that existing formal methods do not offer usable and effective methods to employ in the well-established industrial software process. None of the existing tools are able to support the formal techniques based software-development, although tools are supporting the use of formal methods in limited areas are available in [41, 45, 59]. To make formal methods more practicable and acceptable in industry, some substantial changes must be made.

Although formal methods are part of the standard recommendations [28] for developing and certifying the critical systems, how to integrate formal methods into the certification process is, in large part, unclear. Especially, it is challenging that how to demonstrate the final developed system that behaves safely. This chapter describes formal methods based development process that we have applied to produce evidence for the certification, based on the certification standards [15, 23, 36], of a software based critical system. It also describes the most effective aspects of our methodology for certification and research that could significantly increase the utility of formal methods in software certification.

The main contribution of this chapter is to propose a development life-cycle methodology for developing the highly critical software systems using formal techniques from requirements analysis to code implementation using rigorous safety assessment approach [55]. This new development life-cycle is an extension of the waterfall model [60], which can support formal methods based development using various tools. In this new development life-cycle, we introduce some new steps, which are essential for improving the quality of the system. For example, the real-time animation [53] helps in requirement traceability and to bridge among various stakeholders. There are lacks of supporting tools, which can support for developing critical systems. To realise this new development life-cycle, we use different techniques from the past research related to the field of formal methods and software engineering. For implementation purpose, we use different tools at various level of development.

Some new tools, we have developed according to the requirement of this methodology like real-time animator [53], automatic code generation [54]. There are not exiting a set of supporting tools, which can be used for developing a system using formal methods. Our proposed methodology provide a rigorous framework for developing critical systems, which may give an evidence to obtain certificate from the international standards [15, 23, 36]. We have applied our proposed approach on an industrial-scale case study related to the cardiac pacemaker to show the effectiveness of this new development life-cycle methodology.

4.1.1 Structure of This Chapter

This chapter is organised as follows. Section 4.2 presents related work and Sect. 4.3 describes the heart of the methodology for critical software system development. Section 4.4 presents benefits of proposed approach. Section 4.5 evaluates this development methodology with other existing tools. Finally, Sect. 4.6 summarises this chapter.

4.2 Related Work

During the 1950's and 1960's [31, 60], the main purpose of the software life-cycle was to provide a conceptual idea for managing the development of software systems. The conceptual idea was related to the planning, organising, coordinating, staffing, budgeting and directing the software-development activities. Since the 1960's, different kinds of descriptions and characterisations of the software-development life-cycle have emerged [10, 21, 31, 60, 62, 65].

Mainly, four traditional models of software evolution are very popular from the earliest days of software engineering. These four models are waterfall model, stepwise refinement model, incremental release model and military standards based model. The most familiar software-development model is the waterfall model, which was originated by Royce [60]. This model presents a way for developing a large complex software system using an iterative process. Stepwise refinement model develops the software system through the progressive refinement and helps in enhancement of the high-level system specifications into source code components [56, 68]. The refinement process is undefined, while it is used during the development process, and formalisation is expected to apply heuristically according to the expertise and acquired skills. These two models are effective and widely applied in the current practices of the software engineering [52]. The incremental release model is mostly applied into industrial practices. Developing systems through incremental release provides a foundation level for essential operating functions, then enriching the system functionalities at the regular intervals [5]. This model combines the classic software life-cycle with an iterative enhancement at the level of system development organisation. Periodical software maintenance and services are also supported by this incremental release model.

Military standards based models are the refined form of the classical life-cycle models, which eliminate complications that emerge during large software development. Since 1970's many government contractors use military standards for developing the large software systems [20]. Military software system is not commonly used in the industrial and academic practices. Mainly, it is used for: (1) meeting required military standards; (2) developing complex embedded systems (e.g., airplanes, submarines, missiles, command and control systems), which are mission-critical; and (3) developing under contract to private firms through cumbersome procurement and acquisition procedures that can be subject to public scrutiny and legislative intervention [20].

All these four models are used for coarse-grain characterisations of the software evolution. The primary progressive steps of software evolution are requirements specification, design, and implementation. Moreover, these models are independent of any organisational development setting, software application domain, choice of programming language, etc. However, all of these life-cycle models have been in use for some time, we refer to them as the traditional models, which are used for software evolution [52].

There have been several efforts involving the use of formal methods to verify safety-critical systems. Formal methods have been used to handle complex safety-critical systems, for instance, steam boiler control [2], Siemens Transportation Systems [4], space and avionic system [13, 18, 25, 42, 57] and so on. Various formalisms and rigorous techniques (VDM [9], Z [66], ASTRÉE [18], SCADE [7], Event-B [1], Alloy [37], CSP [29], PVS [19], SPIN [30], etc.) have been used for developing the safety-critical systems. These approaches provide a given level of reliability and confidence to develop an error-free system. Few case studies show that the formal methods have been used to check correctness of operating modes, functions and desired behaviours of the medical devices [12, 24, 39, 40, 48, 49].

C.L. Heitmeyer et al. [26, 27] have presented an approach for software certification using formal methods. They describe how formal methods are used to produce evidence in a certification, based on facts of a safety-critical software system. The evidence includes a top-level specification (TLS) of the safety-relevant software behaviour, a formal statement of required safety properties, proofs that the specification satisfied properties, and a demonstration that the source code, which has been annotated with preconditions and post-conditions, is a refinement of the top-level specification (TLS) [27]. A research report [61] is presented by John Rushby, which is based on certification issues for advanced technology. Its purpose is to explain the use of formal methods in the specification and verification of software and hardware requirements, designs, and implementations, to identify benefits, weaknesses, and difficulties in applying these methods to digital systems used in critical applications, and to suggest factors for consideration when formal methods are offered in support of certification.

Maibaum and Wassyng [50] have proposed that the assessment procedure should focus on activities and as well as a product should be reviewed according to the domain requirements based on profound engineering expertise. Assessment procedure should consider all relevant risks, including suitable activities in the development plan, selected techniques should be appropriate for activities and safety classification, and acquired evidence of software development supports validity of the arguments.

Intermediate steps during the development of the final product require several kinds of methodologies and approaches, which are also useful for providing certain facts that help for certifying the final product. For example, a requirement specification, a design specification, a document describing validation of the design against the requirements, documents relating to testing, and documents proving correctness [28, 33].

Existing development life-cycles are not well integrated with formal methods, which can support domain specific requirements and certification standards. According to the literature survey, different kinds of arguments insist to design a new methodology, which may be able to design a consistent formal model based on domain-specific requirements, and helps to certify the system. In this context, we propose a development life-cycle methodology for developing critical systems using formal techniques. This approach provides certain evidence of correctness at each level of system development from requirement analysis to code implementation. This development approach assists to design a system using *correct-by-construction* [14] and helps to verify all the essential safety properties according to the system requirements. We believe that our methodology adds value with its comprehensiveness; it focuses on correctness by establishing the standards to perform software certification. It uniformly establishes what to check and how to check, and it provides evidence to support the correctness.

4.3 Overview of the Methodology

In recent years, the critical systems have grown more complex and providing certification assurance, is a common crucial issue for certification bodies [23, 28, 35, 36, 43]. Under consideration of all kinds of requirements of certification bodies, we propose a novel development methodology that addresses the issue of certification for all kinds of critical systems, which is an extension of the waterfall model [3, 6, 63, 67] for developing a critical software system using formal methods and standard safety assessment approaches [47] from requirement analysis to final system implementation.

This development process is based on refinement approach, where we have introduced some new steps for designing the complete system using formal verification, validation and real-time animation [53]. All these steps are not only used in the development life-cycle, but they are also validating the correctness of a system, and all these processes are moreover verified by safety assessment techniques, which comply with software standards. Basic architecture of the methodology is depicted in Fig. 4.1, which may be used in the development process of a critical system [55].

In this development methodology, we have considered mainly two types of development: static development and dynamic development. Each phase includes capturing of requirements. The static development refers to the straight-forward process, which produces a program, and dynamic development refers to the activities that improve the quality of the program using refinement approach until it satisfies user requirements. In order to reach the required safety level and gain reliability, we have used standard safety assessment approaches in the development process, and also ensuring traceability between the different stages of the system development in order to reduce the validation effort. Different phases of the methodology are shown in Fig. 4.1 which is used in the development process of a critical system. Seven main phases of proposed methodology are described as follows:

4.3.1 Informal Requirements

The first activity of static development captures user requirements as completely as possible, which is an initial phase of the proposed methodology, presents an informal requirements of a given system. Software requirements specifications are widely used in a restricted form of natural language. Natural language is convenient because it allows non-technical users to understand systems requirements. On the other hand, the lack of precise semantics increases the possibility of errors being introduced due to interpretation mistakes and inherent ambiguities. Under or over specification are also common problems when using a natural language. Software requirements specification consists of the categorisation and structuring of the informal requirements fragment described in the requirements document to produce categorised requirements fragments. The main objective of informal requirements is to provide a precise, yet understandable description of the safety-relevant behaviour

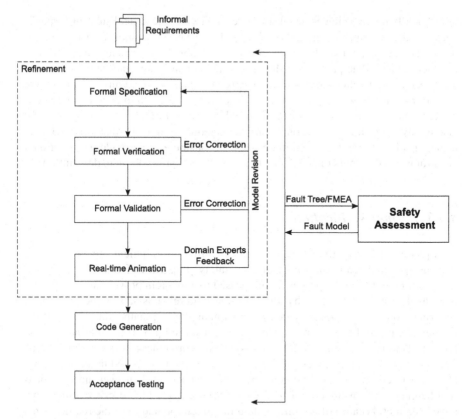

Fig. 4.1 Formal methods based development methodology of critical system

of a system and to make explicit assumptions on which the safety of a system is based. Once the developer reaches a general understanding of the problem, static development proceeds to the formal requirements specification.

4.3.2 Formal Specification

The required security requirements are formally expressed as properties of the state-based model that underlies the informal requirements. The categorised requirements fragments describe through the set of formal notations in any specific modelling language like Event-B [1], Z [66], ASM [11], VDM [9], RAISE [58], TLA$^+$ [44], etc. Formal specification languages have a mathematical (usually formal logic) basis and employ a formal notation to express the system requirements. The formal specification is typically a mathematical based description of the system behaviour, using state tables or mathematical logic. In this stage, more detailed requirements analysis is carried out by building a formal specification. Using the formal notation, precision and conciseness of specifications can be achieved. Formal specification will not normally describe lowest level software, such as mathematical subroutine packages or data structure manipulation, but will describe the response of the system to events and inputs, to a degree, necessary to establish the critical properties. For instance, in a cardiac pacemaker the sensor and actuator are functioning correctly. This specification reflects the primary user requirements derived through successive evolutions, each of which transforms an abstract specification to become more concrete. Evolution steps may involve the usual notion of formal refinement, and may also involve introducing additional constraints required in the final solution. Hence, a specification during the evolution process is considered to provide the functional constraints on the final concrete specification rather than a complete description.

4.3.3 Formal Verification

This phase has a very important role in the formal development. To demonstrate that the informal requirements satisfy the safety properties of interest, the informal requirements and the properties are passed to a theorem prover and then prover is applied to prove formally that the informal requirements satisfy the properties. A formal notation can be analysed and manipulated using mathematical operators, mathematical proof procedures can be used to test (and prove) the internal consistency (including data conservation) and syntactic correctness of the specifications. Furthermore, the completeness of the specification can be checked in the sense that all enumerated options and elements have been specified. However, no specification language can ensure completeness in the sense that all the user's requirements have been met, because of the informal human-intention nature of the requirements specifications [38]. Finally, the implementation of the system will be in a formal language (i.e., the programming language), it is easier to avoid misconceptions and ambiguities in crossing the divide from formal specifications to formal implementations. A formal verification phase is done to ensure that,

- The model is designed correctly
- The algorithms have been implemented properly
- The model does not contain errors, oversights, or bugs

In summary, we can say that verification ensures that the specification is complete and that mistakes have not been made in implementing the model. But verification does not ensure the model,

- Solves an important problem
- Meets a specified set of model requirements
- Correctly reflects the working of a real world process

In Fig. 4.1, this phase provides a feedback to the formalisation phase in case of not satisfying given properties of the system. The feedback approach is allowed to modify the formal model and verify again it through the formal verification phase. The verification process is applied to continue until not to find the correct formal model according to the expected behaviour of the system.

4.3.4 Formal Validation

Formal validation phase is the process of determining the degree to which a model is an accurate representation of the real world from the perspective of the intended uses of the model that is not covered by the formal verification. It consists of the identification of a subset of the formalised requirements fragments for an automatic validation analysis:

- Validation ensures that the model meets its intended requirements in terms of the methods employed and the results obtained.
- The ultimate goal of model validation is to make the model useful in the sense that the model addresses the right problem, provides accurate information about the system being modelled, and to make the model actually used.

Model checking [17] is a complementary technique for validation and verification of a formal specification. Model checkers attempt to make formal techniques easier to use by providing a high degree of automation at the expense of generality. Inputs to a model checker are typically a finite state model of a system, along with a set of properties that are expected to be preserved by the system. Properties to be verified can be usually categorised as one of the following:

1. Correct sequences of events
2. Proper consequences of activities
3. Simultaneous occurrences of particular events
4. Mutual exclusion of particular events
5. Required precedence of activities

The model checker explores all the possible event sequences of a model to determine that system is always holding required safety properties. If properties hold, the model checker confirms the correctness of a system. If a property fails to hold for some possible event sequences, the tool produces counter-examples, i.e., traces of event sequences that lead to failure of the property [46].

In Fig. 4.1, this phase also presents that it provides a feedback information to the formalisation phase when a model is not satisfying expected behaviour of a system. This feedback information helps to modify the developed formal model and verify it through the formal verification phase and validation through a model checker tool [17, 46]. This cyclic process for finding a correct model is applied to continue until not to find the correct formal model according to the expected system behaviour.

4.3.5 Real-Time Animation Phase

This phase is a new validation technique to verify the formal model in the real-time environment using *real-time data* set instead of using a *toy-data* set. A detailed description about the architecture of the real-time animator is available in Chap. 7

[53]. This phase is applied for rigorous testing of the formal model under domain expert's reviews. Real-time animation shows the behaviours of the system using real environment in early phase of the development without generating the source code. Such kind of techniques are very useful when domain experts are also involved in the system development [53]. Formal models are used to animate with the real-time animator [53], in order to verify on given scenarios according to the real system. This model animator is not part of the validation process, as this can be required to qualify as software requirements, but it helps us to check models against reality and to internally verify their suitability.

In Fig. 4.1, this step also presents feedback loop into the formalisation phase to correct an unexpected error of the system. The feedback approach is allowed to modify the formal model and verify it using any theorem prover tool and finally validate it using a model checker tool. In this phase of the formal development, most of the errors are discovered by the domain experts. The verification, validation and real-time animation processes are applied to continue until not find the correct formal model according to the domain experts.

Most simulation researchers agree that animation may be dangerous too, as the analysts and users tend to concentrate on a very short simulation runs so the problems that occur only in long runs go unnoticed. Of course, good analysts, who are aware of this danger, will continue run long enough to create a rare event until not cover all possible events, which is then displayed to the users. Each phase of the methodology is supported by a specific tool.

4.3.6 Code Generation

The final stage of static development is an implementation, in which a program is constructed to realise the design. This involves the realisation of the major executable components, definition of the concrete data structures, and an implementation of any minor auxiliary structures or functions that may be assumed in the design. It is important to verify the design and program against the requirements specification and design through rigorous reviews. Automatic code generation [7] is well known process to get highly verified codes according to the requirements analysis. It is an important part of the software-development process, for implementing the final system. There are several reasons for using an automatic code generator in the development of the safety-critical systems. Automatic code generation techniques produce the executable specification with fewer numbers of implementation errors than a human programmer. Manual translation process can be error prone and time consuming. An iterative process for successive changes in the specification and manual code translation can introduce errors by various ways. The consistency between the specification and code translation is often lost. This is not the case when an automatic code generator is used to obtain a source code from the verified specification. The code generator translates a proved formal model directly into a desired programming language. It ensures that the generated code is always consistent with the formal model. Code generation from the verified formal model is our final objective of this methodology.

4.3.7 Acceptance Testing

In the system development process, acceptance testing are used to determine if the requirements of a specification are met. Acceptance tests represent the customer's interests. The acceptance tests give the customer confidence that the application has the required features and that they behave correctly. In theory when all the acceptance tests pass the project is done [32]. Acceptance testing in software engineering generally involves execution of number of test cases which constitute to a particular functionality based on the requirements specified by the user. In system engineering process it may involve black-box testing performed on a system. It is also known as functional testing, black-box testing, QA testing, application testing, confidence testing, final testing, validation testing, or factory acceptance testing [8].

The dynamic development is the process to discover hidden features of the system through applying several types of tools like formal verification, model checker and real-time animator in the development process. This is an iterative way for acquiring more requirements according to the stakeholders and to verify the correctness of the system. The real-time animator based on formal methods is used here as a prototype model in the early stage of the system development. Prototyping can also be used for risk analysis, but the use of formal methods can improve the quality of prototypes. After code generation, the final system can be used to verify the system against both the informal user requirements (system testing) and the end-user (acceptance testing).

In this proposed methodology, we have used combined approach of formal proofs and rigorous reviews for a system development. The purpose of formal proof and rigorous reviews is to ensure the internal consistency of the specifications at different levels of development, to validate the specification against user requirements and certification standards, and to ensure that the designs and programs satisfy their requirements specifications.

4.4 Benefits of Proposed Approach

In this methodology, we have provided an architecture to develop a critical system (see Fig. 4.1). Our methodology has the potential for improving quality and increasing safety for certifying the highly critical systems. Specific benefits include improving requirements, reducing error introduction, improving error detection, and reducing cost. Secondly, the proposed architecture of methodology allows us to carry out rigorous analyses. Such analyses can verify the useful properties such as consistency, deadlock-freedom, satisfaction of high level requirements, correctness of a proposed system design and expected system behaviour according to the domain experts using real-time environment in early phase of the development without generating the source code.

4.4.1 Improving Requirements

Using our methodology to capture requirements provides a simple validation check in early stage of critical-system development. Requirements expressed in a formal notation can also be analysed early to detect inconsistency and incompleteness for removing errors that are normally found later in the development process.

4.4.2 Reducing Error Introduction

Formalised requirements prevent misunderstandings due to ambiguities that lead to an error introduction. As development proceeds, compliance can be continually checked using a formal analysis to ensure that errors have not been introduced. A further advantage of using our methodology at the requirements level is the ability to derive or refine from these requirements the code itself, thus ensuring that no error is introduced at this stage. Alternatively their use at the requirements level allows formal analysis to establish correctness between requirements and final generated source code of the complex systems.

4.4.3 Improving Error Detection

Out methodology can provide exhaustive verification at whatever levels it is applied: high level requirements or low level requirements. Exhaustive verification means that the whole structure is verified over all the possible inputs and states. This can detect errors that would be difficult or impossible to find using only a test based approach.

4.4.4 Reducing Development Cost

Our proposed methodology is based on formal techniques. In general, software errors are less expensive to correct the earlier in the development life-cycle they are detected in the critical systems. The effort required to generate formal models is generally more than offset by the early identification of errors. That is, when formal methods are used early in the life-cycle, they can reduce the overall cost of the project development. When requirements have been formalised, the costs of downstream activities are reduced. Formal notations also reduce cost by enabling the automation of verification activities.

4.5 Evaluation with Existing Tools

As far as we know, some commercial tools like Rational Rhapsody,[1] helps to realise the goal of Model Driven Architecture (MDA) by facilitating the creation of models of software systems. The models have varying levels of abstraction from very high-level views of the design to very specific, implementation-level views of the code. The ideal MDA tool would allow a model at a given level of abstraction to be transformed into a model at a different level. This tool is used by industries for developing the critical systems. But, this tool is not supporting any formal verification, validation and real-time animation approaches in an iterative way to verify the correctness as well as to discover hidden elements of the systems. Therefore, there are no such a tool, which can support this new methodology. As for our purpose, we have integrated the various existing tools for implementing the prototype [64]. Some new tools, we have developed according to the requirement of this methodology like real-time animator [53] and automatic code generation [54]. The proposed methodology is much superior to other exiting approaches, because they are not able to provide formal techniques based development approaches in the current industrial practices.

4.6 Summary

One valuable by-product of applying formal methods in software certification is that the process produces a formal specification of the required software behaviour. Developing this specification has at least two benefits. First, a formal specification can be valuable when a new version of the software is developed. Second, the process of developing a formal specification by itself may expose errors.

A new methodology for developing a critical system using formal methods, which is an extension of waterfall model [3, 6, 63, 67] has been described to applying formal methods in critical software development process from requirement analysis to automatic source code generation under rigorous analysis of the development process using standard safety assessment techniques. This development methodology combines the refinement approach with a verification tool, model checker tool, real-time animator and finally generates the source code using automatic code generation tool. System development process is concurrently assessed by safety assessment approach [47] to comply with certificate standards. This life-cycle methodology consists of seven main phases: informal requirements, formal specification, formal verification, formal validation, real-time animation, automatic code generation and acceptance testing. This kind of approach is very useful to verify complex properties of a system and to discover the potential problems like deadlock and liveness at early stage of the system development.

---

[1]http://www.ibm.com/software/awdtools/rhapsody/.

Building on existing software certification standards, such as IEC-62304 and the Common Criteria [15, 22, 34], more and improved approaches which use formal methods in software certification are needed. Applying these new approaches for highly critical systems should have many benefits; the exposure of errors which might have not been detected without formal methods. That guidance, as proposed by NITRD, IEEE, and IEC/ISO [28, 35, 36], allows adoption of formal methods into an established set of processes for the development and verification of a critical system to be an evolutionary refinement rather than an abrupt change of methodology. Formal methods might be used in a very selective manner to partially address a small set of objectives, or might be the primary source of evidence for the satisfaction of many of the objectives concerned with development and verification.

Two reliable facts of formal methods have demonstrated by last decades of research and experience—they are not the "*silver bullet*" to eliminate all software failures, but neither are they beyond the budget constraints of software developers. In critical system, formal methods are commonly demonstrating the absence of undesired behaviours and preserving essential properties. Model checkers, theorem provers, real-time animation and automatic code generation make it possible to analyse the complexity of the system and produce the final implemented system. On the other hand, the ability to generate complete test cases from formal specifications can result in overall savings, despite the cost of developing the specification. The process of developing a specification is often the most valuable phase of a formal verification, and "lightweight formal methods" approaches make it possible to formally analyse partial specifications and early requirements definitions. Experience with mandated use of formal techniques and other standards provides empirical evidence that these methods can be successfully incorporated into the development process for the critical systems. Remaining chapters include detailed descriptions of the new associated techniques and tools, which are used in this development methodology for critical system development.

References

1. Abrial, J.-R. (2010). *Modeling in Event-B: System and software engineering* (1st ed.). New York: Cambridge University Press.
2. Abrial, J.-R., Börger, E., & Langmaack, H. (Eds.) (1996). *Lecture notes in computer science: Vol. 1165. Formal methods for industrial applications, specifying and programming the steam boiler control*. Berlin: Springer.
3. Acuña, S. T., & Juristo, N. (2005). *International series in software engineering. Software process modeling*. Berlin: Springer.
4. Badeau, F., & Amelot, A. (2005). Using B as a high level programming language in an industrial project: Roissy VAL. In H. Treharne, S. King, M. Henson, & S. Schneider (Eds.), *Lecture notes in computer science: Vol. 3455. ZB 2005: Formal specification and development in Z and B* (pp. 15–25). Berlin: Springer.
5. Basili, V. R., & Turner, A. J. (1975). Iterative enhancement: A practical technique for software development. *IEEE Transactions on Software Engineering, 4*, 390–396.
6. Bell, R., & Reinert, D. (1993). Risk and system integrity concepts for safety-related control systems. *Microprocessors and Microsystems, 17*, 3–15.

7. Berry, G. (2007). Synchronous design and verification of critical embedded systems using SCADE and Esterel. In *Formal methods for industrial critical systems*, FMICS (p. 2).

8. Bertolino, A., & Strigini, L. (1997). Acceptance criteria for critical software based on testability estimates and test results. In *Lecture notes in computer science. Proceedings of the 15th international conference on computer safety, reliability and security*, SAFECOMP'96 (pp. 83–94). Berlin: Springer.

9. Bjørner, D., & Jones, C. B. (Eds.) (1978). *The Vienna development method: The metalanguage*. London: Springer.

10. Boehm, B. W. (1976). Software engineering. *IEEE Transactions on Computers, 25*, 1226–1241.

11. Börger, E., & Stärk, R. (2003). *Abstract state machines: A method for high-level system design and analysis*. Berlin: Springer.

12. Bowen, J., & Stavridou, V. (1993). Safety-critical systems, formal methods and standards. *Software Engineering Journal, 8*(4), 189–209.

13. Butler, R. W. (1996). *An introduction to requirements capture using PVS: Specification of a simple autopilot* (NASA Technical Memorandum 110255). Hampton: NASA Langley Research Center.

14. Carloni, L. P., McMillan, K. L., Saldanha, A., & Sangiovanni-Vincentelli, A. L. (1999). A methodology for correct-by-construction latency insensitive design. In *Proceedings of the 1999 IEEE/ACM international conference on computer-aided design*, ICCAD'99 (pp. 309–315). Piscataway: IEEE Press.

15. CC. Common criteria. http://www.commoncriteriaportal.org/.

16. CDRH (2006). Safety of marketed medical devices. Center for Devices and Radiological Health, US FDA.

17. Clarke, E. M., Grumberg, O., & Peled, D. (2001). *Model checking*. Cambridge: MIT Press.

18. Cousot, P., Cousot, R., Feret, J., Mauborgne, L., Miné, A., Monniaux, D., et al. (2007). Combination of abstractions in the Astrée static analyzer. In *Lecture notes in computer science. Proceedings of the 11th Asian computing science conference on advances in computer science: Secure software and related issues* (pp. 272–300). Berlin: Springer.

19. Crow, J., Owre, S., Rushby, J., Shankar, N., & Srivas, A. (1995). *A tutorial introduction to PVS*. Computer Science Laboratory, SRI International.

20. De Weese, P. R., Moore, J. W., & Rilling, D. (1997). U.S. software life cycle process standards. *Crosstalk: The DoD Journal of Software Engineering*.

21. Distaso, J. R. (1980). Software management—a survey of the practice in 1980. *Proceedings of the IEEE, 68*(9), 1103–1119.

22. Farn, K.-J., Lin, S.-K., & Fung, A. R.-W. (2004). A study on information security management system evaluation—assets, threat and vulnerability. *Computer Standards & Interfaces, 26*(6), 501–513.

23. FDA. Food and Drug Administration. http://www.fda.gov/.

24. Gomes, A., & Oliveira, M. (2009). Formal specification of a cardiac pacing system. In A. Cavalcanti & D. Dams (Eds.), *Lecture notes in computer science: Vol. 5850. FM 2009: Formal methods* (pp. 692–707). Berlin: Springer.

25. Halbwachs, N., Caspi, P., Raymond, P., & Pilaud, D. (1991). The synchronous dataflow programming language Lustre. In *Proceedings of the IEEE* (pp. 1305–1320).

26. Heitmeyer, C. L. (2009). On the role of formal methods in software certification: An experience report. *Electronic Notes in Theoretical Computer Science, 238*(4), 3–9.

27. Heitmeyer, C. L., Archer, M., Leonard, E. I., & McLean, J. (2008). Applying formal methods to a certifiably secure software system. *IEEE Transactions on Software Engineering, 34*(1), 82–98.

28. High Confidence Software and Systems Coordinating Group (2009). *High-confidence medical devices: Cyber-physical systems for 21st century health care* (Technical report). NITRD. http://www.nitrd.gov/About/MedDevice-FINAL1-web.pdf.

29. Hoare, C. A. R. (1985). *Communicating sequential processes*. Upper Saddle River: Prentice Hall.
30. Holzmann, G. J. (1997). The model checker SPIN. *IEEE Transactions on Software Engineering, 23*, 279–295.
31. Hosier, W. A. (1961). Pitfalls and safeguards in real-time digital systems with emphasis on programming. *IRE Transactions on Engineering Management, EM-8*(2), 99–115.
32. Hsia, P., Kung, D., & Sell, C. (1997). Software requirements and acceptance testing. *Annals of Software Engineering, 3*, 291–317.
33. Huhn, M., & Zechner, A. (2010). Arguing for software quality in an IEC 62304 compliant development process. In T. Margaria & B. Steffen (Eds.), *Lecture notes in computer science: Vol. 6416. Leveraging applications of formal methods, verification, and validation* (pp. 296–311). Berlin: Springer.
34. IEC62304 (2006). International Electrotechnical Commission: Medical device software—software life-cycle processes. http://www.iec.ch/.
35. IEEE-SA. IEEE Standards Association. http://standards.ieee.org/.
36. ISO. International Organization for Standardization. http://www.iso.org/.
37. Jackson, D. (2002). Alloy: A lightweight object modelling notation. *ACM Transactions on Software Engineering and Methodology, 11*(2), 256–290.
38. Jackson, M. (2007). The problem frames approach to software engineering. In *14th Asia-Pacific software engineering conference*, APSEC 2007 (p. 14).
39. Jetley, R., Purushothaman Iyer, S., & Jones, P. (2006). A formal methods approach to medical device review. *Computer, 39*(4), 61–67.
40. Jetley, R. P., Carlos, C., & Purushothaman Iyer, S. (2004). A case study on applying formal methods to medical devices: Computer-aided resuscitation algorithm. *International Journal on Software Tools for Technology Transfer, 5*(4), 320–330.
41. Jones, C. B. (1990). *Systematic software development using VDM* (2nd ed.). Upper Saddle River: Prentice Hall.
42. Joshi, A., & Heimdahl, M. P. E. (2005). Model-based safety analysis of Simulink models using SCADE design verifier. In *SAFECOMP* (pp. 122–135).
43. Keatley, K. L. (1999). A review of the FDA draft guidance document for software validation: Guidance for industry. *Quality Assurance, 7*(1), 49–55.
44. Lamport, L. (1994). The temporal logic of actions. *ACM Transactions on Programming Languages and Systems, 16*, 872–923.
45. Lecomte, T., Servat, T., & Pouzancre, G. (2007). Formal methods in safety-critical railway systems. In *10th Brazilian symposium on formal methods*, Ouro Preto (pp. 29–31).
46. Leuschel, M., & Butler, M. (2003). *Lecture notes in computer science. ProB: A model checker for B* (pp. 855–874). Berlin: Springer.
47. Leveson, N. G. (1991). Software safety in embedded computer systems. *Communications of the ACM, 34*, 34–46.
48. Macedo, H. D., Larsen, P. G., & Fitzgerald, J. (2008). Incremental development of a distributed real-time model of a cardiac pacing system using VDM. In *Lecture notes in computer science. Proceedings of the 15th international symposium on formal methods*, FM'08 (pp. 181–197). Berlin: Springer.
49. Magee, J. H. (2003). Validation of medical modeling & simulation training devices and systems. *Studies in Health Technology and Informatics, 94*, 196–198.
50. Maibaum, T. S. E., & Wassyng, A. (2008). A product-focused approach to software certification. *Computer, 41*(2), 91–93.
51. Maisel, W. H., Sweeney, M. O., Stevenson, W. G., Ellison, K. E., & Epstein, L. M. (2001). Recalls and safety alerts involving pacemakers and implantable cardioverter-defibrillator generators. *Journal of the American Medical Association, 286*(7), 793–799.
52. Marciniak, J. J. (2002). *Encyclopedia of software engineering* (2nd ed.). New York: Wiley.
53. Méry, D., & Singh, N. K. (2010). Real-time animation for formal specification. In M. Aiguier, F. Bretaudeau, & D. Krob (Eds.), *Complex systems design & management* (pp. 49–60). Berlin: Springer.

54. Méry, D., & Singh, N. K. (2011). Automatic code generation from Event-B models. In *Proceedings of the second symposium on information and communication technology*, SoICT'11 (pp. 179–188). New York: ACM.
55. Méry, D., & Singh, N. K. (2012). Critical systems development methodology using formal techniques. In *Proceedings of the third symposium on information and communication technology*, SoICT'12, Ha Long (pp. 3–12). New York: ACM.
56. Mili, A., Desharnais, J., & Gagné, J. R. (1986). Formal models of stepwise refinements of programs. *ACM Computing Surveys, 18*, 231–276.
57. Miller, S. P. (1998). Specifying the mode logic of a flight guidance system in Core and SCR. In *FMSP'98: Proceedings of the second workshop on formal methods in software practice* (pp. 44–53). New York: ACM.
58. Nielsen, M., Havelund, K., Wagner, K. R., & George, C. (1988). The raise language, method and tools. In *Lecture notes in computer science. VDM Europe* (pp. 376–405).
59. Overture. Overture: Formal modelling in VDM. http://www.overturetool.org/.
60. Royce, W. W. (1987). Managing the development of large software systems: Concepts and techniques. In *Proceedings of the 9th international conference on software engineering*, ICSE'87 (pp. 328–338). Los Alamitos: IEEE Comput. Soc.
61. Rushby, J. (1995). *Formal methods and their role in the certification of critical systems* (Technical report). Safety and reliability of software based systems (twelfth annual CSR workshop).
62. Scacchi, W. (1984). Managing software engineering projects: A social analysis. *IEEE Transactions on Software Engineering, SE-10*(1), 49–59.
63. Schumann, J. M. (2001). *Automated theorem proving in software engineering*. New York: Springer.
64. Singh, N. K. (2011). *Reliability and safety of critical device software systems*. PhD thesis, Department of Computing Science, Université Henri Poincaré-Nancy 1.
65. Sommerville, I. (1995). *Software engineering* (5th ed.). Redwood City: Addison-Wesley Longman.
66. Spivey, J. M. (1989). *Prentice Hall international series in computer science. The Z notation—a reference manual*. Upper Saddle River: Prentice Hall.
67. Wichmann, B. A., & British Computer Society (1992). *Software in safety-related systems* (Special report). BCS.
68. Wirth, N. (1971). Program development by stepwise refinement. *Communications of the ACM, 14*, 221–227.
69. Woodcock, J., Larsen, P. G., Bicarregui, J., & Fitzgerald, J. (2009). Formal methods: Practice and experience. *ACM Computing Surveys, 41*, 19:1–19:36.

Chapter 5
Real-Time Animator and Requirements Traceability

Abstract According to the development life-cycle of a critical system, first of all we emphasise on requirements traceability using a real-time animator. Formal modelling of requirements is a challenging task, which is used to reasoning in earlier phases of the system development and to make sure that the completeness, consistency, and automated verification of the requirements. This is an initial step in the proposed development methodology of the critical system development. The real-time animation of a formal model has been recognised to be a promising approach to support the process of validation of requirements specification. It is crucial to get an approval and feedback when domain experts have a lack of knowledge of any specification language, to avoid the cost of changing a specification at the later stage of development. This chapter introduces a new architecture, together with a direct and an efficient method of using real-time data set, in a formal model without generating the source code in any target language. This is a phase for validating a system through domain experts in our development life-cycle methodology. The principle is to simulate the desired behaviours of a given system using formal models in the real-time environment and to visualise the simulation in some form appealing to stakeholders. The real-time environment assists in the construction, clarification, validation and visualisation of a formal specification.

5.1 Introduction

Formal methods aim to improve software quality and to produce *zero-defect* software, by controlling the whole software-development process, from specifications to implementations. In formal model development, they use top-down approaches and start from high-level and abstract specifications, by describing the fundamental properties of the final system. Requirements Engineering (RE) provides a framework for simplifying a complex system to get a better understanding and to develop the quality systems. The role of verification and validation is very important in the development of safety critical systems. Verification starts from the requirements analysis stage where design reviews and checklists are used for validation where functional testing and environmental modelling are done.

N.K. Singh, *Using Event-B for Critical Device Software Systems*,
DOI 10.1007/978-1-4471-5260-6_5, © Springer-Verlag London 2013

There are several ways to validate a specification: to model a prototype of a system, structured walk-through, transformation into a graphical language, animation, and others. Each technique has a common goal, to validate a system according to the operational requirements. Animation focuses on the observable behaviour of the system [51]. The principle is to simulate an executable version of the requirements model and to visualise exact behaviours of the actual system. Animators use finite state machines to generate a simulation process which can be then observed with the help of UML diagrams, textual interfaces, or graphical animations [42]. Animation can be used in the early stage of development during the elaboration of the specification. As a relatively low cost activity, animation can be frequently used during the process to validate important refinement steps.

The final code generation process consists of two stages: final level formal specifications are translated into programs in a given programming language, and then these programs are compiled. Nevertheless, all approaches which support a formal development from specification to code must manage several constraining requirements, particularly in the domain of embedded software where specific properties on the code are expected likes timeliness, concurrency, liveness, reactivity, and heterogeneity [36]. All these properties can be represented abstractly. Finally, it is impossible to use the real-time data in the early stage of formal development without compiling the source code in any target language.

Based on our various research experience using formal tools in industrial requirements (*verification* and *validation*) and our desire to disseminate formal methods, we have imagined a new approach to present an animated model of specification using real-time data set, in the early stage of formal development [41]. Animation of formal specification is not a new idea, but capture the real-time data and perform animation of formal methods in the real environment is a new idea. In this work, we present an architecture which allows to easily develop the visualisations for a given specification with support of existing tool Brama [48]. Here, we describe an approach to extend an animator tool which will be useful to use the real-time data set. Now, present time all the animation tools use a *toy data* set to test the model while we are proposing a *key idea* to use the real-time data set with the model without generating the source code in any target language (C, C++, VHDL, etc.). It can help a specifier to gain confidence that the model that is being specified, refined and implemented, does meet the domain requirements.

This architecture supports state-based animations, using simple pictures to represent a specific state of Event-B [1] specification, and transition-based animations consisting of picture sequences by using real-time data set. A sequence of pictures is controlled by the real-time data set, and it presents an actual view of a system. Before moving on we should also mention that there are scientific and legal applications as well, where the formal model based animation can be used to simulate (or emulate) certain scenarios to glean more information or better understandings of the system requirements. Moreover, this real-time animation technique is very helpful to assist in the certification process to analyse an evidence-based validation in a critical system.

5.1.1 Structure of This Chapter

This chapter is organised as follows. Section 5.2 presents motivations behind this work. Section 5.3 presents basic definition of traceability and Sect. 5.4 presents related work. Section 5.5 presents basic details about animation and their benefits and limitations. Section 5.6 presents the functional architecture which enables the animation of a proved specification with a real-time data set. The functional architecture is then illustrated in Sect. 5.7 for applications and case studies. Section 5.8 presents limitations of this tool and finally Sect. 5.8 summarises the chapter.

5.2 Motivation

To discover the real requirements, discover errors in the early stage of the system development and design a quality system, we need to look beyond the system itself, and into the human activities that it will support. For example, medical systems are mainly used by doctors, physicians, medical practitioners and patients in a more convenient ways for their own purpose. The medical device manufacturing companies are providing safe, secure and profitable services to stakeholders. Such human activities may be complex due to several involvements of many people with different types of conflicts of interests. In this situation, it is hard to handle any problem and to reach final agreement among the stakeholders. Requirements engineering techniques offer ways to handle complex problems by decomposing into simple ones, so that we can understand them better. Complexity of a system classifies it into a specific class of problems known as *wicked problems* [45]. This term was introduced by Rittel and Webber [45] for problems that have the following characteristics:

- There is no proper definition of the problem—such as each stakeholders have their own definition of the same problem.
- Wicked problems have no stopping rule—each solution is likely to extend into a new set of problems, and the problem is never likely to be solved entirely.
- Solutions are not exactly in the form of right or wrong, but it provides for better or worse solutions.
- There is no any fixed standard for a particular solution. Solution results are depended on the judgement of various stakeholders according to their needs.
- For wicked problems, there is no any fixed enumerable solutions. The solutions are discovered during problem analysis.
- Every wicked problem is unique and considered as sufficiently complex and different from others.
- Every wicked problem is a symptom of another problem, which makes difficult to choose an appropriate level of abstraction for describing the problem.
- The designer has no 'right' to be wrong. In other words, designers are liable for the consequences of the actions they generate.

Requirement Engineering (RE) techniques are used at the early stages of the system development life-cycle, which are crucial for successful development of a system. As the computer systems play increasingly important roles in organisations, it seems to pay more attention towards the early stages of Requirement Engineering (e.g., [9]). The cost of the system development increases more when errors are discovered later phases of the system development [8]. The basic beginning objective of stakeholders and the initial requirements statement of requirement engineering are "what the system should do?". Incompleteness, ambiguity, inconsistencies, and vagueness, are the most common problems encountered when eliciting and specifying requirements and to find these common problems are the main goals of any requirement engineering tool [9].

A model captures a view of a physical system. It is an abstraction of the physical system, with a certain purpose. Thus the model completely describes those aspects of the physical system that are relevant to the purpose of the model, at an appropriate level of detail. Not only a system developer is required to view a system from several angles but stakeholders want the same view of the system from different angles according to the requirements. Requirements traceability is a branch of requirements management within software development. Requirements traceability is concerned with documenting the life of a requirement and to provide bi-directional traceability between various associated requirements. It enables users to find the origin of each requirement and track every change, which was made to this requirement.

Validation of the requirements specification is an integral and indispensable part of the Requirements Engineering (RE). Validation is the process of checking, together with the stakeholders, whether the requirements specification meets the stakeholders' intentions and expectations [39]. Animation of a formal specification is one of the well-known approaches in the area of verification and validation, which provides visual animation of the formal models. An architecture of the real-time animation tool is presented in [41], that allows to check the presence of desired functionality and to inspect the behaviour of a specification according to the stakeholders in the real-time environment.

The contribution of this chapter is to propose a new functional architecture, together with a direct and an efficient method of using real-time data set, in a formal model without generating the source code in any target programming language [41]. Real-time animation helps to design a critical system, which helps a specifier to gain confidence that the model is being specified, refined and implemented, does meet the domain expert's requirements. Main objective of this proposed real-time animation framework bridges the gap among different domain experts. For example, in the development of a medical system [34], a formal model that is designed by a software engineer is not understandable by the medical experts like doctors or medical practitioners due to lack of mathematical knowledge. If a software engineer presents a formal specification into animated graphics, based on actual behaviour of the formal specification, then the animated graphics can be simpler and easily understandable by the doctors, physicians and medical practitioners.

5.2.1   Traceability

Gotel et al. [23] have given basic definition of the requirements traceability as follows:

> *The requirements traceability is the ability to describe and follow the life of a requirement, in both a forward and backward direction, i.e. from its origins, through its development and specification, to its subsequent deployment and use, and through periods of ongoing refinement and iteration in any of these phases.*

Requirements traceability has provided twofold value. First of all, using requirements traceability, changes in the context of an application can easily be analysed for their impact on the code and test cases, and vice versa, which heavily shortens the time required for software maintenance. On the other hand, increased accountability simplifies the verification of a system to its requirements and allows better monitoring of the processes. Requirement traceability is also used as to advocate desirable properties of the software development processes [37]. Lots of problems are identified during a system development process. Traceability is used as an optional activity during system development due to limited available resources related to the traceability [6].

A project team always determines the way in which project development process should be performed at the initial phase of the project development. Various kinds of decisions realised for acceptance or rejection about a project plan are made by a project board, whereas all other technical details are determined by others [6]. In this chapter, we have introduced a new technique to use for traceability that helps to find bugs at the early stage of the system development through visual animations of a formal specification. All these approaches, methods, techniques and tools proposed for the requirements traceability are useful as long as its adoption decision is present preferably at the early stages of the projects, and we need to understand how a decision on requirements traceability is made and which factors influence an adoption of the traceability. Here, we present the conceptual treatment of these questions, which eventually provide us with a theoretical lens to examine this adoption in a systematic manner.

The traceability needs of different stakeholders according to the different kinds of goals. The requirements traceability presents a connection between requirements and related artifacts, which are created during the system development using requirements. A set of tools [2, 21, 25, 31] is used for requirement traceability for the different purpose during the software life-cycle. However, we have used real-time animator based on the formal model to trace the hidden requirements of a complex system. In requirements engineering and elicitation phase it is important that the rationales and sources to the requirements are captured in order to understand requirements evolution and verification. During design phase, the requirements traceability allows to keep track of what happens when change request is implemented before a system is redesigned. Traceability can also give information about the justifications, important decisions and assumptions behind requirements [43]. Most important advantage of the requirements traceability is to support validation of the system functionality according to the stakeholder requirements.

5.3 Related Work

Traceability is a necessary system characteristic as it supports software management, software evolution, and validation [21]. Traceability approaches help for understanding the complexity of the problems and assist for capturing, tracking and verification of the actual requirements during the software life-cycle. We believe that the established use of animation approaches should explicitly include traceability support to provide more benefits on developing software for medical and automotive domains. An interesting related work for the traceability is presented in [2, 21], where the authors review the most-recent advances techniques for traceability and also survey on tracing approaches in traditional software engineering.

Prototype refers to an incomplete version of the system development, which simulates only few aspects of the final system when requirements are indefinite and system behaviour is unclear [14]. The prototype is only used to be clarified and validated requirements. The experiences gain from prototypes are helping to produce a quality system and the requirements specification document. The prototypes work very well for only small parts of the complex problems. Various kinds of traditional techniques are used to build a rapid throwaway prototype; these include functional and logic programming languages, simulation techniques, object-oriented languages, and visual programming languages.

A prototype of executable formal specifications is used to bridge the gap between a traditional software prototyping and formal methods. An executable formal specification is considered as an abstract program which enables abstract requirements, designs formulation, explored and validated at an early stage of the system development [20]. Such kinds of prototyping techniques help to discover behaviour of the system interacting with its environment that can be observed before it exists in the actual system. Validation of a system assists to design formal documentation using the specification descriptions of system. In few cases, an executable specification forms only relevant document for all phases of the system development, such as in the use of executable specifications with transformational approaches [4].

Goguen and Meseguer [22] have proposed a novel approach for constructing a prototype using formal specification. They advocated the use of an algebraic specification language named OBJ, which can be executed by interpreting the equations of the OBJ specification as a left-to-right term rewriting system. Since several, attempts have been made to execute formal notations for rapid prototyping. Siddiqi et al. [49] have divided these attempts into three categories. First category belongs to the use of functional and logical programming languages for the construction of the prototypes [27, 35, 38, 50]. Second category is distinguished by "specially designed and specific purpose" executable specification languages that are usually embedded in an existing programming language which provides the execution mechanism [28]. Last category can be characterised as the development of an environment for the automatic prototyping of specifications. Siddiqi et al. [49] have proposed distinct approach for supporting environment, which combines the benefits of a formal system specification and its subsequent execution via rapid prototype model.

Animation is a simulation technique which is used to execute a model and shows the animation in the visual form using a formal model of a given specification. Lots of works have been done over the last few decades in this area while the idea was originally proposed by Balzer et al. [3]. The contributions mainly differ by (a) how far the model is from the underlying requirements, (b) how far the visualisation is from phenomena within the software environment, (c) how the simulation works (through direct execution of the model or preliminary translation to some executable form), and (d) how interactive and controlled the simulation can be [51]. Bloomfield et al. [7] had presented a case study in which a simple prototype for nuclear reactor protection was modelled in VDM [5], whereas a part of the safety assessment process was presented using Prolog [13] animation. Another interesting study of the industrial use of animation in the analysis of a formal model of information flow in dynamic virtual organisations (VOs) is presented by John et al. [19]. VDM tool is used for developing the formal model of virtual organisation (VO) structure. This development also supports interaction with the model without requiring exposure to the formalism. All kinds of simulation tools for Requirements Engineering (RE) with compressive comparison study have been presented by Schmid et al. [47].

A reference model for requirements and specifications is given by Gunter et al. [24]. This model is based on mainly five artifacts W, R, S, P, and M for applying formal methods to the development of user requirements and their reduction to a behavioural system specification. This paper presents the shared phenomena that defines an interface between system and environment.

Run-time technique for monitoring requirements satisfaction is presented in [17, 18], where requirements are monitored for violations, and system behaviour dynamically adapted the new behaviours. New introduced behaviours change the system requirements, which should meet the higher-level goal. Our proposed approach is based on monitoring of the animation, which is controlled by the proved formal specifications and real-time data sets. According to our literature survey, none of the existing approaches discuss to construct a formal specification based prototype, which can use a real-time data set to test the validation of the formal specifications for developing any critical systems like avionic and medical systems. Most of the existing tools are used a *toy-data* set for validating the formal specifications. Limitations of existing tools are that they cannot support real-time environment to capture the data set for testing. We have proposed an architecture for real-time animation using formal specification [41], which can be used for real-time animation for any existing animation tool and formal language. We have given the prototype model of this framework for Event-B specification. This tool is very helpful to show the real-time system behaviour from a formal specification and meets stakeholders requirements. Moreover, it bridges the gap between different kinds of domain experts. It can help a formal model designer to gain confidence that the formal model that is being designed, refined in an incremental way and finally implemented, does meet the domain requirements. The real-time animation tool is very helpful for evidence-based validation as well as in the certification process. This technique uniformly establishes what to check and how to check it and gives certain evidence of correctness.

5.4 Animation

Animation is a well-established technique that is used to check for compilation of the actual requirements of stakeholders with the given software specifications. It shows an actual behaviour of a system through execution of a formal model in the form of animation. An executable model is based on the software specifications; the software behaviour is simulated by executing that model; the simulation is visualised on a textual or graphical model representation by highlighting the current model element being executed. Animation thus allows a software engineer to discover the presence of problems, not their absence. Several kinds of benefits and limitations of animation [26, 47] are given as follows:

5.4.1 Benefits of Animation

- Animation has major benefits of validating a system model through earlier detection and correcting the problems for improving the quality of requirements specification.
- Animation provides behaviour of a system model, which can be used to validate the internal mechanism of the system model by inspection, and it helps to clarify requirements using animated interaction with the specification when requirements are unclear.
- In this prototyping technique, all kinds of tools have their own automatic translation tools, which is used for making formal specifications executable.
- Execution of the formal model in the form of animation helps inspection and formal reasoning as a means of validation for better understanding of the given system. Quite often the stakeholders are not sure about what they exactly want or how to describe their ideas. This technique helps to them to discover real requirements.

5.4.2 Limitations of Animation

- Animation techniques are not for exhaustive testing. In a complex system, there are numerous states, which is impossible to test due to the problem of "states explosion".
- Animation tools are not always stakeholder-friendly due to specific notations of the supported modelling languages, which are not easily understandable by non-technical stakeholders and might be difficult to read and interpret such animations.
- As long as the requirements engineering process is in progress, the requirements engineers have to handle ambiguous and incomplete requirements. Nevertheless, in that case requirements engineers are obliged to define a semantically correct and formal system model in order to run animation.

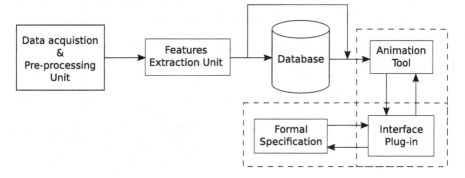

Fig. 5.1   A functional architecture to animate a formal specification using real time data set without generating source code

- Animation always focuses on the behavioural aspects of a system. However, non-functional requirements, such as reliability, cannot be animated from requirements. The mean life function, such as the mean time to failure (MTTF), is widely used as the measurement of a product's reliability and performance. This value is often calculated by dividing the total operating time of the units tested by the total number of failures encountered. Hence, reliability is usually measured by a rate. For example, the reliability of a system is 95 %, then how it is possible to measure that the reliability of that system is 95 % through animation.

5.5 Proposed Architecture

Figure 5.1 depicts a functional architecture that can use the real-time data set to animate a formal model without generating a source code in any target language (C, C++, VHDL, etc.). This architecture has six components: Data acquisition and preprocessing unit; Feature extraction unit; Database; Graphical animations tools; Interfacing plug-in; and formal specification model. All these six components can use any particular tool for building a prototype for realising the concepts of a real-time animator.

We have used some existing tools to build a prototype model of this proposed architecture. Figure 5.2 presents prototype implementations in order to understand the different development phases of the real-time animator. This architecture is applicable to building an animation tool for any formal modelling languages like VDM, Z, TLA$^+$, etc. Here, we present an equivalent architecture of the real-time animator in the context of Event-B formal modelling language. The prototype architecture has six components: Data acquisition and preprocessing unit; Feature extraction unit; Database; Graphical animations dedicated tool: Macromedia Flash; a Formal model animation tool Brama plug-in to interface between Flash animation and Event-B model; and formal specification system Event-B.

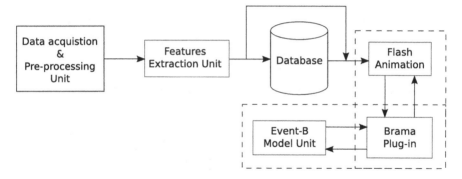

Fig. 5.2 A prototype model of the functional architecture to animate a formal specification

5.5.1 *Data Acquisition & Preprocessing*

Data acquisition and preprocessing begin with the physical phenomenon or physical property to be measured. Examples of this include temperature, light intensity, heart activities and blood pressure [15] and so on. Data acquisition is the process of sampling of real-world physical conditions and conversion of the resulting samples into digital numeric values. The data-acquisition hardware can vary from environment to environment (i.e. camera, sensor, etc.). The components of data-acquisition systems include sensors that convert physical properties. A sensor, which is a type of transducer, that measures a physical quantity and converts it into a signal which can be read by an observer or by an instrument.

Data preprocessing is a next step to perform on the raw data to prepare it for another processing procedure. Data preprocessing transforms the data into a format that will be more easily and effectively processed for the purpose of the user. There are a number of different tools and methods used for preprocessing on different types of raw data, including: sampling, which selects a representative subset from a large population of data; transformation, which manipulates raw data to produce a single input; de-noising, which removes noise from data; normalisation, which organises data for more efficient access.

5.5.2 *Feature Extraction*

The features extraction unit is a set of algorithms that is used to extract the parameters or features from the collected data set. A set of algorithms is implemented in any particular language (Matlab, C, C++, etc.). All these algorithms are different for each system. For example, during prototype implementation of this architecture, we have used a set of algorithms for extracting the ECG features or parameters. These parameters or features are numerical values that are used by animated model at the time of animation. The feature extraction relies on a thorough understanding of the entire system mechanics, the failure mechanisms, and their manifestation in the signatures. The accuracy of the system is fully dependent on the feature or parameter values being used. Feature extraction involves simplifying the amount of resources required to describe a large set of data accurately. When performing analysis of a complex data one of the major problems stems from the number of variables involved. Analysis with numerous variables generally requires a large amount of memory and computation power or a classification algorithm which overfits the training sample and generalises poorly to new samples. Feature extraction is a general term for methods of constructing combinations of the variables to get around these problems while still describing the data with sufficient accuracy. Collecting measured data and processing these data to accurately determine model parameter values is an essential task for the complete characterisation of a formal model.

5.5.3 Database

The database unit is optional. It stores the feature or parameter values in a database file in any specific format. This database file of parameters or features can be used in future to execute the model. Sometimes, feature extraction algorithms take more time to calculate the parameters or the features. In such a situation, modeller can store the parameters or the features in a database file to test the model in the future. A modeller can also use the extracted parameters or features directly in the formal model, without using the database.

5.5.4 Graphical Animations Tool: Macromedia Flash

The animated graphics are designed in the Macromedia Flash tool [44]. Macromedia Flash, a popular authoring software developed by Macromedia, is used to create vector graphics-based animation programs with high graphic illustrations and simple interactivity. Here, we use this tool to create an animated model of the physical environment and to use the Brama plug-in to connect the Flash animation and the Event-B model. This tool also helps to connect the real-time data set to a formal model specification using some intermediate steps and finally makes the animated model closer to the domain expert expectations.

5.5.5 Animator: Brama Plug-in

Brama [48] is an animator for Event-B specification, which is designed by ClearSy. Brama is an Eclipse plug-in suit and Macromedia Flash extension that can be used with Windows, Linux and MacOS for Rodin platform [46]. Brama can be used to create animations at different stages of development of a simulated system. To do so, a modeller may need to create an animation using the Macromedia Flash plug-in for Brama. The use of this plug-in is established through a communication between the animation and the simulation.

Brama is a tool allowing to animate Event-B models on the Rodin platform. It allows animating and inspecting a model using Flash animations. Brama has two objectives: to allow the formal model's designer to ensure that his model is executed in accordance with the system it is supposed to represent; to provide this model with a graphic representation and animate this representation in accordance with the state of the formal model. A modeller can represent the system manually within Rodin [46] or represent the system with the Macromedia Flash tool that allows for communication with the Brama animation engine through a communication server. The graphic representation must be in Macromedia Flash format and requires the use of a separate tool for its elaboration (Flash MX, for example). Once the Event-B model is satisfactory (it has been fully proven, and its animation has demonstrated that the model behaves like its related system), you can create a graphic representation of this system and animate it synchronously with the underlying Event-B Rodin model. Brama does not create this animation. It is up to the modeller to create the representation of the model depending on the part of the model he wants to display. However, Brama provides the elements required to connect your Flash animation and Event-B model [48].

5.5.6 Formal Modelling Language: Event-B

Event-B is a *proof-based* formal methods [1, 10] for system-level modelling and analysis of large reactive and distributed systems. In order to model a system, Event-B represents in terms of *contexts* and *machines*. The set theory and first-order logic are used to define contexts and machines of a given system. Contexts [1, 10] contain the static parts of a model. Each context may consist of carrier sets and constants as well as axioms, which are used to describe the properties of those sets and constants. Machines [1, 10] contain the dynamic parts of an Event-B model. This part is used to provide the behavioural properties of a model. A machine model is a state, which is defined by means of variables, invariants, events and theorems. The use of refinement represents systems at different levels of abstraction and the use of mathematical proof verifies consistency between refinement levels. Event-B is provided with tool support in the form of an open and extensible Eclipse-based IDE called Rodin [46] which is a platform for Event-B specification and verification.

5.6 Applications and Case Studies

We have applied our proposed approach of the real-time animator [41] in the development of cardiac pacemaker [40] (see Chap. 9). A cardiac pacemaker is a high confidence medical device [29, 30, 52] that is implemented to provide proper heart rhythm when the body's natural pacemaker does not function properly. In the development of the cardiac pacemaker, real-time animator of formal specification helps to animate the formal model with a *real-time data* set instead of *toy-data*, and offers a simple way for specifiers to build a domain-specific visualisation that can be used by domain experts to check whether a formal specification corresponds to their expectations. The pacemaker models are validated to make sure that they meet all the functional requirements of the cardiac pacemaker. The validation process is carried out by both logic experts and medical experts.

5.7 Limitations

The proposed architecture of the real-time animator is sufficient to validate refinement-based formal specifications using real-time data set instead of *toy-data* set. The major limitation of this tool is real-time data collection and features extraction for testing the validation of formal specifications of a system, where feature extraction algorithms are not able to calculate required features under real-time (i.e. ECG features extraction). Due to limitation of this algorithm, we proposed off-line validation technique using database. Database is used to store the extracted features in a specific file format for validating the formal models.

Another limitation we have discovered through our experiments that every refinement step is not animatable, specially early development of the formal model (or abstract model), where concrete functional behaviours of the system are not specified yet. Incremental refinement approach builds the system gradually and provides the concrete system behaviour, which may be animatable. Refinement based modelling helps for obtaining stepwise validation for modelling a system [38]. This is consistent with using animation as a kind of quality-assurance activity during development. Early stages of system models are too abstract and not able to present parametric based desired behaviour of the system. So that, this real-time animation is useful to validate later refinement stages of a system or concrete models, when some parametric behaviours are introduced in the system. These parameters are used as features in the formal specifications for real-time validation. We believe that one animation per abstraction level is sufficient. In fact, the first refinement of a level may often have a non-determinism too wide to allow for meaningful animation (concept introduction), but subsequent refinements get the definitions of the new concept precise enough to allow animation.

5.8 Summary

The objective of this proposed architecture is to validate the formal model with real-time data set in the early stage of development without generating the source code in any target language. Here, we focused the attention on the techniques introduced in the architecture for using the real-time data set to achieve the adaptability and confidence on a formal model. Moreover, this architecture may provide validation for the formal model with respect to the high level specifications according to the domain experts (i.e. medical experts). At last, this proposed architecture should be adaptable to various target platforms and formal models techniques (Event-B, Z, Alloy, TLA$^+$, etc.).

Our approach has involved for designing and using of the real-time animator for executing a formal specification to validate actual requirements. The main objectives of our work are to promote the use of such kind of real-time animator [41] to bridge the gap between software engineers and stakeholders to build a quality system, and to discover all ambiguous informations from the requirements. Moreover, this tool helps to verify the correctness of behaviour of a system according to the stakeholders requirements. The formal verification and evidence based testing using an animation offer to obtain that challenge of complying with FDA's QSR, ISO/IEC and IEEE standards quality system directives [11, 12, 16, 32, 33] and help to get certification for highly complex critical systems.

A key feature of this validation as it is full automation and animation of specification in the early stage of formal development. The case study (see Chap. 9) has shown that requirements specifications could be used directly in the real-time environment without modifications for automatic test result evaluation using our approach. Moreover, there are scientific and legal applications as well, where the formal model based animation can be used to simulate (or emulate) certain scenarios to glean more information or better understandings of the system and assist to improve the final given system. Main contributions of proposing this real-time animator tool are,

• to reduce the gap between software engineers and stakeholders requirements using real-time animator and easy to explain model behaviour to the domain experts as well stakeholders;
• a real-time animation of a specification supplements inspection and reasoning as means for validation. This is especially important for the validation of non-functional behaviour;
• a real-time animation technique is available in early phase of the system development life-cycle, which can be used to correct validation errors immediately, without incurring costly redevelopment;
• ambiguous and incomplete requirements can be clarified and completed by hands-on experience with the specifications using our approach;
• the goal-oriented animation for evidence based expectation to verify particular portions of a behaviour model;
• animation can be helpful for incremental model building and analysis of a complex system;
• helps to domain experts to analyse work process guidelines;
• animator assists to regulatory agencies and helps to meet ISO/IEC and IEEE standards;

- ability to monitor a real-time environment using animator at animation time and analyse the requirements, violations of goals, expectations on the environments, and domain properties.

This work has been influenced by guiding principles and technical benefits of the formal system engineering, which offers participation of both software engineers and user stakeholders that helps to move closer towards a quality requirements specification and to develop an error-free system.

References

1. Abrial, J.-R. (2010). *Modeling in Event-B: System and software engineering* (1st ed.). New York: Cambridge University Press.
2. Aizenbud-Reshef, N., Nolan, B. T., Rubin, J., & Shaham-Gafni, Y. (2006). Model traceability. *IBM Systems Journal, 45*(3), 515–526.
3. Balzer, R. M., Goldman, N. M., & Wile, D. S. (1982). Operational specification as the basis for rapid prototyping. *Software Engineering Notes, 7*, 3–16.
4. Berzins, V., Luqi, & Yehudai, A. (1993). Using transformations in specification-based prototyping. *IEEE Transactions on Software Engineering, 19*(5), 436–452.
5. Bjørner, D., & Jones, C. B. (Eds.) (1978). *The Vienna development method: The metalanguage.* London: Springer.
6. Blaauboer, F., Sikkel, K., & Aydin, M. N. (2007). Deciding to adopt requirements traceability in practice. In *Proceedings of the 19th international conference on advanced information systems engineering*, CAiSE'07 (pp. 294–308). Berlin: Springer.
7. Bloomfield, R. E., & Froo, P. K. D. (1986). The application of formal methods to the assessment of high integrity software. *IEEE Transactions on Software Engineering, 12*, 988–993.
8. Boehm, B. W. (1981). *Software engineering economics* (1st ed.). Upper Saddle River: Prentice Hall.
9. Bubenko, J. A., Jr. (1995). Challenges in requirements engineering. In *Proceedings of the second IEEE international symposium on requirements engineering* (pp. 160–162).
10. Cansell, D., & Méry, D. (2008). The Event-B modelling method: Concepts and case studies. In D. Bjørner & M. C. Henson (Eds.), *Monographs in theoretical computer science. Logics of specification languages* (pp. 47–152). Berlin: Springer.
11. CC. Common criteria. http://www.commoncriteriaportal.org/.
12. CDRH (2006). Safety of marketed medical devices. Center for Devices and Radiological Health, US FDA.
13. Clocksin, W. F., & Mellish, C. S. (1987). *Programming in Prolog.* New York: Springer.
14. Davis, A. M. (1992). Operational prototyping: A new development approach. *IEEE Software, 9*, 70–78.
15. Dorticós, F., Quiones, M. A., Tornes, F., Fayad, Y., Zayas, R., Castro, J., et al. (2006). Rate-responsive pacing controlled by the TVI sensor in the treatment of sick sinus syndrome. In A. Raviele (Ed.), *Cardiac arrhythmias 2005* (pp. 581–590). Milan: Springer.
16. FDA. Food and Drug Administration. http://www.fda.gov/.
17. Feather, M. S., Fickas, S., Van Lamsweerde, A., & Ponsard, C. (1998). Reconciling system requirements and runtime behavior. In *Proceedings of the 9th international workshop on software specification and design*, IWSSD'98 (p. 50). Washington: IEEE Comput. Soc.
18. Fickas, S., & Feather, M. S. (1995). Requirements monitoring in dynamic environments. In *Proceedings of the second IEEE international symposium on requirements engineering*, RE'95 (p. 140). Washington: IEEE Comput. Soc.

19. Fitzgerald, J. S., Bryans, J. W., Greathead, D., Jones, C. B., & Payne, R. (2007). Animation-based validation of a formal model of dynamic virtual organisations. In *Proceedings of the 2007 international conference on formal methods in industry*, FACS-FMI'07, London (p. 3). Swinton: British Computer Society.
20. Fuchs, N. E. (1992). Specifications are (preferably) executable. *Software Engineering Journal*, 7(5), 323–334.
21. Galvao, I., & Goknil, A. (2007). Survey of traceability approaches in model-driven engineering. In *Proceedings of the 11th IEEE international enterprise distributed object computing conference* (p. 313). Washington: IEEE Comput. Soc.
22. Goguen, J., & Meseguer, J. (1982). Rapid prototyping in the obj executable specification language. *Software Engineering Notes*, 7, 75–84.
23. Gotel, O. C. Z., & Finkelstein, C. W. (1994). An analysis of the requirements traceability problem. In *Proceedings of the first international conference on requirements engineering* (pp. 94–101).
24. Gunter, C. A., Gunter, E. L., Jackson, M., & Zave, P. (2000). A reference model for requirements and specifications. *IEEE Software*, 17, 37–43.
25. Guo, Y., Yang, M., Wang, J., Yang, P., & Li, F. (2009). An ontology based improved software requirement traceability matrix. In *Proceedings of the 2009 second international symposium on knowledge acquisition and modeling*, KAM'09 (Vol. 01, pp. 160–163). Washington: IEEE Comput. Soc.
26. Hayes, I., & Jones, C. B. (1989). Specifications are not (necessarily) executable. *Software Engineering Journal*, 4, 330–338.
27. Henderson, P. (1986). Functional programming, formal specification, and rapid prototyping. *IEEE Transactions on Software Engineering*, 12, 241–250.
28. Henderson, P., & Minkowitz, C. J. (1986). The me too method of software design. *ICL Technical Journal*, 5(1), 64–95.
29. High Confidence Software and Systems Coordinating Group (2009). *High-confidence medical devices: Cyber-physical systems for 21st century health care* (Technical report). NITRD. http://www.nitrd.gov/About/MedDevice-FINAL1-web.pdf.
30. Hoare, C. A. R., Misra, J., Leavens, G. T., & Shankar, N. (2009). The verified software initiative: A manifesto. *ACM Computing Surveys*, 41(4), 22:1–22:8.
31. Hull, M. E. C., Jackson, K., & Dick, J. (2005). *Requirements engineering* (2nd ed.). London: Springer.
32. IEEE-SA. IEEE Standards Association. http://standards.ieee.org/.
33. ISO. International Organization for Standardization. http://www.iso.org/.
34. Keatley, K. L. (1999). A review of the FDA draft guidance document for software validation: Guidance for industry. *Quality Assurance*, 7(1), 49–55.
35. Kowalski, R. (1985). The relation between logic programming and logic specification. In *Proceedings of a discussion meeting of the Royal Society of London on mathematical logic and programming languages* (pp. 11–27). Upper Saddle River: Prentice Hall.
36. Lee, E. A. (2002). Embedded software. *Advances in Computers*, 56, 56–97.
37. Lindvall, M., & Sandahl, K. (1996). Practical implications of traceability. *Software, Practice & Experience*, 26(10), 1161–1180.
38. Mashkoor, A., Jacquot, J.-P., & Souquières, J. (2009). Transformation heuristics for formal requirements validation by animation. In *2nd international workshop on the certification of safety-critical software controlled systems*, SafeCert 2009, York, UK.
39. McDermid, J. (1991). *Software engineer's reference book*. Boca Raton: CRC Press.
40. Méry, D., & Singh, N. K. (2009). *Pacemaker's functional behaviors in Event-B* (Research report). MOSEL-LORIA-INRIA-CNRS: UMR7503-Université Henri Poincaré-Nancy I-Université Nancy II-Institut National Polytechnique de Lorraine. http://hal.inria.fr/inria-00419973/en/.
41. Méry, D., & Singh, N. K. (2010). Real-time animation for formal specification. In M. Aiguier, F. Bretaudeau, & D. Krob (Eds.), *Complex systems design & management* (pp. 49–60). Berlin: Springer.

42. Ponsard, C., Massonet, P., Rifaut, A., Molderez, J. F., van Lamsweerde, A., & Van, H. T. (2005). Early verification and validation of mission critical systems. *Electronic Notes in Theoretical Computer Science*, *133*, 237–254. Proceedings of the ninth international workshop on formal methods for industrial critical systems, FMICS 2004.

43. Ramesh, B., & Jarke, M. (2001). Toward reference models for requirements traceability. *IEEE Transactions on Software Engineering*, *27*, 58–93.

44. Reinhardt, R., & Dowd, S. (2007). *Adobe Flash CS3 professional bible* (p. 1232). New York: Wiley. ISBN 9780470119372.

45. Rittel, H. W. J., & Webber, M. M. (1973). Dilemmas in a general theory of planning. *Policy Sciences*, *4*(2), 155–169.

46. RODIN (2004). Rigorous open development environment for complex systems. http://rodin-b-sharp.sourceforge.net.

47. Schmid, R., Ryser, J., Berner, S., Glinz, M., Reutemann, R., & Fahr, E. (2000). *A survey of simulation tools for requirements engineering* (Technical report).

48. Servat, T. (2006). *Lecture notes in computer science. Brama: A new graphic animation tool for B models* (pp. 274–276). Berlin: Springer.

49. Siddiqi, J. I., Morrey, I. C., Roast, C. R., & Ozcan, M. B. (1997). Towards quality requirements via animated formal specifications. *Annals of Software Engineering*, *3*, 131–155.

50. Turner, D. A. (1985). Functional programs as executable specifications. In *Proceedings of a discussion meeting of the Royal Society of London on mathematical logic and programming languages* (pp. 29–54). Upper Saddle River: Prentice Hall.

51. Van, H. T., van Lamsweerde, A., Massonet, P., & Ponsard, C. (2004). Goal-oriented requirements animation. In *Proceedings of the 12th IEEE international requirements engineering conference* (pp. 218–228). Washington: IEEE Comput. Soc.

52. Woodcock, J., & Banach, R. (2007). The verification grand challenge. *Journal of Universal Computer Science*, *13*(5), 661–668.

Chapter 6
Refinement Chart

Abstract Refinement techniques serve as a key role for modelling a complex system in an incremental way. This chapter also presents a required technique namely refinement chart for handling the complexity of a system. Refinement chart is a graphical representation of a complex system using layering approach, where functional blocks are divided into multiple simpler blocks in a new refinement level, without changing the original behaviour of the system. The main objective of this refinement chart is to model the whole system using graphical notations and to obtain a concrete specification. The refinement chart offers a clear view of assistance in "system" integration. This approach also gives a clear view about the system assembling based on operating modes and different kinds of features. To show the effectiveness of this approach, we have used this graphical modelling technique to simplifying the complexity of a system in the development of our selected case study: cardiac pacemaker.

6.1 Introduction

High-confidence medical devices (ICD, pacemaker, infusion pump, etc.), automotive and avionic systems are too much error prone in operating due to the complexity of the systems [3, 5, 12]. New methodologies are needed to make critical viable in the future marketplace by simplifying the various design stages. This chapter

---

Sections of this chapter are adapted from the original publication: Méry, D., & Singh, N. K. (2013). Formal specification of medical systems by proof-based refinement. *ACM Transactions on Embedded Computing Systems, 12*(1), 15:1–15:25.

ACM COPYRIGHT NOTICE. Copyright © 2013 by the Association for Computing Machinery, Inc. Permission to make digital or hard copies of part or all of this work for personal or classroom use is granted without fee provided that copies are not made or distributed for profit or commercial advantage and that copies bear this notice and the full citation on the first page. Copyrights for components of this work owned by others than ACM must be honored. Abstracting with credit is permitted. To copy otherwise, to republish, to post on servers, or to redistribute to lists, requires prior specific permission and/or a fee. Request permissions from Publications Dept., ACM, Inc., fax +1 (212) 869-0481, or permissions@acm.org.

proposes a refinement-based graphical technique for designing the complex critical systems. The refinement chart provides an easily manageable representation for different refinement subsystems and offers a clear view of assistance in system integration. This methodology simplifies specification, synthesis, and validation of the systems and enables an efficient creation/customisation of the critical systems at low-cost and development time.

Despite all the efforts of the community, critical system designers still need a new way for modelling the systems and analyse the complexity of the systems. This is mainly because of a set of requirements that is mandatory for an efficient modelling solution, but is still not provided by a single existing environment:

- Infrastructure for critical system integration and inter-operation.
- Introspection features for easier debugging and analysis of complex specifications.
- Model-based development and component-based design frameworks.
- System integration of critical infrastructure.
- Possibility of annotating models for different purposes (e.g., directing the synthesis or hooking to verification tools).
- Decomposition of the complex system into different independent subsystems.

The contribution of this chapter is to propose a new graphical notation based refinement chart for a complex critical system design. This technique provides the solutions for all the requirements enumerated above. The refinement chart is proposed in this methodology for designing a critical system like medical device, automotive and avionic systems.

6.1.1 Structure of This Chapter

This chapter is organised as follows. Section 6.2 presents related work. Section 6.3 depicts a refinement chart and describes basic rules for presenting any system using the refinement chart. Section 6.4 presents assessment of the refinement chart using applications and case study and finally, Sect. 6.5 summarises this chapter.

6.2 Related Work

A *modal system* is a system characterised by *operation modes*, which coordinates system operations. Many systems are *modal systems*, for instance, space and avionic systems [5, 12], steam boiler control [3], transportation and space system and so on. Operation modes explore the actual system behaviour through observation of a system functioning under multiple situations. In this approach, a system is considered as a set of operating modes, where each operating mode is categorised according to the system functionality over different operating conditions.

Modecharts [9] is a graphical technique, which is used to handle mode and mode switching of a system. The authors have given the detailed information about the state space partition, various working conditions of the system and to define the control information in the large state machines. However, modecharts lack adequate support to specifying and reasoning about functional properties. Some papers [7, 13] have also addressed the problem of mode changing in a real-time system. Dotti et al. [6] have proposed both formalisation and a refinement notion for a *modal system*, using existing support for the construction of *modal system*.

According to our literature survey, none of the existing approaches discuss a refinement-based technique for handling the complexity of a system. We have given a technique of the refinement chart for presenting different operating modes under various subsystems. Each subsystem represents an independent function according to the operating modes. This refinement chart technique helps to design complex system structure and relationship between two subsystems using operating modes that helps in system integration using code structuring of the different subsystems.

6.3 Refinement Chart

The purpose of this refinement chart is to specify the modal system requirements in a form that is easily and effectively implementable. During the modelling of modal system, several styles of specification are usually adopted for handling the complex operating modes. Functional blocks are divided into multiple simpler blocks in a new refinement level, without changing the original behaviour of a system. The final goal is to obtain a specification that is detailed enough to be effectively implemented, but also to correctly describe the requirements of a system.

The development of embedded software for the critical system requires significant lower level manual interaction for organising and assembling a complete system. This is inherently error-prone, time-consuming and platform-dependent. To detect the failure cases in a software is not an easy task. Manually reviewing the source code is the only way to trace the cause of a failure. Due to the technological advancement and modern complexity of the critical system software, this is an impossible task for any third party investigator without prior knowledge of the software. Consequently, we have proposed the synthesis of a system using incremental refinements, to synchronise and integrate the different subsystems of a system. This approach also helps in code integration and to test the different subsystems of a system independently.

As the nature of critical systems is often characterisable as *modal systems*, we follow a state-based approach to propose suitable abstractions. We consider that the state of a model is detailed enough to allow one to distinguish its different operating conditions and also to characterise required mode functionality and possible mode switching in terms of state transitions.

Each subsystem that forms the specification is represented into a block diagram as a refinement chart. Figure 6.1 presents the diagrams of the most abstract modal

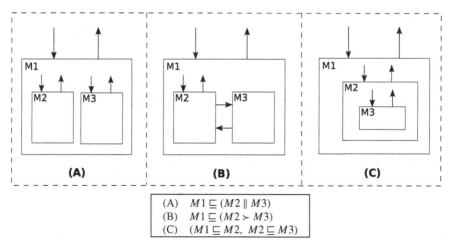

(A)	$M1 \sqsubseteq (M2 \parallel M3)$
(B)	$M1 \sqsubseteq (M2 \succ M3)$
(C)	$(M1 \sqsubseteq M2, \ M2 \sqsubseteq M3)$

Fig. 6.1 Refinement charts

system. The diagrams use a visual notation loosely based on Statechart [8]. A mode is represented by a box with a mode name; a mode transition is an arrow connecting two modes. The direction of an arrow indicates the previous and next modes in a transition. Refinement is expressed by nesting boxes. A refined diagram with an outgoing arrow from an abstract mode is equivalent to outgoing arrows from each of the concrete modes. It is also similar to ingoing arrow. In a refinement, nesting box can be arranged hierarchically and can be represented by basic rules of our refinement chart (see Fig. 6.2). Basic rules of refinements are a parallel refinement $[M1 \sqsubseteq (M2 \parallel M3 \parallel \ldots \parallel M_{n-1} \parallel M_n)]$, sequential refinement $[M1 \sqsubseteq (M2 \succ M3 \succ \cdots \succ M_{n-1} \succ M_n)]$ and nested refinement $[(M1 \sqsubseteq M2, \ M2 \sqsubseteq M3, \ldots, \ M_{n-1} \sqsubseteq M_n)]$. Furthermore, refinement charts, which appears in the hierarchical form can be represented in the sequential or parallel or nesting, or in all sequential, parallel and nesting ways. A complete system can be represented by using mixing of all refinement chart notations, means each subsystem can be refined by any rule that is given in Fig. 6.2.

Figure 6.1 presents for only three modes (M1, M2 and M3) with different kinds of refinements. The parallel relationship among several refinement boxes states that a system operates simultaneously in all the subsystems. For instance, Fig. 6.1(A) represents the abstract mode $M1$ and two parallel refinements are represented by nesting mode boxes $M2$ and $M3$. Transition between these two refinements $M2$ and $M3$ are not allowed. Entry into a parallel refined subsystem requires entry into all of its immediate child refinement. A transition out of one refinement requires an exit out of all the refined subsystems in parallel to it. The sequential relationship among several refinement boxes states that the system operates in at most one of these subsystems at any time. For example, Fig. 6.1(B) represents an abstract mode $M1$ and two sequential refinements are presented by the nesting mode boxes $M2$ and $M3$ in two levels of hierarchy, where $M2$ and $M3$ are embedded in $M1$. The transitions between $M2$ and $M3$ allows the system to go from one refinement to an-

Fig. 6.2 Basic rules of refinement chart

$$M1 \sqsubseteq (M2 \parallel M3 \parallel \ldots \parallel M_{n-1} \parallel M_n)$$
$$M1 \sqsubseteq (M2 \succ M3 \succ \cdots \succ M_{n-1} \succ M_n)$$
$$(M1 \sqsubseteq M2, \; M2 \sqsubseteq M3, \; \ldots, \; M_{n-1} \sqsubseteq M_n)$$

other refinement according to the operating modes. The nesting relationship among several refinement boxes states that the system operates in any subsystems. For example, Fig. 6.1(C) represents an abstract mode $M1$ and the subsystems refinement by a nesting box $M2$ and the subsystem $M2$ is refined by a nesting box $M3$ in three levels of hierarchy, where $M2$ is embedded in $M1$ and $M3$ is embedded in $M2$. A transition is allowed to next level of refined subsystem. A transition out of one refinement requires an exit out of all the refined sub level of refined subsystems.

As an example, Fig. 6.3 presents the diagrams of the most abstract modal system for the one electrode pacemaker system (A) and the resulting models of three successive refinement steps (B to D). The diagrams use a visual notation to represent the bradycardia operating modes of the pacemaker under the functional and parametric requirements. An operating mode is represented by a box with a mode name; an operating mode transition is an arrow connecting two operating modes. The direction of an arrow indicates the previous and next operating modes in a transition. Refinement is expressed by nesting boxes. A detailed description about these refinement blocks related to the one-electrode cardiac pacemaker is given in case study (see Chap. 9).

Refinement based representation is used during the decomposition and synthesis phases of a system. The purpose of the refinement chart is to provide an easily manageable representation for different refinements of a system. The refinement chart offers a clear view of assistance in system integration. This is an important issue not only for being able to derive system-level performance and correctness guarantees, but also for being able to assemble components in a cost-effective manner.

Refinement is a modelling technique that is used to introduce more concrete behaviour of a system in the next level of refinement, where it preserves the safety properties and system behaviour between two refinement levels. This preservation property allows us to model the whole system from initial specification to a concrete level in a form of executable specification using incremental development. The concrete model is considered as that it preserves a system behaviour, thereby establishing that the generated code satisfies the initial specification [15]. Proof of consistency between source and target of a refinement is an intrinsic capability of a refinement process, which can be composed in a similar fashion [14].

A refinement-based system development has a different cost structure than the traditional development life-cycle. The cost of building models and related other required design knowledge may be higher for producing the first system. However, these costs are amortised when reuse these models and designs for developing the other future systems. Thus, the cost of producing first program may be higher, but the cost of development for reproducing advanced version of the products and reuse same codes in other products should be less than the conventional programming [14, 15]. The cost of handling of proof obligations of specifications and refinements should be less than the cost of analysing the final product. It can also help to

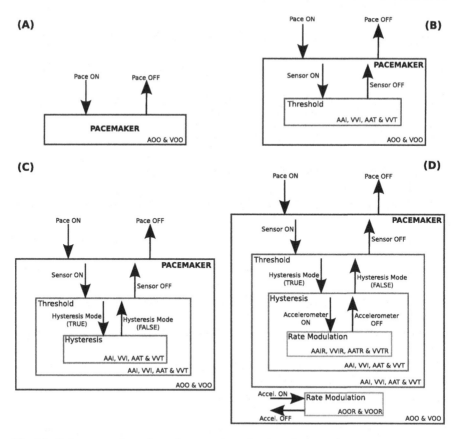

Fig. 6.3 Refinements of one-electrode pacemaker using the refinement chart

a code designer to improve the code structures, code optimisation, and code generation techniques. Every incremental refinement represents additional functionalities.
This refinement-based structure may greatly improve the safety, hardware integration and guidelines to develop the critical systems. We, therefore, propose a simple
methodology of system integration using the refinement chart, that seeks to minimise the effort and overhead.

6.4 Applications and Case Studies

We have applied the refinement chart [11] in the system development of a cardiac
pacemaker for handling the complexity of the system model (see Chap. 9). Refinement chart helps to model the system integration, which also complies with refinement based formal development. The block diagrams of the refinement chart help to
build the complete system and used to handle the complexity of the whole system
through decomposing in multiple independent parts. Here, refinement chart models

different kinds of operating modes, and decompose the whole system based on operational modes. Decomposing using the refinement chart helps to analyse individual component and interaction or switching from one operating mode to other operating modes. Formal verification and validation are carried out by both formal modelling experts and domain experts (medical experts and control engineers), while refinement chart based system integration approach and system development are carried out by industrial people.

6.5 Summary

Today, in order to respect the certifiable assurance and safety, time to market and strict cost constraints, critical system designers need some new modelling and simulation solutions. The solutions must also permit software component modelling, component integration in a distributed environment, easier debugging of complex specifications, and mitigated connection with other, existing or new systems [10].

In this chapter, we would like to stress the original contribution of our work. At each refinement step, some functional blocks are divided into simpler blocks, without changing the behaviour of a system is represented by the refinement chart. We have proposed a technique to synthesis, integrate, and synchronise the subsystems of a system using incremental refinements. This approach helps in code integration and to test the different subsystems independently. The purpose of the refinement chart is to provide an easily manageable representation for different refinement subsystems. The refinement chart offers a clear view of assistance in the system integration. This is an important issue not only for being able to derive system-level performance and correctness guarantees, but also for being able to assemble components in a cost-effective manner. Moreover, the refinement chart represents a block diagram for each subsystems and provides a structure in various refinements to build the complete system. Concrete refinement charts provide system integration information in the form of compose and decompose of software codes according to the blocks diagrams. Composition and decomposition help to improve the code structure and code optimisation. To find a minimum set of events for each independent subsystem is known as code optimisation, and synthesising and synchronising of a set of events are known as code structuring. The refinement chart specially covers component-based design frameworks and decomposition, integration of critical infrastructure and device integration. The complexity of design is reduced by structuring systems using modes and by detailing this design using refinement.

References

1. Abrial, J.-R. (1996). *The B-book: Assigning programs to meanings*. New York: Cambridge University Press.
2. Abrial, J.-R. (2010). *Modeling in Event-B: System and software engineering* (1st ed.). New York: Cambridge University Press.

3. Abrial, J.-R., Börger, E., & Langmaack, H. (Eds.) (1996). *Lecture notes in computer science: Vol. 1165. Formal methods for industrial applications, specifying and programming the steam boiler control.* Berlin: Springer.

4. Back, R. J. R. (1981). On correct refinement of programs. *Journal of Computer and System Sciences, 23*(1), 49–68.

5. Butler, R. W. (1996). *An introduction to requirements capture using PVS: Specification of a simple autopilot* (NASA Technical Memorandum 110255). Hampton: NASA Langley Research Center.

6. Dotti, F., Iliasov, A., Ribeiro, L., & Romanovsky, A. (2009). Modal systems: Specification, refinement and realisation. In K. Breitman & A. Cavalcanti (Eds.), *Lecture notes in computer science: Vol. 5885. Formal methods and software engineering* (pp. 601–619). Berlin: Springer.

7. Fohler, G. (1993). Realizing changes of operational modes with a pre run-time scheduled hard real-time system. In H. Kopetz & Y. Kakuda (Eds.), *Dependable computing and fault-tolerant systems: Vol. 7. Responsive computer systems* (pp. 287–300). Vienna: Springer.

8. Harel, D. (1987). Statecharts: A visual formalism for complex systems. *Science of Computer Programming, 8*(3), 231–274.

9. Jahanian, F., & Mok, A. K. (1994). Modechart: A specification language for real-time systems. *IEEE Transactions on Software Engineering, 20*(12), 933–947.

10. Méry, D., & Singh, N. K. (2010). Trustable formal specification for software certification. In T. Margaria & B. Steffen (Eds.), *Lecture notes in computer science: Vol. 6416. Leveraging applications of formal methods, verification, and validation* (pp. 312–326). Berlin: Springer.

11. Méry, D., & Singh, N. K. (2013). Formal specification of medical systems by proof-based refinement. *ACM Transactions on Embedded Computing Systems, 12*(1), 15:1–15:25.

12. Miller, S. P. (1998). Specifying the mode logic of a flight guidance system in Core and SCR. In *FMSP'98: Proceedings of the second workshop on formal methods in software practice* (pp. 44–53). New York: ACM.

13. Real, J., & Crespo, A. (2004). Mode change protocols for real-time systems: A survey and a new proposal. *Real-Time Systems, 26*(2), 161–197.

14. Smith, D. (2008). Generating programs plus proofs by refinement. In B. Meyer & J. Woodcock (Eds.), *Lecture notes in computer science: Vol. 4171. Verified software: Theories, tools, experiments* (pp. 182–188). Berlin: Springer.

15. Walters, H. (1990). Hybrid implementations of algebraic specifications. In H. Kirchner & W. Wechler (Eds.), *Lecture notes in computer science: Vol. 463. Algebraic and logic programming* (pp. 40–54). Berlin: Springer.

Chapter 7
EB2ALL: An Automatic Code Generation Tool

Abstract The most important step in the software-development life-cycle is the code implementation. This chapter presents a design architecture of an automatic code generation tool, which can generate code into several programming languages (C, C++, Java and C#). This tool is a collection of plug-ins, which are used for translating the Event-B formal specifications into multiple programming languages. The translation tool is rigorously developed with safety properties preservation. This is an essential tool, which supports code implementation phase of our proposed development life-cycle methodology for developing the critical systems.

7.1 Introduction

Formal methods provide a sound mathematical basis for system requirements descriptions and aim to produce zero-defect software, by controlling the whole software-development process, from specification to implementation. The capability of formal and automated verification of safety properties in formal models, before transformation into code, has added real value to industrial systems, including hardware systems and software systems. Several constraining requirements are existing particularly in the embedded domain due to limited size of memory for translating from formal specifications to a given target programming language (C [22, 29],

---

Sections of this chapter are adapted from the original publication: Méry, D., & Singh, N. K. (2011). Automatic code generation from Event-B models. In *Proceedings of the second symposium on information and communication technology*, SoICT'11, Hanoi (pp. 179–188). New York: ACM.

ACM COPYRIGHT NOTICE. Copyright © 2011 by the Association for Computing Machinery, Inc. Permission to make digital or hard copies of part or all of this work for personal or classroom use is granted without fee provided that copies are not made or distributed for profit or commercial advantage and that copies bear this notice and the full citation on the first page. Copyrights for components of this work owned by others than ACM must be honored. Abstracting with credit is permitted. To copy otherwise, to republish, to post on servers, or to redistribute to lists, requires prior specific permission and/or a fee. Request permissions from Publications Dept., ACM, Inc., fax +1 (212) 869-0481, or permissions@acm.org.

N.K. Singh, *Using Event-B for Critical Device Software Systems*,   105
DOI 10.1007/978-1-4471-5260-6_7, © Springer-Verlag London 2013

C++ [37], Java [3, 21] and C# [31]). To overcome such kinds of problems, first, a compromise must be found between the expressiveness of the formal implementation language and the simplicity of the translation process. Another compromise is also necessary between formal models, which generally favour the readability and the simplicity of the verification process, over the code efficiency.

The code generation process consists in several stages: formal implementations are translated into programs in a given programming language using a *tool chain* of a translator, and then these programs are compiled. This approach offers several advantages: the translation process is as simple as possible, and it can be validated in an easy way; secondly having a formal specification of a system suggests as a next step to use it during the testing phase. Software testing tries to check the correctness of a system with respect to its specification in program states that are chosen for the test. The simplicity of the translation ensures the traceability between formal specification and executed code.

This chapter describes a tool translating Event-B specification into any given target programming language. The structure of Event-B and the nature of tool has been developed to support for direct-translation from Event-B formal specification into any target programming language. We provide a rigorous translation tool EB2ALL [17, 25] for Event-B specification to target programming language that can easily be adapted in any domain and gives freedom for developers to adjust at best their integer representation for overcoming memory-related problems.

The EB2ALL code generator supports automatic generation of C, C++, Java and C# code from Event-B [2] formal specifications. The tool EB2ALL is a collection of plug-ins, which are named as EB2C, EB2C++, EB2J and EB2C# [17, 25]. All these tools are used as plug-in features for the Rodin development tool [32]. Rodin development tool is an open and extensible Eclipse-based IDE, which is a platform for Event-B specification and verification.

We present a multi-phased translation process from the Event-B [2] models. The Event-B models support *set-theoretical* notations that are impossible to directly translate into any target programming language. The translator automatically rewrites partially formal notations of Event-B [2], that can be easily translatable into a programming language. Any target programming language source code is then automatically generated from the model via using an appropriate translation phase of the tool. The final translated code is applicable to compile into an executable code using the conventional compilation tools.

A developer can also use translated code to extend the functionality of a system by inserting extra code or some new functionalities that are not included in the Event-B formal development. Some parts of the implementation code are not supported by the code generator, and a user wants to implement some existing components more efficiently are main reasons for inserting extra code into the automatically generated code. Moreover, it offers a flexible way for Event-B designer to generate C, C++, Java and C# codes. Due to manual intervention in the generated source code, we propose a code verification technique using the meta-proof and software model checking tools like BLAST [10] for verifying desired behaviours of the developed system. This tool is freely available for download.[1] The use of this tool is exemplified through the generation of C, C++, Java and C# codes from the specification of a cardiac pacemaker (see Chap. 9).

A code translation from Event-B was relatively easy, but its subsequent use presented more problems. The most important challenging task in the code generation is the code verification. The reason is that the preservation at the code level of the properties proved at the architectural level is guaranteed only if—the underlying platform is correct and—correctness of the final system when filling in the stubs for internal actions into the automatic generated code. Another important challenge is to support all formal notations of Event-B. Few formal notations are used at the abstract level for a system development, those symbols are not directly translatable. We have also faced a specific challenge related to the non-deterministic behaviour of a system. Most of the formal specifications are non-deterministic, which are not safe for an automatic code generation. To make a formal specification deterministic before code generation and to verify that the system behaviours are correct according to the developer, and also comply with non-deterministic system specifications, are challenging tasks in this code generation process. Invariants are used for defining type definition and safety properties of a system. How to use invariants corresponding to the safety properties for verifying generated codes is also one kind of challenge.

7.1.1 Structure of This Chapter

This chapter is organised as follows. Section 7.2 presents related work and Sect. 7.3 depicts an architecture of the translator in a form of a *tool chain* and describes various parts of the translation process. Section 7.4 presents use of code generator plug-ins. Section 7.5 discusses limitations of the tool and finally, Sect. 7.6 summarises the chapter.

7.2 Related Work

Automatic code generation is a standard technique in the area of Software Engineering. Several tools are developed by research community for generating source code from graphical modelling tool like UML [20, 33, 36] to any target programming language like C++ or Java. But automatic source code generation from formal specification to a high-level programming language is supported by few formal

---

[1]Download: http://eb2all.loria.fr/.

techniques like Classic B [2] and Vienna Development Method (VDM) [11, 28]. The VDM [11, 28] is a set of techniques and tools based on formal specification language—the VDM Specification Language (VDM-SL). Extended version of VDM tool (VDM++) supports modelling of object-oriented and concurrent systems. VDM tools attract both industrial and academic people in the area of formal based development. VDM tools provide features for analysing models, testing and proving properties of models, and generating program codes from the validated VDM models.

A tool vMAGIC [30] is based on Java library that is used for automatic code generation for VHDL. According to the paper, this tool is very usable and reliable, but a lot of useful features are not implemented yet. This tool is continued under development for adding new features that will be able to do semantic operations as well. In the area of model-driven software engineering, a tool PADL2Java [13] has been developed that translates PADL models into Java code. PADL is a process algebraic architectural description language equipped with a rigorous semantics and transformation rules into multi-threaded object-oriented software, which is employed in the verification tool TwoTowers [8]. This tool provides the code generation approach and code synthesising techniques.

SPARK [5] is a formally-defined programming language based on a restricted subset of the Ada language [23], intended to be secure and to support the development of high integrity software related to the critical systems. It describes desired behaviour of the system components and to verify the expected runtime requirements. Main features of this language are to support strong static typing, static and run-time checking, object-oriented programming, exception handling, parallel tasks, etc. Static verification tools allow to check the absence of general run-time errors like numerical overflow or division by zero and that the user-specified properties hold. The proofs will either be generated automatically or developed with the programmer's assistance for the more complex cases.

From Classic-B [1] notation to 'C', C++ and ADA language translation tool has been developed by D. Bert et al. [9]. This paper presents a methodology for translating a formal specification based-on Classic-B modelling language. Before generating the 'C' code, the specification model must be restated into an intermediate language 'B0'. The intermediate language 'B0' is restricted set of Classic-B formal notations. This tool is particularly designed for generating a 'C' code for an embedded system. This tool is not able to handle any complex expressions in the specification, so, this tool has very limited use. In the area of code generation from Event-B model to 'C' code is proposed by Stephen Wright [38]. But this tool is particularly designed for MIDAS [38] project. This tool also supports a subset of Event-B formal notations with a very simple expression form. This tool is no more usable for any Event-B formal specification. Edmunds et al. [18, 19] have presented a way for generating code, for concurrent programs, from Event-B specifications. Authors aim to integrate their code generation approach with existing Event-B methodology and tools.

As for as we know that there is no any mature translation tool existing, which can translate directly from Event-B formal specification into any target language

(C, C++, Java and C#). We have developed a tool that supports automatic translation into several target languages (C, C++, Java and C#) from Event-B formal specifications. This tool also supports the only subset of Event-B [2] formal notations, but it is much richer than previously developed tools [9, 38]. This chapter discusses the code generation approach underlying EB2C, EB2C++, EB2J and EB2C# tools [17, 25]. This is our first step toward in the direction of code generation from the Event-B formal specification, and our aim is to improve this tool to meet the industrial requirements.

7.3 A Basic Framework of Translator

A translator tool is developed as a set of plug-ins for the Rodin Tool [32], which can generate the source codes from a formal specification into many programming languages (C, C++, Java and C#). The translation tool is named as EB2ALL, which is a group of four kinds of different plug-ins, called EB2C, EB2C++, EB2J and EB2C#. All these tools have common architecture and a set of protocols for generating a source code. The translation process consists in transforming the concrete part of Event-B project into a semantically equivalent text written in any target programming language. This section proposes an architecture for the Event-B translator; different parts of the translator have been shown in Fig. 7.1 and this architecture supports translation for several target programming languages like C, C++, Java and C#. The translator tool is customised for each new target programming language to generate an efficient code, which can support various types of execution platforms. The proposed architecture is able to generate a verified code, which also comply with the behaviour of formal specifications. The translation tool is implemented in the Eclipse framework as a set of plug-ins for Event-B. The basic description of translation process is given as follows:

7.3.1 Selection of a Rodin Project

Formal development of a system in Event-B modelling language is provided by an open and extensible Eclipse-based IDE called Rodin [32], which supports system specifications and verification. A visual interface and a set of plug-ins help to specify and to prove a system under logico-mathematical theory. A proof manager is integrated in Rodin tool. Event-B models and all proof-related informations of a system project are always stored in the Rodin database. The translator tool is implemented as a set of plug-ins under the Eclipse development framework, using the recommended interfaces to traverse the statically checked internal database, thus decoupling the tool from the syntax of the Event-B notation by accessing its underlying meaning. The syntax of the mathematical notation, that is, expressions, predicates, and assignments, are maintained in the form of an abstract syntax tree.

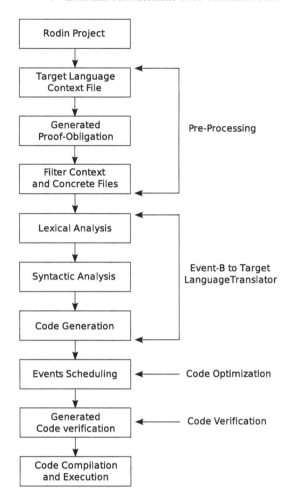

Fig. 7.1 A general architecture of a translation tool

This is the first phase of the translation process, which presents an explicit selection of a Rodin [32] project from all the loaded projects into the workspace. The selected project is passed to the next phase of the translation process for generating the source code.

7.3.2 Introduction of a Context File

Motivation

Failure of a critical system can be a cause of loss of life, financial loss, environmental damage and injury, where the cost of failure is not tolerable or affordable. For a critical system *run-time* error may be just as hazardous as any other logical error. For instance, overflow and underflow of bounded integer are run-time errors that should be addressed in the proof process. For developing a critical system, an automated technique based on formal methods have been matured to provide a high degree of confidence. Introduction of a context file is a very important phase of the code generation process, which provides one more level of refinement to make a system specification deterministic. The deterministic model is known as concrete well formed specification, which shows correct system behaviour before generating the source code. New context file consists of all *primary data types* corresponding to the programming languages (C, C++, Java and C#).

The papers [15, 16, 35] address a solution for the proof of clean termination that provides the facts that a program is totally correct. Clean termination means that a program terminates normally without any execution-time semantic errors like integer overflow, use of undefined variables, subscript out of range, etc. [16, 35]. We propose a pre-processing stage for obtaining a deterministic model using one more level of refinement through introduction of a new context that is similar to the clean termination approach [15, 35]. This refinement phase provides the deterministic definitions of constants and variables. This new refinement generates a lot of proof obligations. Types of generated proof obligations and proof details are similar to the papers [15, 16, 35]. This level of refinement complies system specification abstractly. The generated proof obligations are discharged by automatic as well as manual, and all proofs that are necessary to verify the specification in order to guarantee the consistency and correctness of the system. Therefore, this phase is very important to maintain all safety properties in the automatic code generation process.

Selection of a Context File

This phase provides many context files, to add into a current project according to a target programming language choice (C, C++, Java and C#). Table 7.1 shows bounded integer data types for all target programming languages. In the Event-B language, there are two kinds of constants and variables (*data*): abstract data and concrete data. Abstract data consists in all the elements and sets that can be used in set theory, as defined in Event-B (integers, enumerated sets, Cartesian products, power sets, relations, and so on). They are mainly used at the higher levels of specification (machines and in top level refinements) [2].

Concrete data are those which may be used in the final translation process, each time the data thus introduced will not be further refined in the development. It is the case for constants and variables at the implementation level but also for parameters and results of operations, which cannot be refined in Event-B [2]. Concrete data must match ordinary data types in a usual programming language because they should be "implemented" directly in the target programming language. So, the correspondence between concrete data and data types must be obvious. In standard Event-B, they are the following ones:

Table 7.1 Integer bounded data type declaration in different context files

Event-B type	Formal range	C & C++ type	Java type	C# type
*tl_int*16	$-2^{15}..2^{15}-1$	int	short	short
*tl_uint*16	$0..2^{16}-1$	unsigned int	–	ushort
*tl_int*32	$-2^{31}..2^{31}-1$	long int	int	int
*tl_uint*32	$0..2^{32}-1$	unsigned long int	–	uint
*tl_int*64	$-2^{63}..2^{63}-1$	–	long	long
*tl_uint*64	$0..2^{64}-1$	–	–	ulong

- enumerated types (including the boolean type)
- bounded integer type (from MININT to MAXINT)
- arrays on finite index intervals where the type of elements is a concrete type (in set theory, they are similar for total functions)

Refinement Using a New Context File

A new context file consists of a new data type definition equivalent to the primary data type (see Table 7.1). This new context file helps to model a system more deterministic through transforming abstract data types into concrete data types. Here, we consider the Event-B data types as the abstract data types, and the programming language data type as the concrete data types. A refinement technique is used to introduce a set of new concrete data types in the formal model. In this new refinement process, a developer can replace all the Event-B abstract data types of the contexts and the last concrete machine models, corresponding to the concrete data types according to the selected target programming language. The following figure presents an example for transforming an abstract data type into concrete data type.

$$var1 \in \mathbb{Z}$$

$$var2 \in \mathbb{N}$$

$$var1 \in tl\_int16$$
$$var1 \in tl\_int32$$
$$var1 \in tl\_int64$$

$$var2 \in tl\_uint16$$
$$var2 \in tl\_uint32$$
$$var2 \in tl\_uint64$$

A developer can skip this refinement level. In case of skipping of this refinement level in the translation process, the translator generates default maximum bounded integer primitive data type for all the variables and constants. New redefined deterministic ranges using refinement generates a lot of proof obligations.

7.3.3 Generated Proof Obligations

Introduction of a new context file is used as a data refinement of the system through removing all the abstract data types into a selected target programming language using concrete data types. The refinement is supported by the Rodin [4, 32] platform guarantees the preservation of safety properties. Thus, the behaviour of the final system is preserved by an abstract model as well as in the correctly refined models. A lot of proof obligations are generated, which can prove automatically as well as through manual intervention using interactive proof procedures [2, 4]. A model developer can discharge all the generated proof obligations with the help of the Rodin proof tool [32]. For example, when a set of constants and variables based on abstract data types changes into the concrete data types in a new refinement level, then some proof obligations are generated due to restrictive set of data ranges according to the predefined system behaviours. All these new generated proof obligations are required to discharge before continue the process. There is no guarantee to preserve all the safety properties (related to overflow or underflow) of the proved system unless all proof obligations are discharged.

Refinement using a context file provides proof of absence of run time errors into the generated code. Such kind of approach is also known as formal code verification [14]. Formal code verification techniques are used to demonstrate that at every point in the code where a run time error may occur like numeric overflow or underflow. A set of required conditions as in the form of predicates guarantees that the run time error will not occur. One more level of refinement approach is a very valuable step in the translation process to save from run time error, which demonstrates that especially in systems where the occurrence of an undesired run time error is unrecoverable.

7.3.4 Filter Context and Concrete Machine Modules

Refinement is a key feature of a formal development that supports incremental development for specifying a complex system. Event-B modelling language supports refinement based incremental development of a system, where a formal model is a series of development starting with a very abstract model of the system under development. Details are gradually added to this first model by building a sequence of more concrete events and ending with the implementation of machine as a final concrete system. The relationship between two successive models in this sequence is *refinement* [2, 4]. Relations between modules are only relations *sees* and *refines*.

This stage of the automatic translation process is used to filter all context and concrete machine files from the selected project. The context files consist of static properties as *sets, constants, functions* and *enumerated sets* of a system, while the machine files contain dynamic properties as *variables, functions* and *events* of a system. A set of filtered context and concrete files contains concrete *sets*, concrete *constants*, concrete *variables*, concrete *functions* and concrete *events*, which are used for implementation of a system. A selected project always contains some concrete models, which are refinements of the abstract models. The translation tool automatically filters a set of context and concrete files. If the translation tool is not able to filter all context and concrete files from the selected project, then immediately the translation process terminates with an error message, else all the filtered context and concrete files are passed to the next translation phase for continuing translation process.

7.3.5 Basic Principles of Code Generation

This phase is the heart of the translation tool. Before this level, all phases are used as preprocessing steps for obtaining the run-time errors free codes through data refinement of the formal specification. Main objective of this phase is to translate statically checked and proved formal specifications of Event-B model into *observationally equivalent* standard programming languages (C, C++, Java and C#). A set of rules has been generated for producing a source code, which is applicable to all context and concrete machine modules (i.e. those found to have no further refinement).

The translation tool generates source files as equivalent to the number of concrete machine files [2]. Source code generated file has a similar name corresponding to the concrete machine file, and a file extension generates according to the choice of a programming language. Source code generated files are saved in the folder of a particular language (C, C++, Java and C#) in the workspace of the selected Rodin project. Source code generated file begins with insertion of header comments containing a time-stamp and the name of selected Rodin project. Some required header informations are also inserted in the header of the source file according to the target programming language requirements. For instance, in C++ and C# source files contain all required header files related to the standard template library (STL) and Collection class of .NET Framework [12, 37], respectively. A Java source file contains *sets* definition of the set operations for handling the *sets* based notations of Event-B using standard class of Java utilities.

Main cause of failure of this translation tool is unable to parse any predicate. For example, the current tool is not able to handle relational operator ($\leftrightarrow$) and quantifiers ($\exists$ and $\forall$). If any predicate expression contains any quantifiers or relational operators, then the translation process is unable to translate it into a selected programming language, and the translation process fails. In case of translation failure, the tool immediately proceeds with translation of the next module. For avoiding the errors in the translation process, we have considered mainly two approaches:

- To model a system specification using a set of symbols (see Table 7.2 and Table 7.3), which is supported by the translation tool.
- Transformation of the final concrete models into a supported symbol list (see Table 7.2 and Table 7.3) through the refinement process.

Table 7.2 Event-B to C & C++ translation syntax

Event-B	'C' & 'C++' language	Comment
n..m	int	Integer type
$x \in Y$	Y x;	Scalar declaration
$x \in$ tl_int16	int x;	'C' & 'C++' contexts
$x \in n..m \rightarrow Y$	Y x [m + 1];	Array declaration
$x :\in Y$	/* No action */	Indeterminate init.
$x : \mid Y$	/* No action */	Indeterminate init.
$x = y$	if(x == y) {	Conditional
$x \neq y$	if(x! = y) {	Conditional
$x < y$	if(x < y) {	Conditional
$x \leq y$	if(x <= y) {	Conditional
$x > y$	if(x > y) {	Conditional
$x \geq y$	if(x >= y) {	Conditional
$(x > y) \wedge (x \geq z)$	if ((x > y) && (x >= z)) {	Conditional
$(x > y) \vee (x \geq z)$	if ((x > y) || (x >= z)) {	Conditional
$x := y + z$	x = y + z;	Arithmetic assignment
$x := y - z$	x = y − z;	Arithmetic assignment
$x := y * z$	x = y * z;	Arithmetic assignment
$x := y \div z$	x = y / z;	Arithmetic assignment
$x := F(y)$	x = F(y);	Function assignment
$a := F(x \mapsto y)$	a = F(x, y);	Function assignment
$x := a(y)$	x = a[y];	Array assignment
$x := y$	x = y;	Scalar action
$a := a \mathbin{\vartriangleleft\mkern-14mu-} \{x \mapsto y\}$	a[x] = y;	Array action
$a := a \mathbin{\vartriangleleft\mkern-14mu-} \{x \mapsto y\} \mathbin{\vartriangleleft\mkern-14mu-} \{i \mapsto j\}$	a[x] = y; a[i] = j;	Array action
$X \Rightarrow Y$	if(!X || Y){	Logical implication
$X \Leftrightarrow Y$	if((!X || Y) && (!Y || X)){	Logical equivalence
$\neg x < y$	if(!(x < y)){	Logical not
$x \in \mathbb{N}$	unsigned long int x	Natural numbers
$x \in \mathbb{Z}$	signed long int x	Integer numbers
$\forall$	/* No action */	Quantifier
$\exists$	/* No action */	Quantifier
$fun \in \mathbb{N} \times \mathbb{N} \rightarrow \mathbb{N}$	unsigned long int fun(unsigned long int *arg*1, unsigned long int *arg*2) { //TODO: Add your Code return; }	Function definition

Table 7.3 Event-B to Java & C# translation syntax

Event-B	'Java' & 'C#'	Comment
n..m	short	Integer type
x ∈ Y	Y x;	Scalar declaration
x ∈ tl_int16	short x; (Java) & ushort x; (C#)	'Java' & 'C#' contexts
x ∈ n..m → Y	Y [ ]x = new Y[m + 1];	Array declaration
x :∈ Y	/* No action */	Indeterminate init.
x : ∣ Y	/* No action */	Indeterminate init.
x = y	if(x == y) {	Conditional
x ≠ y	if(x! = y) {	Conditional
x < y	if(x <y) {	Conditional
x ≤ y	if(x <= y) {	Conditional
x > y	if(x > y) {	Conditional
x ≥ y	if(x >= y) {	Conditional
(x>y) ∧ (x ≥ z)	if ((x > y) && (x >= z)) {	Conditional
(x>y) ∨ (x ≥ z)	if ((x > y) ∥ (x >= z)) {	Conditional
x := y + z	x = y + z;	Arithmetic assignment
x := y − z	x = y − z;	Arithmetic assignment
x := y * z	x = y * z;	Arithmetic assignment
x := y ÷ z	x = y / z;	Arithmetic assignment
x := F(y)	x = F(y);	Function assignment
a := F(x↦y)	a = F(x, y);	Function assignment
x := a(y)	x = a[y];	Array assignment
x := y	x = y;	Scalar action
a := a ⩤ {x↦y}	a[x] = y;	Array action
a := a ⩤ {x↦y} ⩤ {i↦j}	a[x] = y; a[i] = j;	Array action
X⇒Y	if(!X ∥ Y){	Logical implication
X⇔Y	if((!X ∥ Y) && (!Y ∥ X)){	Logical equivalence
¬x < y	if(!(x < y)){	Logical not
x ∈ ℕ	unsigned long int x	Natural numbers
x ∈ ℤ	signed long int x	Integer numbers
∀	/* No Action */	Quantifier
∃	/* No Action */	Quantifier
fun ∈ ℕ × ℕ → ℕ	public long fun(long *arg*1, long *arg*2) { //TODO: Add your Code return; }	Function definition

Table 7.4 Event-B to Java & C# Sets translation syntax

Event-B	'C++'	Comment
set_var	set *<data type>* set_var	STL library
∪	set_union(...)	STL library
∩	set_intersection(...)	STL library
\	set_difference(...)	STL library
⊆	includes(...)	STL library
⊂	includes(...) && !(equal(...))	STL library
⊈	!(includes(...))	STL library
⊄	!(includes(...)) && !(equal(...))	STL library

Event-B	'Java'	Comment
set_var	Set *<data type>* set_var = new HashSet*<data type>*()	Java Utilities
∪	unionSet(...)	Java Utilities
∩	intersectionSet(...)	Java Utilities
\	differenceSet(...)	Java Utilities
⊆	isSubset(...)	Java Utilities
⊂	isSubset(...) && !(isEqualSet(...)) {	Java Utilities
⊈	!(isSubset(...))	Java Utilities
⊄	!(isSubset(...)) && !(isEqualSet(...))	Java Utilities

Event-B	'C#'	Comment
set_var	HashSet *<data type>* set_var = new HashSet*<data type>*()	.NET Framework 4
∪	UnionWith(...)	.NET Framework 4
∩	IntersectWith(...)	.NET Framework 4
\	ExceptWith(...)	.NET Framework 4
⊆	IsSubsetOf(...)	.NET Framework 4
⊂	IsProperSubsetOf(...)	.NET Framework 4
⊈	!(IsSubsetOf(...))	.NET Framework 4
⊄	!(IsProperSubsetOf(...))	.NET Framework 4

Before generating a source code from a model, a user is required to refine a system using a subset of Event-B symbols (see Tables 7.2, 7.3 and 7.4), which can restate the model in a more translatable form. Supported symbols are available in Tables 7.2, 7.3 and 7.4. These tables show a set of Event-B syntax to the equivalent C, C++, Java and C# programming languages. All constants defined in a model's context must be replaced with their literal values. This translation tool supports *Sets* theory notations (not in 'C'), conditional, arithmetical and logical expressions of a formal specification. The formal notations and expressions are translated into equivalent programming language code. A detailed translation process of the context and concrete machine files are given in the following sections.

Process Context and Machine Files Using Lexical and Syntax Analysis

Context and machine files consist of static and dynamic properties of a system in the form of modular architecture, which represents a system behaviour using formal notations. To generate a source code into any programming language, it is required to process the context and machine files separately using lexical and syntactic analysis. Usually, the parsing of a formal model is divided into two stages: lexical analysis and syntactic analysis. In real-world problem like code generation, lexical analysis and syntactic analysis stages may be intertwined with each other [34]. We are very thankful to the Rodin development team for providing source code of Rodin tool. Source code of the Rodin tool is well-written and developed as in the form of a set of plug-ins to design a complete tool. The Rodin tool has a set of library files of an Abstract Syntax Tree (AST) which is mainly used for lexical and syntactic analysis for Event-B notations at the time of modelling. We have used same library for lexical and syntactic analysis of Event-B model for generating a source code into any programming language (C, C++, Java and C#). To generate a source code into any target programming language, input source (Event-B formal model) is always same. Therefore, we have similar kinds of procedures to process context and machine files using existing AST library of the Rodin tool.

Process Context Files

The context of Event-B model consists of *sets*, *enumerated sets*, *constants*, *arrays* and *constant functions*, associated with their respective type. The translation tool supports all kinds of context components to generate a constant type with respect to a programming language. An instance of the context consists in associating to each name a value consistent with its declared type. The observational equivalence is based on equivalence between Event-B values and target programming language values. This equivalence on values is naturally extended on instances of context. The observational equivalence between Event-B sets and target programming language types is given in Table 7.5.

Mapping Event-B Constant Types to Programming Language

- *Enumerated Sets*
  Event-B enumerated sets is semantically equivalent to a target programming language enumerated type. It is very easy to translate into a target programming language equivalent form due to equivalent semantical structure.

Table 7.5 Equivalence between Event-B and programming language

Event-B types	Target language types
Enumerated sets	Enumerated types
Basic integer sets	Predefined integer types
Event-B array types	Target programming language array type
Function	Target programming language function structure
Sets theory	Set theory implementation using advanced library function in target language (not in 'C')

```
Event-B
partition(ESet, {On}, {Off})
```

```
C and C++
    enum ESet{On, Off};

Java and C#
    public enum ESet{On, Off};
```

- *The Numeric Types*

  The links between Event-B and target programming languages for integer values have been considered as crucial for the efficiency of a generated code and for the correctness of the translation process. So, the solution is provided in the second phase by introducing target programming language context, and it is able to interface very tightly between Event-B types and a target programming language type. The Event-B numeric types ($\mathbb{N}$, $\mathbb{N}_1$ and $\mathbb{Z}$) are either all mapped to the predefined context files (see second phase of the translation process) or defined the maximum integer range according to a programming language. For translating constant data type in C, C++ and C# programming languages use *const* keyword, while Java uses *static final* keyword for defining a constant.

```
Event-B
Lnum ∈ ℕ
```

```
C, and C++
    const long int Lnum;

C#
    const long Lnum;

Java
    static final long Lnum;
```

- *The Array Type*

  The links between Event-B arrays and target programming language arrays are not straightforward. In Event-B, an array corresponds to a total function whereas in the target programming language, an array corresponds to a contiguous zone of memory (coded as the beginning address of the array and its size). However, it is easy to do a semantic correspondence between an array element *arr(i)* in Event-B and a value at the location *arr[i]* in target programming languages (see Tables 7.2, 7.3).

Event-B
$ARR \in 1..10 \to \mathbb{N}$

> **C, and C++**
> *const long int ARR*[11];
>
> **C#**
> *const* [ ]*long* = *new long*[11];
>
> **Java**
> *static final* [ ]*long* = *new long*[11];

- *The Function Type*

  The links between Event-B function and target programming language function is also very ambiguous. The Event-B functions are generated explicitly into a target language code, and function definitions are placed in the corresponding source file. The translation tools only supports total function of Event-B into equivalent corresponding target programming language function. However, it is an easy way to do a semantical correspondence between function passing parameters in a target programming language is equivalent to the elements of left side of the total functions symbol ($\to$) and output of a target programming language function corresponds to the right-hand side of the total functions symbol ($\to$) in Event-B. So, this step of function translation generates a function structure into a target programming language (see Tables 7.2, 7.3).

Event-B
$fun \in \mathbb{N} \times \mathbb{N} \to \mathbb{N}$

> **C, and C++**
> *unsigned long int* (*unsigned long int arg*1,
> *unsigned long int arg*2)
> {
>   *//TODO* : *Add your Code*
>   *return*;
> }
>
> **Java**
> *public long* (*long arg*1, *long arg*2)
> {
>   *//TODO* : *Add your Code*
>   *return*;
> }

- *The Set Type*

  The translation tool is a set of plug-ins, in which C++, Java and C# languages plug-ins can support *Sets* formal notation for translation. The Event-B sets type is translated into a programming language using the standard template library (STL) in C++, advanced Java class utilities in Java and Generic Collection of .NET Framework in C#. We have developed some functions with the help of existing library functions in C++, Java and C#, which are equivalent to Event-B sets operations (see Tables 7.2, 7.3 and 7.4). We have given the following snap shot of sets operations, which are by default generated in every source code of Java file.

```java
public static <T> Set<T>
unionSet(Set<T> setA, Set<T> setB)
{
Set<T> tmp = new HashSet<T>(setA);
tmp.addAll(setB);
return tmp;
}

public static <T> Set<T>
intersectionSet(Set<T> setA, Set<T> setB)
{
Set<T> tmp = new HashSet<T>(setA);
tmp.retainAll(setB);
return tmp;
}

public static <T> Set<T>
differenceSet(Set<T> setA, Set<T> setB)
{
Set<T> tmp = new HashSet<T>(setA);
tmp.removeAll(setB);
return tmp;
}

public static <T> boolean
isSubset(Set<T> setA, Set<T> setB)
{
return setB.containsAll(setA);
}

public static <T> boolean
isEqualSet(Set<T> setA, Set<T> setB)
{
return (setB.containsAll(setA)&& setA.containsAll(setB));
}
...
```

- *Set Definition*: To define a set type into C++, Java and C#, the translation tool uses some fixed code structures to define a *sets* type with the help of STL library, Java utilities and .NET Framework (when set type is unknown). The following structures are excerpted from a translated code to understand the set definition of a context model:
  In the C++ language...

```cpp
class DATASet{
private:
        string element;
```

```
public:
    DATASet() {element="";}
    DATASet(string elem) {element = elem; }
    string outElement() const { return element; }
    bool operator <(DATASet temp) const {
        return (element<temp.outElement());
    }
    bool operator ==(DATASet temp) const {
        return (element==temp.outElement());
    }
};
/* Sets definition */
set <DATASet> DATA;
```

In the Java language...

```
public static class DATASet{
    private String element;
    public DATASet() {element="";}
    public DATASet(String elem) {element = elem; }
    public String outElement() { return element; }
};

/* Sets definition */
Set <DATASet> DATA = new HashSet<DATASet>();
```

In the C# language...

```
public static class DATASet{
    private string element;
    public DATASet() {element="";}
    public DATASet(string elem) {element = elem; }
    public string outElement() { return element; }
};
/* Sets definition */
HashSet <DATASet> DATA = new HashSet<DATASet>();
```

To define a set of numbers are very simple, which can be defined as follows:
In C++ language...

```
set <int> A; /* Sets definition */
```

In the Java language...

```
Set <Long> A= new HashSet<Long>(); /* Sets definition */
```

In the Java language...

```
HashSet <int> A= new HashSet<int>(); /* Sets definition */
```

A set of context files is used as an input to declare all kinds of data-types in form of global constants on top of the source code file. All elements of the context files are declared as global. Context element type information is derived from the type-defining *AXIOM* statement within the context, which may express as integer ranges, specially supported bit-map types or arrays of these defined by mapping functions.

Process Machine Files

Machine file contains dynamic behaviour of a system, which is denoted by generally *variables*, *arrays*, *functions* and *events*. All these components of a machine file model a system. In the following section, we present automatic transformation of a machine model into any programming language (C, C++, Java and C#).

Mapping Event-B Variable Types to Programming Language

A machine file contains *functions*, *arrays* and *variables* for representing a system state. All these elements are declared as global. Global element's type information is derived from the type-defining *INVARIANT* statements within the machine, which may be expressed as integer ranges, function structure, or arrays. Event-B to target language code generator generates target language function definitions corresponding to the invariants. Event-B functions are generated explicitly into the target language code and function definitions are placed in the corresponding source file. The translation tool translates all those into target programming language code according to the same rules, which are defined in the last section for defining a constant type. Static and dynamic type definitions have only difference between context and machine modules data types. For instance, constants and variables have the same definition using primitive data types but C, C++ and C# language constants use *const* keyword and Java uses *static final* keyword with a constant data type declaration, and variables are defined in all languages without using *const* and *static final* keywords.

More than one invariants or axioms may be defined in a single invariant or axiom using and ($\wedge$) logical operator. This translation tool automatically parses an invariant or axioms at the time of constant or variable data type declaration during the translation process.

C, and C++
int var;

Event-B
var ∈ tl_int16

C#
short var;

Java
short var;

Table 7.6 Event B events

Event e	Before-after predicate $BA(e)(x, x')$
BEGIN 　$x : \vert(P(x, x'))$ END	$P(x, x')$
WHEN 　$G(x)$ THEN 　$x : \vert(Q(x, x'))$ END	$G(x) \wedge Q(x, x')$
ANY WHEN 　t WHERE 　$G(t, x)$ THEN 　$x : \vert(R(x, x', t))$ END	$\exists t \cdot (G(t, x) \wedge R(x, x', t))$

Mapping Event-B Events to Programming Language

The translation tool provides a recursive process to generate a source code for each event of the Event-B specification into a target programming language. The translation tool always checks for *null* event (i.e. guard of a false condition), never generates a source code for that event, and inserts suitable comment into the source code for the traceability purpose. This automatic reduction is performed to avoid generation of an unreachable *run-time* code.

- *To Process Event's Variable*
  In Event-B specification, there are two kinds of variables: global variables and local variables. Global variables are derived directly from *VARIABLES* statements of a concrete machine, and all these variables have global scope. Local variables are derived from the *ANY* statement of the particular event, and these are entirely local to the corresponding event function (see Table 7.6). The type of this local variable is declared into the event's guards. Once the guards of an event have been classified, and that conferring local variable type information are used for variable declaration in a function. Remaining guards are used to generate local assignment and conditional statements in the guard section. Local variable type information is derived in a similar fashion as the global variables from the guard predicates instead of using INVARIANTS. A recursive process is used to find a type of Event-B local variable corresponding to the programming language. Each event of Event-B is generated in equivalent to the programming language function. After generation of a function header, all local variables, array declarations are inserted at the beginning of the function, giving them scope across the whole function body.

```
EVENT Sum
  ANY a
  WHEN
    grd1 : a ∈ N
  ⋮
```

```
/ * In the 'C' Language * /
BOOL Sum() {
    long int a;
    ⋮

/ * In the Java language * /
private boolean Sum() {
    long a;
    ⋮
```

- *To Process Event's Guard*

In the Event-B, guard handling is very ambiguous due to contain several kinds of modelling notations, such that local variable type definition, conditions and use of different kinds of logical operators ($\wedge$, $\vee$, $\neg$, $\Rightarrow$, $\Leftrightarrow$). Therefore, for handling so many complex situations, we have designed a recursive algorithm for parsing a complex guard and to separate different kinds of predicates in the form of formal notations for generating a programming language code using guards. Thus, each guard must be automatically analysed to resolve this ambiguity from the context information. In a formal model, the guards are known as pre-conditions and action predicates are known as post-conditions. In an event, all pre-conditions must be true for executing the post-conditions or action predicates. For translating an event of a formal model into a programming language, we translate it into corresponding target language function (C, C++, Java and C#).

Pre-conditions of a guard are translated into equivalent *if* condition statement. A group of guards is translated in the form of *nested-if* conditions, and are placed into an event function as a set of nested conditional statements, using directly translated conditional and local variables declared within nested scope ranges. A suitable comment is also inserted with each guard condition to understand the different elements of the guards like local variables and pre-conditions.

```
EVENT Sum
  . . .
  WHEN
    . . .
    grd3 : a < n
    grd4 : a > m
  ⋮
```

```
/ * In the 'C' Language * /
BOOL Sum() {
    . . .
    if(a < n){
        if(b > m){
        ⋮
```

```
/ * In the Java language * /
private boolean Sum() {
    . . .
    if(a < n){
        if(b > m){
        ⋮
```

A set of guards can be represented through logical operators, which are simply in the form of propositions calculus. In the account of code generation, we want to explore the possibility of logical operators in the translation process. An important goal is to handle the various kinds of logical operators in terms of providing a large class of a set of symbols supported for the code generation and to support various kinds of modelling structures. A key part of a structuralist approach is to define the various logical operators as special functions defined on implication structures. It will be helpful in what follows to use Conjunction, Negation, and Disjunction as examples of the way these characterisations work. Universal and existential quantifications are also part of the guards but these are not defined or discussed here due to restricted in the current version of translation tools.

Conjunction ($\wedge$): The conjunction operator ($\wedge$) in a guard predicate is a function of two arguments, such that for any two predicates connected with a conjunction operator ($\wedge$) is translated as follows:

EVENT Sum

. . .

  WHEN

   . . .

   grd3 : $a < b \wedge P\_State = FALSE$

    $\vdots$

/ ∗ **In the 'C' Language** ∗ /
BOOL Sum() {

  . . .

  if$((a < b)$ && $(P\_State == FALSE))${

    $\vdots$

/ ∗ **In the Java language** ∗ /
private boolean Sum() {

  . . .

  if$((a < b)$ && $(P\_State == FALSE))${

    $\vdots$

Disjunction ($\vee$): The disjunction operator ($\vee$) in a guard predicate is a function of two arguments. Any two predicates connected with a disjunction operator ($\vee$) is translated as follows:

EVENT Sum

 . . .

  WHEN

   . . .

   grd3 : $a < b \vee P\_State = FALSE$

    $\vdots$

/ ∗ **In the 'C' Language** ∗ /
BOOL Sum() {

  . . .

  if$((a < b)$ || $(P\_State == FALSE))${

    $\vdots$

/ ∗ **In the Java language** ∗ /
private boolean Sum() {

  . . .

  if$((a < b)$ || $(P\_State == FALSE))${

    $\vdots$

Negation (¬): The negation operator (¬) in a guard predicate is a function of single argument, such that for any predicate with a negation operator (¬) in a guard is translated as follows:

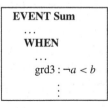

```
/ * In the 'C' Language * /
BOOL Sum() {
    ...
    if (! (a < b)){
         :
```

```
/ * In the Java language * /
private boolean Sum() {
    ...
    if (! (a < b)){
         :
```

Some more logical operators are like implication (⇒) and equivalence (⇔), which can be easily rewritten using logical conjunction (∧), disjunction (∨) and negation (¬) operators. For example, the implication (⇒) and equivalence (⇔) operators, the translator tool automatically rewrite a predicate in an equivalent form using conjunction (∧), disjunction (∨) and negation (¬) operators, an equal relation may signify an assignment or equality comparison, and the precise meaning (and hence the resulting translation) deduced from the type and scope of its operands.

Implication (⇒): The implication operator (⇒) in a guard predicate is a function of two arguments, such that for any predicate connected with an implication operator (⇒) is translated as follows:

EVENT Sum
...
WHEN
...
   grd3 : $a < b \Rightarrow P\_State = FALSE$
   :

```
/ * In the 'C' Language * /
BOOL Sum() {
    ...
    if (! (a < b) || (P_State == FALSE)){
         :
```

```
/ * In the Java language * /
private boolean Sum() {
    ...
    if (! (a < b) || (P_State == FALSE)){
         :
```

Equivalence ($\Leftrightarrow$): The equivalence operator ($\Leftrightarrow$) in a guard predicate is a function of two arguments, such that for any predicate connected with an equivalence operator ($\Leftrightarrow$) is translated as follows:

EVENT Sum

. . .
WHEN

. . .
grd3 : $a < b \Leftrightarrow P\_State = FALSE$
$\vdots$

```
/ * In the 'C' Language * /
BOOL Sum() {

    . . .
    if((! (a < b) || (P_State == FALSE)) ||
       (! (P_State == FALSE) || (a < b))){
    ⋮

/ * In the Java language * /
private boolean Sum() {

    . . .
    if((! (a < b) || (P_State == FALSE)) ||
       (! (P_State == FALSE) || (a < b))){
    ⋮
```

Arithmetical expressions, calling functions and set operations (see Tables 7.2, 7.3) are also supported by Event-B formal notations in the guards, which are all translatable into any target programming language. Event-B expressions and statements are code generated, such that the generated code behaves like it is expected from the specification. A set of translation rules with a basic syntactic architecture is defined in Table 7.2 and Table 7.3. Translation tool follows the similar set of rules for generating a source code. A special kind of ambiguity of a functional-image relation is resolved during the translation process, which may be used to model a data array or an external function. The meaning of functional-image statements within a model is automatically resolved to an array if the mapping is a global variable, otherwise to call an uninterpreted function. A complete set of guards of an event is translated into equivalent programming language code in the form of pre-conditions in an event. During the code translation process, a run-time exception function is generated if an undefined expression or an error statement is occurred. This call of exception function terminates the code translation and reports that an undefined expression into a code generation log file.

The translation tool can support a very complex predicate, where more than one predicate are defined in a single guard. The translation tool is able to automatically parse the whole predicate into a set of predicates, separately for translation purpose.

Set operations: The set operators ($\cup$, $\cap$, $\backslash$) in a guard predicate is a function of two arguments, which uses some intermediate steps according to the C++, Java and C# programming languages. The translation of set based expression is translated as follows:

```
/ * In the 'C++' Language * /
BOOL SetFun() {

    ...

    set < int > tset2;
    set_union(A.begin(), A.end(), B.begin(), B.end(),
    inserter(tset2, tset2.begin()));

    if((includes(C.begin(), C.end(), tset2.begin(),
    tset2.end())))){

        ⋮

/ * In the Java language * /
private boolean SetFun() {

    ...

    if(isSubset(unionSet(A, B), C)){

        ⋮


/ * In the C# language * /
private boolean SetFun() {

    ...

    A.UnionWith(B);
    if(A.IsSubsetOf(C)){

        ⋮
```

```
EVENT SetFun

    ...

    WHEN

    ...

        grd3 : A ∪ B ⊆ C

        ⋮
```

- *To Process Event's Action*
  The next sub-stage of an event translation presents the action translation. In EVENT-B, all action predicates of an event are considered as in the form of concurrent execution. The set of action predicates are post-conditions in the Event-B events, which state that all action predicates only valid when all pre-conditions or guards are satisfied [1, 2]. Event-B modelling approach supports that any state variable is not allowed to be modified by different action expressions, means Event-B ensures that any state variable used as an action assignee is not modified by any prior post conditions or action predicate. In the code translation process, all action predicates are generated into equivalent programming expression. In a programming language, all action expressions are executed in a sequential order of what they have defined in a formal specification. But all action expressions are executed only when all *if* conditions become *true*. Event-B supports three kinds of assignment operators *becomes equal to* (:=), *becomes in* (:∈) and *becomes such that* (: |), where *becomes in* (:∈) and *become such that* (: |) are used basically in an abstract model, and through the refinement process, it is represented in a concrete form as *becomes equal to* (:=). The translation tools only supports *becomes equal to* (:=). If a concrete model uses any *becomes such that* (: |) and *becomes in* (:∈) assignment operators, then the translation tool does not generate action predicates into programming expressions and move to the next action predicate to continue processing. A similar way of parsing is applied on Event-B action statement like a guard statement. The translation tool translates all Event-B actions into an equivalent target programming language source code.

```
                                    / * In the 'C' Language * /
                                    BOOL Sum() {

  ┌─────────────────────────────┐      ...
  │  EVENT Sum                  │      Ans = a + 10 − 6 * 8;
  │  ...                        │
  │  WHEN                       │        ⋮
  │                             │
  │  ...                        │
  │  THEN                       │    / * In the Java language * /
  │    act1 : Ans := a + 10 − 6 * 8│    private boolean Sum() {
  │                             │
  │        ⋮                    │      ...
  └─────────────────────────────┘      Ans = a + 10 − 6 * 8;

                                        ⋮
```

An action translation supports assignments to scalar variables, override statements acting on array-type variables, arithmetic complex expressions and set operations. The Event-B supports a special form of the action predicates, which shows that a state variable can be used in the right side of the assignment operator (:=). To handle such kinds of action predicates, the translation tool automatically modifies the action predicates through a re-write phase and store the value in an intermediate local variable, and finally translate into programming language expression with an assignee in the action expression.

```
                                    / * In the 'C' Language * /
                                    BOOL Sum() {

                                      ...
                                      OvrVar[3] = 67;
  ┌─────────────────────────────┐      OvrVar[4] = 88;
  │  EVENT Sum                  │      OvrVar[t] = 56;
  │  ...                        │      Arr[i] = 5;
  │  WHEN                       │
  │                             │        ⋮
  │  ...                        │
  │  THEN                       │    / * In the Java language * /
  │    act1 : OvrVar := OvrVar◁─ │    private boolean Sum() {
  │          {3 ↦ 67, 4 ↦ 88, t ↦ 56}│
  │    act1 : Arr(i) := 5       │      ...
  │                             │      OvrVar[3] = 67;
  │        ⋮                    │      OvrVar[4] = 88;
  └─────────────────────────────┘      OvrVar[t] = 56;
                                      Arr[i] = 5;

                                        ⋮
```

After insertion of all kinds of action predicates through the translation process into a generated code event function, adds an extra statement returning a boolean *true*, which express run-time traceability and states that an event function is triggered successfully. After insertion of returning boolean statement, inserts all curly braces (}) according to the total number of guards except those guards, who represents local variable data types. Finally, a returning boolean *false* statement again inserts before closing the final braces of an event function. The main objective of this *false* boolean returning statement at a time of execution is that, when this event function executes and any guard of this event is *false*, then this function returns *false* to indicate that this event function is not executed.

```
/ * In the 'C' Language * /
BOOL EventFun() {
    if(Cond₁){
        if(Cond₂){

        ...
        Assignment Expr.
        ...
            return TRUE;
        }
    }
            return FALSE;
}
```

```
/ * In the Java language * /
private boolean EventFun() {
    if(Cond₁){
        if(Cond₂){

        ...
        Assignment Expr.
        ...
            return true;
        }
    }
            return false;
}
```

Set expression: The set operators ($\cup$, $\cap$, $\backslash$) in the action predicate is also function of two arguments similar to the guards predicates, which use some intermediate steps according to the C++, Java and C# programming languages. The translation of set based expression is translated as follows in the action's part:

```
EVENT SetFun

...
WHEN

...
THEN
    act1 : C := A ∪ B
    :
```

```
/ * In the 'C++' Language * /
BOOL SetFun() {

    ...
    set < int > tset4;
    set_union(A.begin(), A.end(), B.begin(), B.end(),
    inserter(tset4, tset4.begin()));

    C.clear(); / * clear data of assignee set C * /
    C = tset4; / * Transfer all sets elements into C * /

    :
```

```
/ * In the Java language * /
private boolean SetFun() {

    ...
    C.clear(); //clear data of assignee set C
    //Transfer all sets elements into C
    C = unionSet(A, B);

    :
```

```
/ * In the C# language * /
private boolean SetFun() {

    ...
    C.clear(); //clear data of assignee set C
    //Transfer all sets elements into C
    C = A.UnionWith(B);

    :
```

The translation tool uses a similar kind of fashion to translate each event of the Event-B model. Event-B is a very rich modelling language for representing formal notation of a specification, but translation tool supports only subset of formal notations of Event-B. Event-B expressions and statements are code generated, such that the generated code behaves like it is expected from the specification. A set of translation rules and basic syntactic architecture is defined in Tables 7.2, 7.3 and 7.4. During the code translation process, a run-time exception function is generated if an undefined expression or an error statement is occurred. A generated error invokes an exception function, which terminates the code translation process and reports that an undefined expression into a code generation log file. The next level of the translation tool presents the scheduling techniques to produce an executable code.

7.3.6   Events Scheduling

This phase is not producing any translation part of the translation tool. This section introduces to generate a function for organising all event functions. There are two ways to organise all the event functions:

1. *Optimise*: An optimised code is used to make a group of calling event functions into a new function. An incremental refinement-based structure of events within an Event-B model provides grouping information about the events. A recursive algorithm is used in the translation tool to discover structuring information from current Rodin project, and could exploit it to recursively generate nesting calling a set of functions corresponding to the abstract events. Merging of common event guards is currently avoided in order to preserve direct mapping between Event-B statements and translated code, at the cost of possible performance optimisations. However, if translatable guards are already placed in an abstract level, then guards are forming a group of concrete events. An event group is inserted for execution in place of multiple events for improving the run-time performance.

    Figure 7.2 shows a basic architecture of event scheduling using optimisation approach. This figure represents a tree structure of the refinement development, where an abstract model is represented as AM and refinement models are represented through $RM_1, RM_2 \ldots$, and finally concrete models are represented by CM. All refinement models (RM_i) are parts of the single abstract refinement (AM). This figure has two groups G_1 and G_2. G_1 makes a group of a set of events at first refinement level and G_2 makes a group of events at the second refinement level. A user can select the refinement level for making a group of events before code generation. Each group has a set of events, which are only executable when abstract guards are *true*. If a user select higher number of refinement level for optimisation then the number of groups may be increased. For instance, in Fig. 7.2 group G_1 has refinement level 1, therefore there are three possible number of groups, while in the group G_2 has refinement level 2 and possible number of maximum groups are five corresponding to the number of blocks in each refinement level.

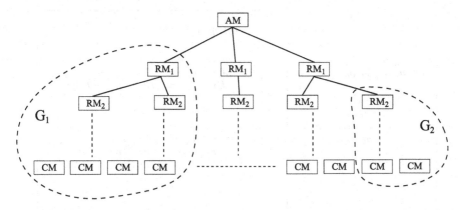

Fig. 7.2 Event scheduling

2. *Sequential*: A sequential organisation of the event functions is used to call event functions into a new function, in the same order, defined by their position in the Event-B model. It is not providing any kind of optimisation in the calling function.

Event scheduling phase is used to synthesise all target language functions. All these target language functions are equivalent to Event-B events. We propose two techniques to trigger all the translated events. First is calling a function *"Iterate"* that implements a continuous iteration of translated target programming language functions of the Event-B model, in the same order, defined by their position in the Event-B model. Second technique is to optimise the calling order of the events. Optimisation approach schedules calling target language functions using a refinement approach. An incremental refinement-based structure of events within the Event-B models exploits to recursively generate nesting calling functions corresponding to the abstract events. Abstract level guards are forming a group of concrete events. Each group of events are triggered by a main *"Iterate"* function. This technique is used to improve run-time performance wherever at the concrete level has several events. In the sequential order of calling event functions in the *"Iterate"* function invokes every calling function in a sequential order. Whenever guards are satisfied by invoked event function, then the function executes and when guards are not *true*, then the next calling function invokes in a sequential way. Main disadvantage of this technique is that, when a translated code has a lot of calling functions (> 50), then the every function consumes some memory as well as time for invoking a function. While in an optimised way, to make a group of calling functions, which automatically reduces time and memory consumption during invocation of the *"Iterate"* function. A scheduling structure (see Fig. 7.3) shows a calling order of event functions in the *"Iterate"* function.

Finally, top-level *main function* of a target programming language is generated to call the generated functions "INITIALISATION" and "Iterate". The only procedural requirement is the calling of "INITIALISATION" prior to "Iterate". All other

```
BOOL Iterate(void)
{
    if(Event₁() == TRUE)
        return TRUE;
    if(Event₂() == TRUE)
        return TRUE;
    .
    .
    .
    if(Eventₙ() == TRUE)
        return TRUE;

    / * Signal deadlock * /
    return FALSE;
}
```

```
BOOL Iterate(void)
{
    if(Condition₁ ...){
    if(Event₁() == TRUE) return TRUE;
    if(Event₂() == TRUE) return TRUE;
    . . .
    }

    if(Condition₂ ...){
    if(Event₄() == TRUE) return TRUE;
    if(Event₅() == TRUE) return TRUE;
    . . .
    }
    .
    .
    if(Conditionₘ ...){
    if(Eventₙ₋₁() == TRUE) return TRUE;
    if(Eventₙ() == TRUE) return TRUE;
    . . .
    }
    / * Signal deadlock * /
    return FALSE;
}
```

Fig. 7.3 Scheduling architecture

behaviour regarding iteration control may be selected. The INITIALISATION function is exposed to allow later calls to it by the execution environment, providing a
mechanism for run-time reset of the Event-B machine if required. In the particular
example, the machine is invoked only once and, after initialisation, is iterated continuously without any scheduling constraints until either implicit or explicit deadlock
(i.e. an event having no actions) is detected. Implicit deadlock is flagged as an error
condition, explicit deadlock is treated as normal execution.

In the C and C++ languages. . .

```
void  main ( void )
  {
     if (  INITIALISATION ()==TRUE  ){
     do {
     Iterate ();
     } while (! kbhit ());
     }
}
```

In the C# language. . .

```
public  static  void  Main ()
  {
M1_VOOR objM1_VOOR  =  new  M1_VOOR ();
     if (  objM1_VOOR . INITIALISATION ()== true  ){
     for ( int  n=0;n<=1000;n++){
```

```
    objM1_VOOR. Iterate ();
    }
    }
}
```

In the Java language...

```
public static void main(String[] args)
  {
M1_VOOR objM1_VOOR = new M1_VOOR();
    if( objM1_VOOR.INITIALISATION()==true ){
    try{
    for(int n=0;n<=1000;n++){
    objM1_VOOR. Iterate ();
    }
    }catch(Exception e){
    e.printStackTrace();
    }
    }
}
```

7.3.7 *External Code Injection and Code Verification*

This is also an important phase of the code generating process, where the source code files have been generated from Event-B specification. This phase provides a way to introduce some handwritten code or introduction of implicit functions in the form of an interface in order to compile and run the application in target languages (C, C++, Java, C#). For example, when a function is defined abstractly and function returns output value using a set of calculation or algorithms. In that case, a user requires to write a function body, which is generated by the translator. Thus, the user has to write a target language function definition for the operation and add it to the function body of the generated file. To provide some code interface through user intervention, we have introduced code verification step. The code verification is a very important step to verify the correctness of an automatic generated code. This step is required due to manual insertion of an external code. We have considered following two main objectives for adding external codes in the generated codes:

- If some part of the implementation code is not supported by the code generator;
- The user wants to implement some existing components more efficiently.

Due to the complex architecture of the software-development process, it is impossible that any modelling tool can generate directly an executable application. In large software, different kinds of languages are used for designing final software. So, we have provided a facility of code injection. For instance, addition of hardware specific code (i.e. assembly code) into Event-B generated code. For example, in pacemaker case study, Sensor and Actuator are specific hardware units,

Fig. 7.4 Generated code
verification

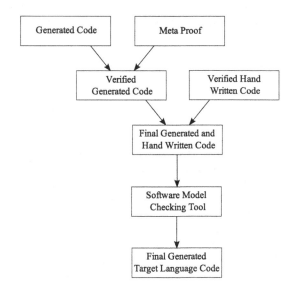

which control by specific hardware codes. The hardware code is provided by the
third-party and pacemaker manufacturing company assumes that this hardware dependent codes are already corrected and verified. So, simple they inject this code
directly into the generated code.

Due to injection of the external code and code addition into a complex function
body, we have proposed a generated code verification technique, which provides
certification of the generated code using this tool. Figure 7.4 shows an approach to
verify a source code of the final developed system. Our idea is to verify the correctness of generated code with respect to Event-B formal specification to give a *meta-
proof* that for all Event-B models, and target language translation, the execution
of the target language program satisfies the execution (abstractly) of the Event-B
model.

In fact, as can be expected, the translation of Event-B descriptions into a target
language software cannot be complete, and hence will require an intervention of
a software developer in specific positions of the generated code, e.g. for inserting
the target language statements corresponding to the internal actions. Hence, next
level of code verification injects hand-written code corresponding to the internal
actions. Further, we have used software model checking tools according to the different target languages. The software model checking tools are complemented of the
analysis conducted on Event-B specification by making it possible the verification
of property preservation at the code level. In fact, although property preservation
is guaranteed under certain constraints [6, 7, 10], an inappropriate intervention of
software developer on the generated code may lead to the violation of properties
proved at an architectural level.

7.3.8 *Compiling and Running the Code*

Once automatic translation and verification of the Event-B model is completed, all additional requirements are added, an execution environment must be provided and compiled by a suitable target programming language compiler. This final step of the translation tool is to produce generated files for compiling on-target platform (Windows, Linux and Mac).

7.4 How to Use Code Generator Plug-ins

To get started using the code generator you should require an Event-B specification. The code generator requires that all files of the Event-B specifications are syntax checked in order to generate correct code. Before generating a source code, it has to ensure that specification is proved and one more level of refinement has been done to make a deterministic model. The code generator tool box will automatically type checked for data types and generates a code according to the programming language.

Figure 7.5 represents a screen shot of translator tools (EB2C, EB2C++, EB2J and EB2C#)[2] under the Rodin environment [17, 24–26]. All these tools are developed as a set of plug-ins under the Eclipse framework. After installation of the EB2C, EB2C++, EB2J and EB2C# plug-ins, menus *Translator/EB2C, /EB2C++, /EB2J, /EB2C#* and tool buttons on the toolbar, will appear. To generate a source code in any target language of any formal model, a user can click on any menu (EB2C, EB2C++, EB2J and EB2C#) or a tool button, then a dialog box will appear (see Fig. 7.5). This dialog box presents a list of active projects. A user can select any project for generating a source code. These tools generate a target language code for all concrete models of the selected project and also generate a log file for the code generating process.

7.4.1 *Assessment of the Translation Tool*

Assessment of this translation tool is given through the code generation of verified formal specifications of a cardiac pacemaker (see Chap. 9). We have illustrated the use of EB2C, EB2C++, EB2J and EB2C# tools [17, 24–26] by means of the automatic generation of C, C++, Java and C# codes for the cardiac pacemaker. These codes are automatically generated in C, C++, Java and C# codes from the verified specification in less than five seconds. To find a detail process of code generation from formal specifications in [27].

---

[2]Download: http://eb2all.loria.fr/.

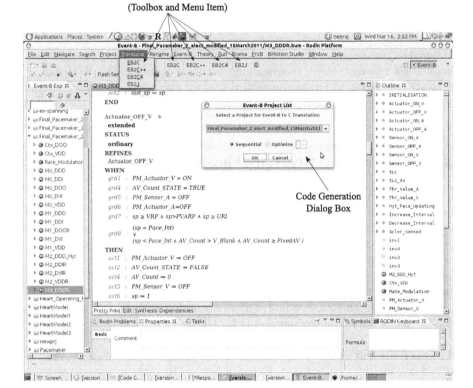

Fig. 7.5   Screen shots of code generation tool

7.5 Limitations

This is our primary version of the code generator from Event-B formal specifications to any programming language (C, C++, Java and C#). In this version of the
code generator can support only that symbols, which are given in Tables 7.2, 7.3 and
7.4. Event-B language is very rich in the area of modelling, and it supports different
kinds of formal notations [2]. All formal notations are not translatable directly into a
programming language. A lot of formal notations are applicable at the abstract level
of modelling, which may be transformed into another formal notation at the concrete level and that can be easily translatable into any programming language. For
instance, relational predicates are usually used for abstract representation, which
can be transformed into array or total function representation, and array and total function both are translatable into current version of this tool. Present time the
translation tools only supports a subset of formal notations, on behalf of modelling
expertise, we believe that these set of Event-B notations are sufficient for modelling
any kind of problems and using these symbols any formal specification can be easily
translatable into any programming language. In this version of the code generator,

the Event-B constructs are not supported except formal notations of Tables 7.2, 7.3 and 7.4. This is our first step toward in the direction of code translation, and it is our ongoing research work. So in future we will provide more and more Event-B symbols, that will be supported by this translation tool.

7.6 Summary

This chapter has introduced the main principles, rules and implementation solutions for the translation tools and code verification techniques for generating the target programming languages (C, C++, Java and C#) code from the Event-B specifications [17, 24–27]. The syntax adopted is restrictive, but it already covers most numeric applications, supports powerful static-analysis methods and generates fast and safe source code in a target programming language. This chapter is to demonstrate an architecture of the translators and their formal verification. Many algorithms (e.g. embedded system, distributed system) are subject to further refinement. The translator provides useful assistance to human programmers by automatically adding comments, generating code for each process, optimising expressions and partitioning event as well as data structures. The translator generates a separate code for all events of concrete modules. Systematic studies on partitioning methods using a refinement structure in target programming languages (C, C++, Java and C#) style is an interesting area of future research. This approach may be applicable to massively parallel processing.

The benefits of developing and enhancing the translation tool presented stem primarily from their increased support for automated translation between the two components of a formal model and a target programming language [17, 24–26]. It has been shown that the Event-B models have been transformed into a deterministic model [35] for automatically translated to the source code using one more level of data refinement. The final concrete model provides sufficient refinement for introducing full determinism and use an easily translatable subset of the notations [9]. The Rodin tool supports the development of the translation tool under the Eclipse framework using all required model information via supported interfaces. The Rodin tool uses an internal database to handle model information, which allows model generation is based on underlying meaning of a model and reduces the syntax dependency.

References

1. Abrial, J.-R. (1996). *The B-book: Assigning programs to meanings*. New York: Cambridge University Press.
2. Abrial, J.-R. (2010). *Modeling in Event-B: System and software engineering* (1st ed.). New York: Cambridge University Press.
3. Arnold, K., Gosling, J., & Holmes, D. (2005). *The Java programming language* (4th ed.). Reading: Addison-Wesley.

4. Back, R. J. R. (1981). On correct refinement of programs. *Journal of Computer and System Sciences, 23*(1), 49–68.
5. Barnes, J. (2003). *High integrity software: The SPARK approach to safety and security.* Boston: Addison-Wesley Longman.
6. Bernardo, M., & Bonta, E. (2004). Generating well-synchronized multithreaded programs from software architecture descriptions. In *Proceedings, Fourth working IEEE/IFIP conference on software architecture*, WICSA 2004 (pp. 167–176).
7. Bernardo, M., & Bontà, E. (2005). Preserving architectural properties in multithreaded code generation. In J.-M. Jacquet & G. Picco (Eds.), *Lecture notes in computer science: Vol. 3454. Coordination models and languages* (pp. 188–203). Berlin: Springer.
8. Bernardo, M., Cleaveland, R., Sims, S., & Stewart, W. (1998). TwoTowers: A tool integrating functional and performance analysis of concurrent systems. In *International conference on formal techniques for networked and distributed systems*, FORTE (pp. 457–467).
9. Bert, D., Boulmé, S., Potet, M.-L., Requet, A., & Voisin, L. (2003). Adaptable translator of B specifications to embedded C programs. In *Lecture notes in computer science: Vol. 2805. International symposium of formal methods Europe* (pp. 94–113).
10. Beyer, D., Henzinger, T., Jhala, R., & Majumdar, R. (2007). The software model checker BLAST, applications to software engineering. *International Journal on Software Tools for Technology Transfer, 9*, 505–525.
11. Bjørner, D., & Jones, C. B. (Eds.) (1978). *The Vienna development method: The meta-language.* London: Springer.
12. Blanc, N., Groce, A., & Kroening, D. (2007). Verifying C++ with STL containers via predicate abstraction. In *Proceedings of the twenty-second IEEE/ACM international conference on automated software engineering*, ASE'07 (pp. 521–524). New York: ACM.
13. Bonta, E., & Bernardo, M. (2009). PADL2Java: A Java code generator for process algebraic architectural descriptions. In *Joint working IEEE/IFIP conference on software architecture, 2009 European conference on software architecture*, WICSA/ECSA 2009 (pp. 161–170).
14. Burns, A., Dobbing, B., & Vardanega, T. (2004). Guide for the use of the Ada Ravenscar profile in high integrity systems. *Ada Letters, XXIV*(2), 1–74.
15. Coleman, D., & Hughes, J. W. (1979). The clean termination of Pascal programs. *Acta Informatica, 11*, 195–210.
16. Cousot, P., Cousot, R., Feret, J., Mauborgne, L., Miné, A., Monniaux, D., et al. (2007). Combination of abstractions in the Astrée static analyzer. In *Lecture notes in computer science. Proceedings of the 11th Asian computing science conference on advances in computer science: Secure software and related issues* (pp. 272–300). Berlin: Springer.
17. EB2ALL (2011). Automatic code generation from Event-B to many programming languages. http://eb2all.loria.fr/.
18. Edmunds, A., & Butler, M. (2010). *Tool support for Event-B code generation.* Presented at WS-TBFM 2010.
19. Edmunds, A., & Butler, M. (2011). *Tasking Event-B: An extension to Event-B for generating concurrent code.* Presented at PLACES 2011.
20. Georg, G., Bieman, J., & France, R. B. (2001). Using alloy and UML/OCL to specify run-time configuration management: A case study. In A. Evans, R. France, A. Moreira, & B. Rumpe (Eds.), *LNI: Vol. P-7. Practical UML-based rigorous development methods—countering or integrating the eXtremists. Workshop of the pUML-group held together with the UML 2001, October 1st, 2001 in Toronto, Canada* (pp. 128–141). German Informatics Society.
21. Gosling, J., Joy, B., Steele, G., & Bracha, G. (2005). *Java(TM) language specification* (3rd ed.). Reading: Addison-Wesley.
22. Kernighan, B. W., & Ritchie, D. M. (1978). *The C programming language.* Upper Saddle River: Prentice Hall. ISBN 0-13-110163-3.
23. Ledgard, H. (1983). *Reference manual for the ADA programming language.* Secaucus: Springer.
24. Méry, D., & Singh, N. K. (2010). *EB2C: A tool for Event-B to C conversion support.* Poster and tool demo submission, published in a CNR technical report in SEFM.

25. Méry, D., & Singh, N. K. (2011). Automatic code generation from Event-B models. In *Proceedings of the second symposium on information and communication technology*, SoICT'11, Hanoi (pp. 179–188). New York: ACM.
26. Méry, D., & Singh, N. K. (2011). *EB2J: Code generation from Event-B to Java*. Short paper presented at the 14th Brazilian symposium on formal methods, SBMF'11.
27. Méry, D., & Singh, N. K. (2012). *Formal development and automatic code generation: Cardiac pacemaker*. New York: ASME Press.
28. Overture. Overture: Formal modelling in VDM. http://www.overturetool.org/.
29. Pearce, D. J., Kelly, P. H. J., & Hankin, C. (2007). Efficient field-sensitive pointer analysis of C. *ACM Transactions on Programming Languages and Systems*, *30*(1), 4.
30. Pohl, C., Paiz, C., & Porrmann, M. (2009). vMAGIC—automatic code generation for VHDL. *International Journal of Reconfigurable Computing*. doi:10.1155/2009/205149.
31. Richter, J. (2006). *CLR via C#* (2nd ed.). Redmond: Microsoft Press.
32. RODIN (2004). Rigorous open development environment for complex systems. http://rodin-b-sharp.sourceforge.net.
33. Rumbaugh, J., Jacobson, I., & Booch, G. (Eds.) (1999). *The unified modeling language reference manual*. Essex: Addison-Wesley Longman.
34. Sebesta, R. W. (2009). *Concepts of programming languages* (9th ed.). Reading: Addison-Wesley.
35. Sites, R. L. (1974). *Clean termination of computer programs*. PhD dissertation, Stanford University, Stanford.
36. Smith, J. E., Kokar, M. K., & Baclawski, K. (2001). Formal verification of UML diagrams: A first step towards code generation. In *Practical UML-based rigorous development methods—countering or integrating the extremists* (pp. 224–240).
37. Stroustrup, B. (1994). *The C++ programming language* (3rd ed.). Reading: Addison-Wesley. ISBN 0-201-88954-4.
38. Wright, S. (2009). *Automatic generation of C from Event-B*. Presented at the workshop on integration of model-based formal methods and tools, IM_FMT'2009, Düsseldorf.

Chapter 8
Formal Logic Based Heart-Model

Abstract A closed-loop model of a system is considered as a *de facto* standard in the area of system engineering for validating a system model. Cardiac pacemakers and implantable cardioverter-defibrillators (ICDs) are the most critical of these medical devices, requiring closed-loop modelling (integrated system and environment modelling) for verification purposes before obtaining a certificate from the certification bodies. This chapter presents a methodology for modelling a biological system, such as the heart, to enable modelling in a biological environment. The heart model is based mainly on electrocardiography analysis, which models the heart system at the cellular level. This heart model will be used for modelling the closed-loop system of a cardiac pacemaker.

8.1 Introduction

The human heart is well known as a mechanical device of amazing efficiency that pumps blood via the circulatory system continuously throughout the person's lifetime. It is one of the most complex and important biological systems, providing oxygen and nutrients to the body to sustain life [30]. The regular impulses generated by the heart result in rhythmic contractions through a sequence of muscles in the heart, beginning at the natural pacemaker known as the sinoatrial (SA) node, which produces an action potential that travels across the atrioventricular (AV) node, the bundle of His and the Purkinje fibres distributed throughout the ventricles. The pattern and the timing of these impulses determine the heart rhythm. Variable time intervals and conduction speeds during the heartbeat generate abnormal heart rhythms, which are also known as heart rhythm impairments. Heart rhythm impairment is the principal source of several diseases. Electrocardiography analysis is frequently used to diagnose various types of heart disease [24] by presenting the timing properties of the electrical system of the heart. These are the most fundamental properties of the heart.

Cardiac pacemakers and ICDs are the two main types among the remarkable range of medical and technological devices recommended by doctors in cases of abnormal heart rhythm. These devices are used to maintain the heart rhythm, and are life-saving in many instances. In the last few years, the use of cardiac pacemakers and cardioverter-defibrillators has increased. However, these devices may sometimes malfunction. Device related problems have been responsible for a large number of serious injuries. Many deaths and injuries caused by device failure have been reported by the FDA [28], which advocates safety and security guidelines for using these devices. FDA officials have found that many deaths and injuries related to the devices are caused by product design and engineering flaws, which can be considered as firmware problems [10, 17].

Providing assurance guarantees for medical devices makes formal approaches appealing. Formal model based methods have been successful in targeted applications of medical devices [9, 20, 21, 25, 31, 32]. Over the past decade, there has been considerable progress in the development of formal methods for improving confidence in complex software-based systems [1, 13, 14]. Although formal methods are part of the standard recommendations for developing and certifying medical systems, the integration of formal methods into the certification process is, in large part, unclear. In particular, it is a very challenging task to ensure that the end product of the software-development system behaves securely.

8.1.1 Motivation

The most challenging problem is environment modelling. That is, to validate and to verify the correct behaviour of a system model requires an interactive formal model of the environment. For example, a formal model of a cardiac pacemaker or ICD requires a heart model to verify the correctness of the developed system (see Fig. 8.1). No tools and techniques are available to provide environment modelling that would enable verification of the developed system model. Medical devices are tightly coupled with their biological environment (i.e., the heart) and use actuators and sensors to interact with the biological environment. Because of this strong relationship between the medical device (e.g., a pacemaker) and the related biological environment (i.e., the heart), it is necessary to model the functioning of the medical device within the biological environment.

The environment model will be independent of the device model, which is helpful in creating an environment for medical devices that simulates the actual behaviour of the system. The medical device model will be dependent on the biological environment. Whenever an undesired state occurs in the biological environment, the device model must act according to the requirements. The main objective is to use a formal approach to modelling the medical device and the biological environment to verify the correctness of the medical system.

To model the biological environment (the heart) for a cardiac pacemaker or ICD, we propose a method for modelling the heart using logico-mathematical theory [33–35]. The heart model is based on electrocardiography analysis [6, 15, 24], which models the heart system at the cellular level [40]. In this investigation, we present a methodology for modelling a heart that involves extracting a set of biological nodes (SA node, AV node, etc.), impulse propagation speeds between nodes, impulse propagation times between nodes and cellular automata (CA) for propagating impulses

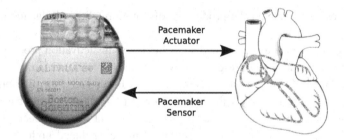

Fig. 8.1 Cardiac pacemaker and heart interaction

at the cellular level. This model is developed through incremental refinement, which introduces several properties in an incremental way and verifies the correctness of the heart model. A key feature of this heart model is the representation of all possible morphological states of the (ECG) [3, 6]. These morphological states represent both the normal and the abnormal states of the ECG. The morphological representation can generate any kind of heart model (a patient's model or a normal heart model) using the ECG. This model can observe both the failure of impulse generation and the failure of impulse propagation. The mathematical heart model, based on logico-mathematical theory, is verified using the RODIN [38] proof tool and the model checker ProB [26]. The model is also verified by electro-physiology and cardiac experts. The main objective of this heart model is to provide a biological environment (the heart) for formalising a closed-loop system (a combined model of a cardiac pacemaker and the heart).

8.1.2 Structure of This Chapter

The outline of the remaining chapter is as follows. Section 8.2 presents related work. A brief outline of the heart system is introduced in Sect. 8.3. Section 8.4 explains the proposed approach. Section 8.5 gives an outline of the formal development of the heart model. Section 8.6 discusses the results of lessons learnt from this experience, and Sect. 8.7 summarises the chapter.

8.2 Related Work

Heart modelling is a challenging problem in the area of real-time simulation for clinical purposes. It is handled by the research community using a variety of different methods. The ECG is an important diagnostic method for measuring the heart's electrical activities, and was invented by Willem Einthoven in 1903 [36]. In this study, the ECG is used in modelling the heart [36]. At the present time, technological advances have enabled the production of a high-quality cellular model of an entire heart.

K.R. Jun et al. [37] have produced a CA model of the activation process in ventricular muscle tissue. They presented a two-dimensional (2D) CA model that accounts for the local orientation of the myocardial fibres and their distributed velocity and refractory period. A three-dimensional (3D) finite-volume-based computer mesh model of human atrial activation and current flow has been presented by Harrild et al. [15]. This cellular-level-based model included both the left and right atria and the major muscle bundles of the atria. The results of using this model demonstrate a normal sinus rhythm and can extract the patterns of the septum's activation. Because of memory and time complexity in the computation of a 3D model, an empirical approach is used in modelling the whole heart. The empirical approach implies a simpler representation of the complex process at a cellular level. In this new approach, researchers have adopted some approximations in modelling the whole heart without compromising the actual behaviour of the heart. Berenfeld et al. [8] have developed a model that can give insight into the local and global complex dynamics of the heart in the transition from normal to abnormal myocardial activity, which helps to estimate myocardial properties. Adam [2] has analysed wave activities during depolarisation in his cardiac model, which is represented by a simplification of the heart tissue.

Recently, a real-time Virtual Heart Model (VHM) has been developed by Jiang et al. [22] to model the electro-physiological operation of proper functioning and malfunctioning. They used a time-automaton model to define the timing properties of the heart. Simulink Design Verifier[1] was used as the main tool for designing the VHM. A heart model based on Uppaal Model checker [7] is developed by Jee et al. [19] for developing the cardiac pacemaker model. This is a very simple heart model, which provides an environment to simulate and verify the pacemaker software in modelling phase.

Our approach is based purely on formal techniques for modelling the heart using electrocardiography analysis. To model the heart for a cardiac pacemaker or ICD, we propose a method based on logico-mathematical theory, which can be implemented using any formal-methods-based tools (Z, TLA$^+$, VDM, etc.). In this chapter, the model is developed using a maximal refinement approach at the cellular level. The incremental refinement approach helps both to introduce several properties in an incremental way and to verify the correctness of the heart model [33–35]. The key feature of this heart model is the representation of all possible morphological states of the ECG, which is used to represent both normal and abnormal states through observation of the failure of impulse generation and the failure of impulse propagation in the heart [3, 6, 24, 30].

---

[1] http://www.mathworks.com/products/sldesignverifier/.

8.3 Background

8.3.1 The Heart System

The human heart is wondrous in its ability to pump blood to the circulatory system continuously throughout a lifetime. The heart comprises four chambers: right atrium, right ventricle, left atrium and left ventricle, each of which contract and relax periodically. The atria form one unit and the ventricles another. The heart's mechanical system (the pump) requires impulses from its electrical system to function. An electrical stimulus is generated by the sinus node (see Fig. 8.2), which is a small mass of specialised tissue located in the right atrium of the heart. The electrical stimulus travels down through the conduction pathways and causes the heart's lower chambers to contract and pump out the blood. The right and left atria are stimulated first and contract for a short period of time before the right and left ventricles. Each contraction of the ventricles represents one heartbeat. The atria contract for a fraction of a second before the ventricles, so their blood empties into the ventricles before the ventricles contract.

Arrhythmias are caused by cardiac problems that produce abnormal heart rhythms. In general, arrhythmias reduce haemodynamic performance, including situations where the heart develops an abnormal rate or rhythm or when normal conduction pathways are interrupted, and a different part of the heart takes over control of the rhythm. An arrhythmia can involve an abnormal rhythm increase (tachycardia: > 100 bpm) or decrease (bradycardia: < 60 bpm), or it may be characterised by an irregular cardiac rhythm, such as that caused by asynchrony of the cardiac chambers. Irregularities in the heartbeat are called bradycardia and tachycardia. Bradycardia indicates that the heart rate falls below the expected level whereas tachycardia indicates that the heart rate goes above the expected heart rate. An artificial pacemaker can restore synchrony between the atria and the ventricles [5, 12, 16, 25, 27, 30]. Beats per minute (bpm) is the basic unit used to measure the rate of heart activity.

8.3.2 Basic Overview of Electrocardiogram (ECG)

The ECG (or EKG) [16, 24] is a diagnostic tool that measures and records precisely the electrical activity of the heart in the form of signals. Clinicians can evaluate the conditions of a patient's heart from the ECG and perform further diagnosis. Analysis of these signals can be used to diagnose a wide range of heart conditions and to predict the related diseases. ECG records are obtained by sampling the bioelectric currents sensed by several electrodes, known as leads. A normal ECG is depicted in Fig. 8.3. Electrocardiogram term is introduced by Willem Einthoven in 1893 at a meeting of the Dutch Medical Society. In 1924, Einthoven received the Nobel Prize for his life's work in developing the ECG [5, 24, 27, 30].

Fig. 8.2 Heart or natural
pacemaker

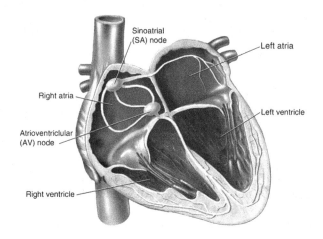

All the segments and intervals used by clinicians are represented in this ECG diagram. Depolarisation and repolarisation of the ventricular and atrial chambers are presented by deflection in the ECG signal. These deflections are labelled in alphabetic order: P-QRS-T. Letter P indicates atrial depolarisation, and the ventricular depolarisation is represented by the QRS complex. The ventricular repolarisation is represented by T-wave. Atrial repolarisation appears during the QRS complex and generates a very low amplitude signal which cannot be uncovered from the normal ECG signal.

8.3.3 ECG Morphology

Sequential activation, depolarisation, and repolarisation are distinct deflections in the ECG, caused by anatomical differences between the atria and the ventricles. The sequences are even distinguishable when they are not in the correct sequence (P-QRS-T). Each beat of the heart can be observed as a series of deflections, which reflects the time evolution of electrical activity in the heart [3, 6, 24]. A single cycle of the ECG is considered as one heartbeat. The ECG may be divided into the following sections.

- *P-wave:* A small low-voltage deflection caused by the depolarisation of the atria prior to atrial contraction as the activation (depolarisation) wave front propagates from the SA node through the atria.
- *PQ-interval:* The time between the beginning of atrial depolarisation and the beginning of ventricular depolarisation.
- *QRS-complex:* The QRS-complex is easily identifiable between the P- and T-waves because it has a characteristic waveform and dominating amplitude. The dominating amplitude is caused by currents generated when the ventricles depolarise prior to their contraction. Although atrial repolarisation occurs before ven-

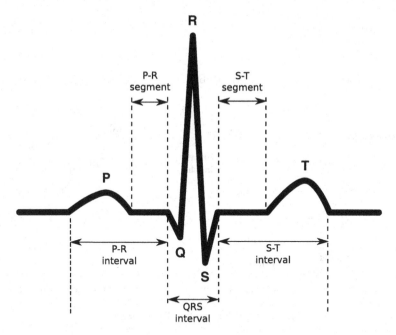

Fig. 8.3 A typical one-cycle ECG tracing

tricular depolarisation, the latter waveform (i.e., the QRS-complex) is of much greater amplitude, and atrial repolarisation is therefore not seen on the ECG.

- *QT-interval:* The time between the onset of ventricular depolarisation and the end of ventricular repolarisation. Clinical studies have demonstrated that the QT interval increases linearly as the RR-interval increases. A prolonged QT-interval may be associated with delayed ventricular repolarisation, which may cause ventricular tachyarrhythmias leading to sudden cardiac death.
- *ST-interval:* The time between the end of the S-wave and the beginning of the T-wave. Significantly elevated or depressed amplitudes away from the baseline are often associated with cardiac illness.
- *T-wave:* Ventricular repolarisation, whereby the cardiac muscle is prepared for the next cycle of the ECG.

8.4 Proposed Idea

Our proposed method exploits a heart model based on logico-mathematics to help the formal methods community to verify the correctness of a developed model of medical devices such as cardiac pacemakers. The heart model is based mainly on the impulse propagation time and conduction speed at a cellular level [33–35]. This method uses the advanced capabilities of a combined approach of formal verification

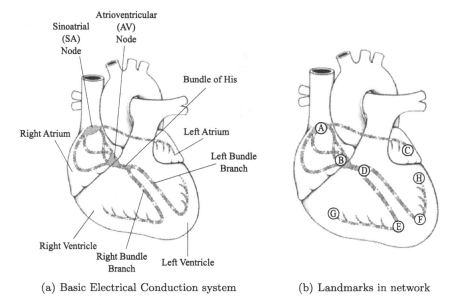

(a) Basic Electrical Conduction system   (b) Landmarks in network

Fig. 8.4 The electrical conduction and landmarks of the heart system

and model validation using a model checker to achieve considerable advantages in heart system modelling.

Figure 8.4(a) shows the more significant components and the impulse conduction path in the entire heart system. The heart is a muscle with a special electrical conduction system. The system comprises two nodes (special conduction cells) and a series of conduction fibres or bundles (pathways). For modelling the heart system, we have assumed eight landmark nodes (A, B, C, D, E, F, G, H) in the whole conduction network, as shown in Fig. 8.4(b), which control the whole heart system. These landmarks were identified via a literature survey [24, 30] and extensive discussions with a cardiologist and a physiologist. Centimetres per second (cm/sec) is a basic unit to measure the conduction speed and milliseconds (ms) is a basic unit to measure the conduction time.

We now introduce the necessary elements we use to define the heart system formally.

Definition 1 (The heart system) Given a set of nodes N, a transition (conduction) t is a pair (i, j), with $i, j \in N$. A transition is denoted by $i \rightsquigarrow j$. The heart system is a tuple $\text{HSys} = (N, T, N_0, TW_{time}, CW_{speed})$ where:

- $N = \{\text{A}, \text{B}, \text{C}, \text{D}, \text{E}, \text{F}, \text{G}, \text{H}\}$ is a finite set of landmark nodes in the conduction pathways of the heart system;
- $T \subseteq N \times N = \{\text{A} \mapsto \text{B}, \text{A} \mapsto \text{C}, \text{B} \mapsto \text{D}, \text{D} \mapsto \text{E}, \text{D} \mapsto \text{F}, \text{E} \mapsto \text{G}, \text{F} \mapsto \text{H}\}$ is a set of transitions to represent electrical impulse propagation between two landmark nodes;
- $N_0 = \text{A}$ is the initial landmark node (SA node);

- $TW_{time} \in N \rightarrow$ TIME is a weight function for the time delay of each node, where TIME is a range of time delays;
- $CW_{speed} \in T \rightarrow$ SPEED is a weight function for the impulse propagation speed of each transition, where SPEED is a range of propagation speeds.

Property 1 (Impulse propagation time) In the heart system, the electrical impulse originates from SA node (node A), travels through the entire conduction network and terminates at the atrial muscle fibres (node C) and at the end of Purkinje fibres in both sides of the ventricular chambers (node G and node H). The impulse propagation time delay differs for each landmark node (N). The impulse propagation time is represented as the total function $TW_{time} \in N \rightarrow \mathbb{P}(0..230)$. The impulse propagation time delay for each node (N) is represented as: $TW_{time}(A) = 0..10$, $TW_{time}(B) = 50..70$, $TW_{time}(C) = 70..90$, $TW_{time}(D) = 125..160$, $TW_{time}(E) = 145..180$, $TW_{time}(F) = 145..180$, $TW_{time}(G) = 150..210$ and $TW_{time}(H) = 150..230$.

Property 2 (Impulse propagation speed) The impulse propagation speed also differs for each transition ($i \rightsquigarrow j$, where $i, j \in N$). The impulse propagation speed is represented as the total function $CW_{speed} \in T \rightarrow \mathbb{P}(5..400)$. The impulse propagation speed for each transition is represented as: $CW_{speed}(A \mapsto B) = 30..50$, $CW_{speed}(A \mapsto C) = 30..50$, $CW_{speed}(B \mapsto D) = 100..200$, $CW_{speed}(D \mapsto E) = 100..200$, $CW_{speed}(E \mapsto G) = 300..400$ and $CW_{speed}(F \mapsto H) = 300..400$.

Electrical activity is spontaneously generated by the SA node, located high in the right atrium, shown as node A in Fig. 8.5(a). The SA node is the physiological pacemaker of the normal heart, responsible for setting its rate and rhythm. The electrical impulse spreads through the walls of the atria, causing them to contract. The conduction of the electrical impulse throughout the left and right atria is seen on the ECG as the P-wave (see Fig. 8.3). From the sinus node, the electrical impulse propagates throughout the atria and reaches nodes B and C, but cannot propagate directly across the boundary between the atria and ventricles. The electrical impulse travels outward into the atrial muscle fibres and reaches the end of the fibres, shown as node C in the conduction network (see Fig. 8.5(b)).

Normally, the only pathway available for the electrical impulse is to enter the ventricles through a specialised region of cells called the AV node. The AV node is located at the boundary between the atria and ventricles, shown as node B in Fig. 8.4(b). The AV node provides the only conducting path from the atria to the ventricles. The AV node functions as a critical delay in the conduction system. Without this delay, the atria and ventricles would contract at the same time, and blood would not flow effectively from the atria to the ventricles. The delay in the AV node forms much of the PR segment on the ECG. Part of the atrial repolarisation can be represented by the PR segment (see Fig. 8.3).

Propagation from the AV node (A) to the ventricles is provided by a specialised conduction system. The distal portion of the AV node is composed of a common bundle called the Bundle of His, shown as landmark node D in Fig. 8.4(b). The

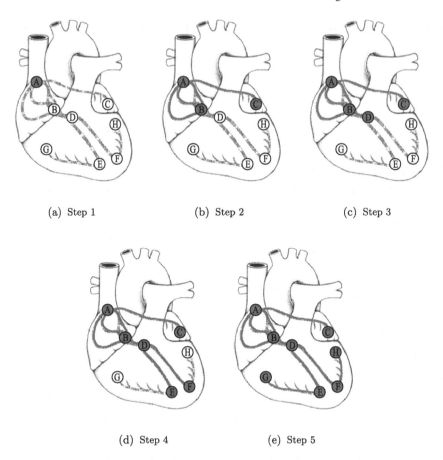

(a) Step 1   (b) Step 2   (c) Step 3

(d) Step 4   (e) Step 5

Fig. 8.5 Impulse propagation through landmarks of the heart system

Bundle of His splits into two branches in the inter-ventricular septum, namely the left bundle branch and the right bundle branch. The electrical impulses then enter the base of the ventricle at the Bundle of His (node D) and follow the left and right bundle branches along the inter-ventricular septum (see Fig. 8.5(c)).

The two separate bundle branches propagating along each side of the septum constitute the left and right bundle branches.We have identified two landmark nodes E and F (see Fig. 8.4(b)) in the lower part of the heart for the left and right bundle branches. These specialised fibres conduct the impulses at a very rapid velocity (see Tables 8.1 and 8.2). The left bundle branch activates the left ventricle, whereas the right bundle branch activates the right ventricle (see Fig. 8.5(d)).

The bundle branches then divide into an extensive system of Purkinje fibres that conduct the impulses at high velocity (see Tables 8.1 and 8.2) throughout the ventricles. The Purkinje fibres stimulate individual groups of myocardial cells to contract. We have identified two final landmark nodes G and H (see Fig. 8.4(b)) at the end of the Purkinje fibres in both sides of the ventricles. These two nodes represent the end

Table 8.1 Cardiac activation time in the heart

Location in the heart	Cardiac activation time (ms)
SA node (A)	0..10
Left atria muscle fibres (C)	70..90
AV node (B)	50..70
Bundle of His (D)	125..160
Right bundle branch (E)	145..180
Left bundle branch (F)	145..180
Right Purkinje fibres (G)	150..210
Left Purkinje fibres (H)	150..230

Table 8.2 Cardiac activation velocity in the heart

Location in the heart	Conduction velocity (cm/sec)
A $\mapsto$ B	30..50
A $\mapsto$ C	30..50
B $\mapsto$ D	100..200
D $\mapsto$ E	100..200
D $\mapsto$ F	100..200
E $\mapsto$ G	300..400
F $\mapsto$ H	300..400

of the conduction network in the heart system. The bundles branch into the Purkinje fibres that diverge across the inner sides of the ventricular walls (see Fig. 8.5(e)). On reaching the end of the Purkinje fibres, the electrical impulse is transmitted through the ventricular muscle mass by the ventricular muscle fibres themselves. Propagation along the conduction system takes place at a relatively high speed once it is within the ventricular region, but prior to this (through the AV node), the velocity is extremely slow [24, 30].

The electrical system provides a synchronised system from atria to ventricles, which aids the contraction of the heart muscle and optimises the haemodynamics. Changed time intervals or conducting speeds between landmarks (see Fig. 8.4(b) and Fig. 8.6) are a major cause of abnormalities in the heart system. Abnormalities in electrical signals in the heart can generate various kinds of arrhythmias. A slow conduction speed generates bradycardia and a fast conduction speed generates tachycardia. In this model, we consider the ranges of all possible values for conduction speeds and conduction times for each landmark node and conduction path. This model represents the morphological structure of the ECG signal through the conduction network (see Fig. 8.6).

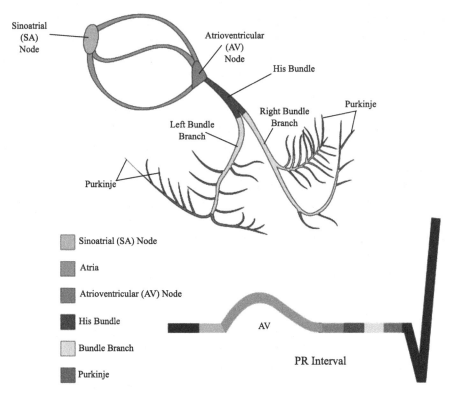

Fig. 8.6 Time intervals and impulse propagation in the ECG signal (adapted from [30])

8.4.1 Heart Block

In this section, we explain the basic heart blocks in the heart conduction system. We have formalised these basic heart blocks in the proposed methodology. Heart block is the term given to a disorder of conduction of the impulse that stimulates heart muscle contraction. The normal cardiac impulse arises in the SA node (A), situated in the right atrium, and spreads to the AV node (B), whence it is conducted by specialised tissue known as the Bundle of His (D), which divides into the left and right bundle branches in the ventricles (see Fig. 8.4(a)). Disturbances in conduction may appear as slow conduction, intermittent conduction failure or complete conduction failure. These three kinds of conduction failure are also known as 1st, 2nd and 3rd degree blocks. We can show these different kinds of heart block throughout the conduction network in terms of our set of landmark nodes (see Fig. 8.7).

SA Block

This block occurs within the SA node (A) and is described as an SA nodal block or sick sinus syndrome. The SA node fails to originate an impulse, and the heart misses one or two beats at regular or irregular intervals (see Fig. 8.7(a)).

AV Block

For an AV block, the sinus rhythm is normal, but there is a conduction defect between the atria and the ventricles. The main cause of this block may be in the AV node (B) or the Bundle of His (D), or both (see Fig. 8.7(b)).

Infra-Hisian Block

Blocks that occur below the AV node (B) are known as Infra-Hisian blocks (see Fig. 8.7(c)). This block describes block of the distal conduction system and it includes Type 2 second degree heart block.

Left Bundle Branch Block

In the normal heart, activation of both ventricles takes place simultaneously. A left bundle branch block occurs when conduction into the left branch of the Bundle of His is interrupted. Blocks that occur within the fascicles of the left bundle branch are known as hemiblocks (see Fig. 8.7(d)).

Right Bundle Branch Block

A right bundle branch block occurs when conduction into the right branch of the Bundle of His is interrupted (see Fig. 8.7(e)).

8.4.2 Cellular Automata Model

A set of spatially distributed cells form a CA model, which contains a uniform connection pattern among neighbouring cells and local computation laws. CA were originally proposed by Ulam and von Neumann [40] in the 1940s to provide a formal framework for investigating the behaviour of complex, spatially distributed systems. CA are discrete dynamic systems corresponding to space and time. CA modelling involves uniform properties for state transitions and interconnection patterns. The model components are specified by a single property caused by the same patterns

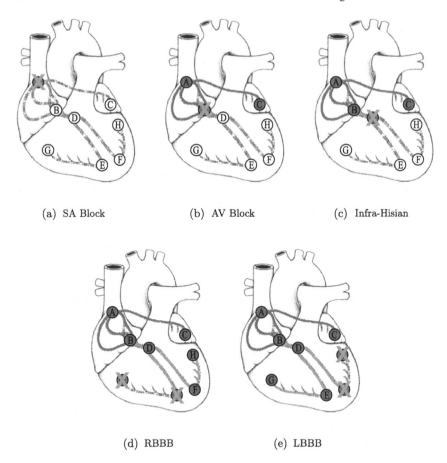

(a) SA Block   (b) AV Block   (c) Infra-Hisian

(d) RBBB   (e) LBBB

Fig. 8.7 Impairments in impulse propagation due to the heart blocks

instead of specifying each component separately. CA models help to visualise a system's dynamics [15, 29, 30, 39]. A CA model can have an infinite number of cells along any dimension. Here, we consider a finite number of cells in two dimensions, as shown in Fig. 8.8. A 2D CA model is defined as:

Definition 2 (The CA model)

$$(CA) = \langle S, N, T \rangle: \text{discrete time system}$$

S: the set of states

N: the neighbouring patterns at $(0, 0)$

T: the transition function

Fig. 8.8 A two-dimensional cellular automata model

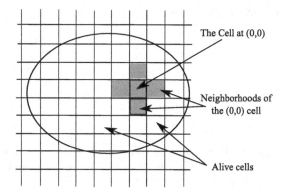

The Cell at (0,0)

Neighborhoods of the (0,0) cell

Alive cells

In the usual case of CA realised on a D-dimensional grid, N consists of D-tuples of indices from a coordinate set:

$$I: N \subseteq I^D$$

The 2D cellular model therefore becomes

$$N \subseteq I^2$$
$$T : S^{|N|} \to S$$

To consider an automaton specified as a CA, let λ and α be the global state and the global transition function of the CA, respectively. Then, $\lambda = \{\tau | \tau : I^2 \to S\}$ and $\alpha(\lambda(i, j)) = T(\tau | N + (i, j))$ for all τ in λ and (i, j) in I^2.

Definition 3 (State transition of a cell) The heart muscle system is composed of heterogeneous cells, the CA model of the muscle system, CAM_{CA}, is characterised by having no dependency on the type of cells. CAM_{CA} is defined as follows:

$$CAM_{CA} = \langle S, N, T \rangle$$
$$S = \{Active, Passive, Refractory\}$$
$$N = \{(0, 0), (1, 0), (-1, 0), (0, 1), (0, -1)\}$$
$$s'_{m,n} = s_{m,n}(t + 1)$$
$$s'_{m,n} = T(s_{m,n}, s_{m+1,n}, s_{m-1,n}, s_{m,n+1}, s_{m,n-1})$$

where, $s_{m,n}$ denotes the state of the cell located at (m, n) and T is a transition function for CAM_{CA} that specifies the next state, as shown in Fig. 8.9.

Each cell in the heart muscle should be in one of the states *Active*, *Passive* or *Refractory*. Initially, all cells are *Passive*. In this state, the cell is discharged electrically and has no influence on its neighbouring cells. When an electrical impulse propagates, the cell becomes charged and eventually activated (*Active* state). The cell then transmits an electrical impulse to its neighbour cells. The electrical impulse is propagated to all the cells in the heart muscle. After activation, the cell

Fig. 8.9 State transition of
a cell

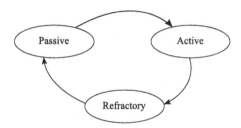

becomes discharged and enters the *Refractory* state within which the cell cannot be
reactivated. After a time, the cell changes its state to the *Passive* state to await the
next impulse.

8.5 Functional Formal Modelling of the Heart

To formalise the heart model, we have used the Event-B modelling language [1, 38],
although the proposed idea can be formalised using any kind of formal-methods
tool such as Z, ASM, TLA$^+$ or VDM. Event-B modelling language supports the
refinement approach [4] that helps to verify the correctness of the system in an
incremental way.

The heart model development is expressed in an abstract and general way. The
initial model formalises the system requirements and environmental assumptions,
whereas the subsequent models introduce design decisions for the resulting system.
Following summary informations present global view of the heart system development, which help to understand the whole modelling approach.

Initial model: This is an observation model, which specifies a heart state in the form
    of *true* and *false*, where *true* represents a normal rhythm and *false* represents an
    abnormal rhythm of the heart.
Refinement 1: This is a conduction model of the heart, which specifies beginning
    of the impulse propagation at SA node and ending of the impulse propagation at
    Purkinje fibres in both left and right ventricles.
Refinement 2: This model specifies impulse propagation between landmark nodes
    with global clock counter to model a real-time system to satisfy the temporal
    properties of impulse propagation.
Refinement 3: This is a perturbation model of the heart, which specifies perturbation
    in the heart conduction system and helps to discover exact block into the heart
    conduction system.
Refinement 4: This is a simulation model of the heart, which introduces impulse
    propagation at the cellular level using cellular automata.

8.5.1 *The Context and Initial Model*

Event-B models are described in terms of two major components: *context* and *machine*. The context contains the static part of the model, whereas the machine con-

tains the dynamic part. The context uses sets and constants to define axioms and theorems. Axioms and theorems represent the logical theory of the elements of a system. The logical theory lists the static properties of constants related to the system and provides an axiomatisation of the system environment. The context can be extended by other contexts and referenced by a set of machines, while a machine can be refined by other machines.

We need to choose electrical features for modelling the heart system. To model the heart system, we identify a set of electrical impulse propagation nodes *ConductionNode* of the heart conduction network (see Fig. 8.4(a)). These nodes are basic landmarks, which enable expression of the normal and abnormal behaviour of the heart system. These landmarks were identified through a literature survey [24, 30] and fruitful discussions with a cardiologist and a physiologist. Three constants define the impulse propagation time, namely *ConductionTime*, impulse propagation path *ConductionPath* and impulse propagation velocity *ConductionSpeed*. Static properties are defined in the context model to specify the electrical impulse propagation network of the heart system, the impulse propagation time for each landmark node and the impulse propagation speed for every path. Paths are represented by a set of pairs of landmark nodes (see Definition 1, Properties 1 and 2 and Tables 8.1 and 8.2).

$$axm1 : partition(ConductionNode, \{A\}, \{B\}, \{C\}, \{D\}, \{E\}, \{F\}, \{G\}, \{H\})$$
$$axm2 : ConductionTime \in ConductionNode \rightarrow \mathbb{P}(0..230)$$
$$axm3 : ConductionPath \subseteq ConductionNode \times ConductionNode$$
$$axm4 : ConductionSpeed \in ConductionPath \rightarrow \mathbb{P}(5..400)$$

As you see axioms are extracted from the definitions and are validated by cardiologist and physiologist.

8.5.2 Abstract Model

We define an abstract model for indicating the heart state according to the observation impulse propagation on the conduction nodes. The machine model represents a dynamic behaviour of the heart system through the step-wise impulse propagation into the atria and ventricular chambers. To define the dynamic properties, we have introduced four variables *ConductionNodeState*, *CConductionTime*, *CConductionSpeed* and *HeartState* in invariants. The variable *ConductionNodeState* is defined as a function, which shows boolean states of the landmark nodes. When the electrical impulse passes through the landmark nodes (see Fig. 8.4(b)), then the visited nodes become *TRUE* and the unvisited landmark nodes are represented by *FALSE*. The variables *CConductionTime* and *CConductionSpeed* represent current impulse propagation time and velocity in the conduction network. The last variable *HeartState* represents a boolean state *TRUE* or *FALSE*. *TRUE* represents the normal condition of the heart while *FALSE* represents an abnormal condition of the heart.

$inv1 : ConductionNodeState \in ConductionNode \rightarrow BOOL$
$inv2 : CConductionTime \in ConductionNode \rightarrow 0..300$
$inv3 : CConductionSpeed \in ConductionPath \rightarrow 0..500$
$inv4 : HeartState \in BOOL$

In the abstract specification of the heart model, there are three events, namely *HeartOK* to represent a normal state of the heart, *HeartKO* to express abnormal state of the heart and *HeartConduction* to update the value of each landmark node of the conduction network in terms of visited landmark nodes (*ConductionNodeState*), impulse propagation intervals (*CConductionTime*) and impulse propagation velocities (*CConductionSpeed*).

The event *HeartOK* specifies a set of required conditions for a normal state of the heart system. The first guard *grd*1 states that all landmark nodes should be visited in a single cycle of impulse propagation. The second guard states that the current impulse propagation time of each landmark node should lie within the pre-specified range of the impulse propagation times. The final guard states that the current impulse propagation velocity of each path should lie between pre-defined impulse propagation velocities. If all guards are satisfied then the heart state indicates the normal condition as being *TRUE*.

EVENT HeartOK
   WHEN
      grd1 : $\forall i \cdot i \in ConductionNode \Rightarrow ConductionNodeState(i) = TRUE$
      grd2 : $\forall i \cdot i \in ConductionNode \Rightarrow$
            $CConductionTime(i) \in ConductionTime(i)$
      grd3 : $\forall i, j \cdot i \mapsto j \in ConductionPath \Rightarrow$
            $CConductionSpeed(i \mapsto j) \in ConductionSpeed(i \mapsto j)$
   THEN
      act1 : $HeartState := TRUE$
   END

The event *HeartKO* specifies as an opposite set of guards to those for the normal state of the heart system to specify abnormal conditions of the heart. These guards state that if any landmark node is not visited in a single cycle of the impulse propagation, or if any the current impulse propagation time of any landmark node does not lie within the pre-specified range of the impulse propagation times, or if the current impulse propagation velocity of any path does not lie within the pre-defined range of impulse propagation velocities, then the heart system is in an abnormal state represents by its normal condition being *FALSE*. Different kinds of heart diseases affect the electrical impulse propagation time and velocity in the heart system [24]. These changes affect the actual heart rhythm and help to identify the possible abnormal behaviours of the heart.

```
EVENT HeartKO
  WHEN
    grd1 : ∃i · i ∈ ConductionNode ∧ ConductionNodeState(i) = FALSE)
               ∨
            (∃j · j ∈ ConductionNode ∧
            CConductionTime(j) ∉ ConductionTime(j))
               ∨
            (∃m, n · m ↦ n ∈ ConductionPath ∧ CConductionSpeed(m ↦ n)
            ∉ ConductionSpeed(m ↦ n))
  THEN
    act1 : HeartState := FALSE
  END
```

The event *HeartConduction* formalises the heart behaviour in an abstract manner by updating the values for impulse propagation time, impulse propagation velocity and visited state of the landmark nodes non-deterministically. This event is used to model more concrete behaviour of the heart system at the next level of refinement.

```
EVENT HeartConduction
  BEGIN
    act1 : ConductionNodeState :∈ ConductionNode → BOOL
    act2 : CConductionTime :∈ ConductionNode → 0 .. 300
    act3 : CConductionSpeed :∈ ConductionPath → 0 .. 500
    act4 : HeartState :∈ BOOL
  END
```

8.5.3 Refinement 1: Introducing Steps in the Propagation

In the abstract model, we have presented that the impulse propagation time, velocity and visited landmark nodes have been updated in an atomic step when electrical impulse fire from the sinus (SA) node and moves towards the Purkinje fibres into ventricles (G, H nodes) and in the left atria muscle fibres (C node). Our main objective is to model step by step impulse propagation through all landmark nodes, where the electrical impulse must pass through a number of intermediate landmark nodes before reaching to the terminal nodes (C, G, H). This refinement is a very simple refinement, where we introduce two extra events *SinusNodeFire* and *HeartConductionEnd* as the refinement of the event *HeartConduction*. The event *SinusNodeFire* models the behaviour of a sinoatrial (SA) node, which originates electrical impulse for traversing throughout the heart system using the conduction network (see Fig. 8.4). The guards of this event state that if all landmark nodes are unvisited (means FALSE state) and current impulse propagation time of each node is 0, and impulse propagation velocity of each path is 0, then the conduction node state *ConductionNodeState* of a landmark node A (SA node) sets TRUE and current impulse propagation time of SA node (A) sets to 0.

EVENT SinusNodeFire Refines HeartConduction
  WHEN
    grd1 : $\forall n \cdot n \in ConductionNode \Rightarrow ConductionNodeState(n) = FALSE$
    grd2 : $\forall n \cdot n \in ConductionNode \Rightarrow CConductionTime(n) = 0$
    grd3 : $\forall n, m \cdot n \in ConductionNode \land m \in ConductionNode \land$
             $n \mapsto m \in ConductionPath \Rightarrow CConductionSpeed(n \mapsto m) = 0$
  THEN
    act1 : $ConductionNodeState(A) := TRUE$
    act2 : $CConductionTime(A) := 0$
  END

The next event *HeartConductionEnd* represents end state of the impulse propagation into Purkinje fibres of ventricles (G, H nodes) and left atria muscle (node C). This event resets all variables for generating next impulse at the SA node. The actions of this event reset all conduction node state as *FALSE*, current impulse propagation time of all landmark nodes reset to 0, current impulse propagation velocity of all landmark nodes reset to 0, and the heart state sets as *FALSE*. All these actions are required before originating the next electrical impulse from the SA node (A).

EVENT HeartConductionEnd Refines HeartConduction
  BEGIN
    act1 : $ConductionNodeState := \{A \mapsto FALSE, B \mapsto FALSE,$
         $C \mapsto FALSE, D \mapsto FALSE, E \mapsto FALSE, F \mapsto FALSE,$
         $G \mapsto FALSE, H \mapsto FALSE\}$
    act2 : $CConductionTime := \{A \mapsto 0, B \mapsto 0, C \mapsto 0, D \mapsto 0,$
         $E \mapsto 0, F \mapsto 0, G \mapsto 0, H \mapsto 0\}$
    act3 : $CConductionSpeed := \{A \mapsto B \mapsto 0, A \mapsto C \mapsto 0, B \mapsto D \mapsto 0,$
         $D \mapsto E \mapsto 0, D \mapsto F \mapsto 0, E \mapsto G \mapsto 0, F \mapsto H \mapsto 0\}$
    act4 : $HeartState := FALSE$
  END

8.5.4 Refinement 2: Impulse Propagation

In the second refinement, we introduce several events as a refinement of the event *HeartConduction* to model the impulse propagation into the heart conduction network. New events formalise impulse flow between two landmark nodes separately; for instance, electrical impulse moves from SA node (A) to AV node (B). This level of refinement introduces seven events for modelling the whole conduction path from originating nodes (A) to the ending nodes (C, G, H). A variable *CCSpeed_CCTime_Flag* is introduced as a boolean type to capture the value of current impulse propagation time and current impulse propagation velocity. A new variable *Cycle_Length* declares a time interval for the single heart beat, which may change in every cycle of an electrocardiogram (ECG). This refinement also introduces a logical clock to synchronise all states of the heart system and checks the heart states under a required time length in the conduction network. A new variable *tic* is defined as current *clock counter*. Invariants (*inv4–inv10*) are introduced as safety properties, which define that if the heart state is *TRUE* then the impulse propagation time and the impulse propagation velocity be within the standard range of time and velocity during the impulse conduction throughout the conduction network (see Fig. 8.4(b)).

$inv1 : CCSpeed\_CCTime\_Flag \in BOOL$
$inv2 : Cycle\_Length \in 500..2000$
$inv3 : tic \in \mathbb{N}$

$inv4 : HeartState = TRUE \Rightarrow CConductionTime(B) \in ConductionTime(B)$
$\quad \wedge CConductionSpeed(A \mapsto B) \in ConductionSpeed(A \mapsto B)$
$inv5 : HeartState = TRUE \Rightarrow CConductionTime(C) \in ConductionTime(C)$
$\quad \wedge CConductionSpeed(A \mapsto C) \in ConductionSpeed(A \mapsto C)$
$inv6 : HeartState = TRUE \Rightarrow CConductionTime(D) \in ConductionTime(D)$
$\quad \wedge CConductionSpeed(B \mapsto D) \in ConductionSpeed(B \mapsto D)$
$inv7 : HeartState = TRUE \Rightarrow CConductionTime(E) \in ConductionTime(E)$
$\quad \wedge CConductionSpeed(D \mapsto E) \in ConductionSpeed(D \mapsto E)$
$inv8 : HeartState = TRUE \Rightarrow CConductionTime(F) \in ConductionTime(F)$
$\quad \wedge CConductionSpeed(D \mapsto F) \in ConductionSpeed(D \mapsto F)$
$inv9 : HeartState = TRUE \Rightarrow CConductionTime(G) \in ConductionTime(G)$
$\quad \wedge CConductionSpeed(E \mapsto G) \in ConductionSpeed(E \mapsto G)$
$inv10 : HeartState = TRUE \Rightarrow CConductionTime(H) \in ConductionTime(H)$
$\quad \wedge CConductionSpeed(F \mapsto H) \in ConductionSpeed(F \mapsto H)$

Events are introduced in this refinement to model the impulse propagation from SA node towards the Purkinje fibres landmark nodes (G, H) and atria fibres nodes (C). Each event is synchronised through progressive electrical impulse propagation in the conduction network. We have given formalisation of only one event *HeartConduction_A_B* to understand the basic formalisation steps of all other events. All other events of impulse propagation in the conduction network among landmark nodes have been modelled in a similar fashion.

EVENT HeartConduction_A_B Refines HeartConduction
  WHEN
    $grd1 : ConductionNodeState(A) = TRUE$
    $grd2 : ConductionNodeState(B) = FALSE$
    $grd3 : CConductionTime(B) \in ConductionTime(B)$
    $grd4 : CConductionSpeed(A \mapsto B) \in ConductionSpeed(A \mapsto B)$
    $grd5 : CCSpeed\_CCTime\_Flag = FALSE$
  THEN
    $act1 : ConductionNodeState(B) := TRUE$
    $act2 : CCSpeed\_CCTime\_Flag := TRUE$
  END

A new event *Update_CCSpeed_CCtime* is a refinement of the event *HeartConduction*. This event is used to capture the current electrical impulse propagation time *CConductionTime* and the current electrical impulse propagation speed *CC-conductionSpeed* during a progressive conduction flow into the heart system in the conduction network.

EVENT Update_CCSpeed_CCtime Refines HeartConduction
  ANY   *i, j, CSpeed, CTime*
  WHERE
    grd1 : $i \in ConductionNode$
    grd2 : $j \in ConductionNode$
    grd3 : $i \mapsto j \in ConductionPath$
    grd4 : $CSpeed \in 0 .. 500$
    grd5 : $CTime \in 0 .. 300$
    grd6 : $CCSpeed\_CCTime\_Flag = TRUE$
    grd7 : $HeartState = FALSE$
    grd8 : $tic = CTime$
  THEN
    act1 : $CConductionTime(j) := CTime$
    act2 : $CConductionSpeed(i \mapsto j) := CSpeed$
    act3 : $CCSpeed\_CCTime\_Flag := FALSE$
  END

The electrical impulse propagates at every millisecond. But the impulse propagation time and velocity are different for each landmark node. The progressive increment of the independent logical clock is modelled through event *tic*, that increments time in 1 ms. The event *Clock_Counter* progressively increases the current clock counter *tic* under pre-defined cycle length *Cycle_Length*. The predicate in guard (grd1) of event *Clock_Counter* represents an upper bound time limit. The current clock counter *tic* is reset to 0 by the event *HeartConductionEnd*. An extra guard is added in the event *HeartConductionEnd* as $tic = Cycle\_Length$ to reset all the parametric values of the heart system for starting a fresh new impulse propagation cycle.

EVENT Clock_Counter
  WHEN
    grd1 : $tic < Cycle\_Length$
  THEN
    act1 : $tic := tic + 1$
  END

We have defined the event *Clock_Counter* as a type of *Convergent* and the system variant is defined as $Cycle\_length - tic$, which generates the convergence proof obligations to verify that the time is progressing with the electrical impulse propagation. It means that the electrical impulse is propagating in the conduction network corresponding to the clock counter.

8.5.5 Refinement 3: Perturbation in the Conduction

It introduces a set of possible blocks in the heart conducting system. These blocks can occur in the conduction network and give trouble in electrical impulse propagation. A set of landmark nodes partition the different regions for all possible heart blocks. For introducing the heart blocks, we introduce an enumerated set *Heart-BlockSets* in a new context model as a static property of the heart system.

$axm1 : partition(HeartBlockSets, \{SA\_nodal\_blocks\}, \{AV\_nodal\_blocks\},$
$\{Infra\_Hisian\_blocks\}, \{LBBB\_blocks\}, \{RBBB\_blocks\}, \{None\})$

To model the heart block system, we define a variable *HeartBlocks* as *Heart-Blocks* $\in$ *HeartBlockSets*. New events are introduced to show different kinds of heart blocks during impulse propagation into the conduction network. Events are *Heart-Conduction_Block_A_B_C* to formalise the sinoatrial (SA) nodal block, *Heart-Conduction_Block_B* to represent atrioventricular (AV) nodal block, *HeartConduction_Block_B_D* to specify Infra-Hisian block, *HeartConduction_Block_D_E_G* to present Left bundle branch block, and *HeartConduction_Block_D_F_H* to specify the Right bundle branch block.

Conduction disturbance in the heart during which an impulse formed within the sinus node (A) is blocked or delayed from depolarising the atria. There are different kinds of SA blocks [24, 30]. To model SA block, we introduce an event *HeartConduction_Block_A_B_C*, which formalises the SA block. In this event, guard (*grd1*) represents that the landmark nodes (A or C) are not visited means FALSE state, or the current impulse propagation time of B and C nodes are not lain within the standard range, or the current impulse propagation velocity of the pairs $A \mapsto B$ and $A \mapsto C$ are not lain within the standard range. When a guard is triggered, then actions of this event state that the heart state is FALSE, and the heart block is a sinoatrial (SA) nodal block.

EVENT HeartConduction_Block_A_B_C Refines HeartKO
  WHEN
    grd1 : $(ConductionNodeState(A) = FALSE) \vee$
          $(ConductionNodeState(C) = FALSE) \vee$
          $(CConductionTime(B) \notin ConductionTime(B)) \vee$
          $(CConductionTime(C) \notin ConductionTime(C)) \vee$
          $(CConductionSpeed(A \mapsto B) \notin ConductionSpeed(A \mapsto B)) \vee$
          $(CConductionSpeed(A \mapsto C) \notin ConductionSpeed(A \mapsto C))$
  THEN
    act1 : $HeartState := FALSE$
    act2 : $HeartBlocks := SA\_nodal\_blocks$
  END

Any interruption in the conduction of electrical impulses from the atria to the ventricles; it can occur at the level of atria, atrioventricular node, bundle of His, or Purkinje system. It is a type of heart block in which a blocking is at the atrioventricular (AV) junction. It is known as first degree when atrioventricular (AV) conduction time is prolonged; it is called second degree or partial when some but not all atrial impulses reach at the ventricle; and it is called third degree or complete when no atrial impulses at all reach the ventricle, so that the atria and ventricles act independently of each other. There are different kinds of AV blocks [24, 30]. To model the AV block, we introduce an event *HeartConduction_Block_B*, which formalises the AV block. The conduction node state *ConductionNodeState* of a landmark node (B) is *FALSE*, which represents a condition for the AV block using guard (grd1) and actions state that the heart state is *FALSE* and such kind of heart block is known as the atrioventricular (AV) nodal block.

EVENT HeartConduction_Block_B Refines HeartKO
  WHEN
    grd1 : $(ConductionNodeState(B) = FALSE)$
  THEN
    act1 : $HeartState := FALSE$
    act2 : $HeartBlocks := AV\_nodal\_blocks$
  END

Infra-Hisian block describes a block of the distal conduction system (node D). There are different kinds of Infra-Hisian blocks [24, 30]. To model Infra-Hisian block, an event *HeartConduction_Block_B_D* is used to formalise the desired conditions for a such kind of blocks through landmark nodes (B, D). Guard (grd1) represents that the landmark node (D) is *FALSE*, means it is not visited, or the current impulse propagation time of a node D is not lain within the standard range, or the current propagation velocity of a pair $B \mapsto D$ is not lain within the standard range. The actions of this event state that the heart state is FALSE, and the heart block is the Infra-Hisian block.

EVENT HeartConduction_Block_B_D Refines HeartKO
  WHEN
    grd1 : $(ConductionNodeState(D) = FALSE) \vee$
        $(CConductionTime(D) \notin ConductionTime(D)) \vee$
        $(CConductionSpeed(B \mapsto D) \notin ConductionSpeed(B \mapsto D))$
  THEN
    act1 : $HeartState := FALSE$
    act2 : $HeartBlocks := Infra\_Hisian\_blocks$
  END

The bundle of His divides into a right bundle branch and a left bundle branch, which lead to the heart's lower chambers (the ventricles). For the left and right ventricles to contract at the same time, an electrical impulse must travel down the right and left bundle branches at the same speed. If there is a block in one of these branches, the electrical impulse must travel to the ventricle by a different route. When this happens, the rate and rhythm of your heartbeat are not affected, but the impulse is slowed. Even ventricle will still contract, but it will take longer because of the slowed impulse. This slowed impulse causes one ventricle to contract a fraction of a second slower than the other [24, 30]. The medical terms for bundle branch block are derived from which branch is affected. If the block is located in the right bundle branch, it is called Right bundle branch block. If the block is located in the left bundle branch, it is called Left bundle branch block.

To model the Right bundle branch block, we introduce an event in a similar fashion like past events. A new event *HeartConduction_Block_D_E_G* formalises the Right bundle branch; guard of this event states that the landmark nodes (E or G) are not visited means FALSE state, or the current impulse propagation time of E and G nodes are not lain within the standard ranges, or the current impulse propagation velocity of the pairs $D \mapsto E$ and $E \mapsto G$ are not lain within the standard range; then the actions of this event state that the heart state is FALSE and the heart block is the Right bundle branch block.

EVENT HeartConduction_Block_D_E_G Refines HeartKO
  WHEN
    grd1 : $(ConductionNodeState(E) = FALSE) \lor$
           $(ConductionNodeState(G) = FALSE) \lor$
           $(CConductionTime(E) \notin ConductionTime(E)) \lor$
           $(CConductionTime(C) \notin ConductionTime(C)) \lor$
           $(CConductionSpeed(D \mapsto E) \notin ConductionSpeed(D \mapsto E)) \lor$
           $(CConductionSpeed(E \mapsto G) \notin ConductionSpeed(E \mapsto G))$
  THEN
    act1 : $HeartState := FALSE$
    act2 : $HeartBlocks := RBBB\_blocks$
  END

To model the Left bundle branch block, we introduce an event like Right bundle branch event. This new event *HeartConduction_Block_D_F_H* formalises the Left bundle branch. Guard of this event states that the landmark nodes (F or H) are not visited means FALSE state, or the current impulse propagation time of F and H nodes are not lain within the standard range, or the current impulse propagation velocity of the pairs $D \mapsto F$ and $F \mapsto H$ are not lain within the standard range. Then the actions of this event state that the heart state is FALSE, and the heart block is the Left bundle branch block.

EVENT HeartConduction_Block_D_F_H Refines HeartKO
  WHEN
    grd1 : $(ConductionNodeState(F) = FALSE) \vee$
          $(ConductionNodeState(H) = FALSE) \vee$
          $(CConductionTime(F) \notin ConductionTime(F)) \vee$
          $(CConductionTime(H) \notin ConductionTime(H)) \vee$
          $(CConductionSpeed(D \mapsto F) \notin ConductionSpeed(D \mapsto F)) \vee$
          $(CConductionSpeed(F \mapsto H) \notin ConductionSpeed(F \mapsto H))$
  THEN
    act1 : $HeartState := FALSE$
    act2 : $HeartBlocks := LBBB\_blocks$
  END

8.5.6 Refinement 4: Getting a Cellular Model

This last refinement introduces cellular level modelling into the heart model. The cellular level modelling is used to model the electrical impulse propagation at the cell level. The formalisation uses cellular automata theory to model the microstructure based cell model. To formalise the cellular automata, we introduce mathematical properties (see Definitions 2 and 3) in a context model. In a biological system, each cell has one of the following states: *Active*, *Passive* or *Refractory*. To define cell states, we declare an enumerated set *CellStates*. We have assumed grid of cells in a square format. Due to square geometry of the cells, we define a constant *NeighbouringCells* to represent a set of coordinated positions of the neighbouring cells. A new function *NEXT* is used to define neighbouring cell's state. This function maps from the power-set of *NeighbouringCells* to a cell's state *CellStates*. A new function *CellS* is defined as to map from *NeighbouringCells* to *CellStates*. This function maps various states like *Active*, *Passive* and *Refractory* to the neighbouring cells.

$axm1 : partition(CellStates, \{PASSIVE\}, \{ACTIVE\}, \{REFRACTORY\})$
$axm2 : x \in \mathbb{Z}$
$axm3 : y \in \mathbb{Z}$
$axm4 : NeighbouringCells =$
        $\{\{x, y\}, \{x + 1, y\}, \{x - 1, y\}, \{x, y + 1\}, \{x, y - 1\}\}$
$axm5 : NEXT \in \mathbb{P}(NeighbouringCells) \rightarrow CellStates$
$axm6 : CellS \in NeighbouringCells \rightarrow CellStates$

A set of properties ($axm7$–$axm10$) is introduced to specify the desired behaviour of the biological cell automata in two-dimensions. All these properties implement the state transition of a cell and formalise the transitions automaton (see Fig. 8.9). The first property ($axm1$) states that if the neighbouring cells are in *Active* state, then the NEXT state of the cell must be *Refractory*. The second property ($axm8$) represents that if the neighbouring cells are in the *Refractory* state, then the NEXT state of the cell must be *Passive*. Third property ($axm9$) states that if a cell at (x, y) is *Passive*, then if all the neighbouring cells in 2D is *Active*, then a set of neighbouring cells must be in *Active*. Similarly, the last property (*axm10*) presents that if a cell at (x, y) is *Passive*, then and if all the neighbouring cells in 2D is not *Active*, then a set of neighbouring cells must be in *Passive*.

$$
\begin{aligned}
axm7 : &\ \forall\, param \cdot param \in \mathbb{P}(NeighbouringCells) \wedge CellS(\{x, y\}) = ACTIVE \\
&\Rightarrow NEXT(param) = REFRACTORY \\
axm8 : &\ \forall\, param \cdot param \in \mathbb{P}(NeighbouringCells) \wedge CellS(\{x, y\}) = \\
&REFRACTORY \Rightarrow NEXT(param) = PASSIVE \\
axm9 : &\ \forall\, param \cdot param \in \mathbb{P}(NeighbouringCells) \wedge \{x, y\} \in param \wedge \\
&CellS(\{x, y\}) = PASSIVE \Rightarrow ((CellS(\{x + 1, y\}) = ACTIVE \vee \\
&CellS(\{x - 1, y\}) = ACTIVE \vee CellS(\{x, y + 1\}) = ACTIVE \vee \\
&CellS(\{x, y - 1\}) = ACTIVE) \Rightarrow NEXT(param) = ACTIVE) \\
axm10 : &\ \forall\, param \cdot param \in \mathbb{P}(NeighbouringCells) \wedge \{x, y\} \in param \wedge \\
&CellS(\{x, y\}) = PASSIVE \Rightarrow ((CellS(\{x + 1, y\}) \neq ACTIVE \wedge \\
&CellS(\{x - 1, y\}) \neq ACTIVE \wedge CellS(\{x, y + 1\}) \neq ACTIVE \wedge \\
&CellS(\{x, y - 1\}) \neq ACTIVE \Rightarrow NEXT(param) = PASSIVE)
\end{aligned}
$$

Each cell in the heart muscle must have one of the states: *Active*, *Passive* or *Refractory*. Initially, all cells have *Passive* state. In this state, a cell is discharged electrically and has no influences on its neighbouring cells. When electrical impulse propagates, then the cell would be charged and eventually activated (*Active* state). Now, the cell transmits the electrical impulse to its neighbour cells. The electrical impulse is propagated to all cells in the heart muscle. After an activation, the cell would be discharged and enter into the *Refractory* state in which a cell cannot be reactivated after a moment, a cell changes its state to the *Passive* state, in which the cell awaits next impulse (see Fig. 8.9).

To model the dynamic behaviour of the cell automata, we declare four variables m, n, *Transition* and *NextCellState*. Two variables m and n represent current position of the active cell during impulse propagation. The variable *Transition* is defined as boolean to set the transition state *TRUE* or *FALSE* to model the behaviour of a tissue. Last variable *NextCellState* is used to store the values of next neighbouring positions after every transition.

$$
\begin{aligned}
inv1 &: m \in \mathbb{Z} \\
inv2 &: n \in \mathbb{Z} \\
inv3 &: Transition \in BOOL \\
inv4 &: NextCellState \in CellStates
\end{aligned}
$$

To implement the dynamic behaviour of a cell in two-dimensions, we introduce two events *HeartConduction_Cellular* to make transition TRUE for the electrical conduction at the cell level and *HeartConduction_Next_UpdateCell* to calculate status of the neighbouring cells and update the current position (m, n) of the cell. The event *HeartConduction_Cellular* is used to set the boolean states of the variable *Transition*. The first guard of this event states that any path $(p \mapsto q)$ is one of the pair from a set of pairs of the conduction network. The next guard (grd2) states that the current impulse propagation speed and velocity flag *CCSpeed_CCTime_Flag* is

TRUE and a set of coordinate positions (*param*) of neighbouring cells is represented in third guard. Fourth guard states that the current cell position (m, n) is *Passive* and last guard represents that the cell transition state *Transition* is *FALSE*. If all guards satisfy, then the transition state of a cell becomes *TRUE*.

```
EVENT HeartConduction_Cellular
   ANY   p, q, param
   WHERE
      grd1 : p ↦ q ∈ ConductionPath
      grd2 : CCSpeed_CCTime_Flag = TRUE
      grd3 : param = {{m, n}, {m + 1, n}, {m − 1, n}, {m, n + 1}, {m, n − 1}}
      grd4 : {m, n} ∈ dom(CellS) ∧ CellS({m, n}) = PASSIVE
      grd5 : NextCellState = CellS({m, n})
      grd6 : Transition = FALSE
   THEN
      act1 : Transition := TRUE
   END
```

The event *HeartConduction_Next_UpdateCell* is used to calculate the state of neighbouring cells and to update the position of the current cell (m, n). The first guard of this event represents a set of coordinate positions (*param*) of neighbouring cells and the next guard (grd2) states that the selected neighbouring cells are a set of cells (*dom(NEXT)*). The last guard presents a transition state *Transition* is *TRUE*. Action of this event calculates a set of the next neighbouring cells in act1. The next action (act2) sets *FALSE* of a transition state. The last two actions update the value of the current cell (m, n) to continuously impulse propagating in the heart using the conduction network.

```
EVENT HeartConduction_Next_UpdateCell
   ANY   param
   WHERE
      grd1 : param = {{m, n}, {m + 1, n}, {m − 1, n}, {m, n + 1}, {m, n − 1}}
      grd2 : param ∈ dom(NEXT)
      grd3 : Transition = TRUE
   THEN
      act1 : NextCellState := NEXT(param)
      act2 : Transition := FALSE
      act3 : m :∈ {m − 1, m, m + 1}
      act4 : n :∈ {n − 1, n, n + 1}
   END
```

Finally, we have completed the formal specifications of the heart modelling. In the next section, we present model validation of the heart model using Event-B model checker ProB tool.

Table 8.3 Proof statistics

Model	Total number of POs	Automatic proof	Interactive proof
Abstract model	29	22 (76 %)	7 (24 %)
First refinement	9	6 (67 %)	3 (33 %)
Second refinement	159	155 (97 %)	4 (3 %)
Third refinement	10	1 (10 %)	9 (90 %)
Fourth refinement	11	10 (91 %)	1 (9 %)
Total	218	194 (89 %)	24 (11 %)

8.5.7 Model Validation and Analysis

There are two main validation activities in Event-B, and both are complementary for designing a consistent system in the medical domain; *consistency checking* and *model analysis*. This section validates the model by using ProB tool [26] and proof statistics. "Validation" refers to the activity of gaining confidence that the developed formal models are consistent with the requirements. We have used the ProB tool that supports *automated consistency checking* of Event-B machines via model checking [11] and constraint-based checking [18]. This tool assists us to validate the heart model according to the conduction network and a set of landmark nodes. It is the complementary use of both techniques to develop formal models of critical systems, where high safety and security are required. The heart model is carefully verified through animations and under supervision of physiologist and cardiologist. We have validated various scenario cases of normal and abnormal heart conditions, and we have also tested morphological behaviour [3, 6] of the ECG during impulse propagation from the SA node (A) to the Purkinje fibres (F, H) in the ventricles. The logic-based mathematical model of the heart can generate all possible scenarios of normal and abnormal heart conditions in the ECG caused by changes in time and velocity among landmark nodes. ProB was very useful in animating all models and in verifying the absence of error (no counter-examples exist) and deadlock.

Table 8.3 expresses the proof statistics of the development using the Rodin tool. These statistics measure the size of the model, the proof obligations generated and discharged by the Rodin prover and those are interactively proved. The complete development of the heart model results in 218 (100 %) proof obligations, within which 194 (89 %) are proved automatically by the Rodin tool. The remaining 24 (11 %) proof obligations are proved interactively using Rodin tool. For the heart model, many proof obligations are generated because of the introduction of the new functional behaviours. To guarantee the correctness of these functional behaviours, we have established various invariants in the incremental refinements. Most of the proofs are interactively discharged in the third refinement of the heart model. These proofs are quite simple, and have been discharged with the help of simplifying predicates. Few proof obligations are proved interactively in other refinements. The incremental refinement of the heart system helps to achieve a high degree of automatic proof.

8.6 Discussion

This chapter presents a methodology for modelling a biological system, such as the heart, by modelling a biological environment. The main objective of this methodology is to model the heart system and integrate it with the model of a medical device such as a cardiac pacemaker, thereby modelling the closed-loop system to enable certification of the medical system via the certification bodies [17, 23] for safe operation. To build a closed-loop model using both environment and device modelling is considered as a standard approach in the area validation, given that designing an environment model is a challenging problem in the real world. Industry has long sought such an approach to validating system models in a biological environment. We have discovered much information via a literature survey and long discussions with experts in cardiology and physiology, and have concluded how best to model the heart system as a cellular-level architecture in an efficient and optimum way. Because of the complexity of the cellular-level calculations (see Sect. 8.2), previous models have failed to model the heart system.

We have proposed modelling the heart in an abstract way to simulate the desired behaviour of the heart system while avoiding the complexity. More importantly, the heart model is based on logico-mathematical theory. Our primary objective was to model the heart system using only simple logico-mathematical methods. The heart model is an environmental model for medical devices that may improve their development in the early phases. As such, it will contribute only one element of the verification process. Other verification steps will also be required. Medical experts have elaborated every minor detail in an effort to understand the complexity of the biological system, particularly because the heart system is the most complex organ in the body. The proposed approach contains only a main part of the specification of the system behaviour, with the remaining information being hidden. We have spent much time identifying an exact abstract model of the heart system that satisfies medical experts. We have used the EVENT B modelling language to model and verify the system. The ProB model checker was used to verify the correctness of the heart model via animation. Any other formal specification language and model checker could be used to model the heart system based on our proposed methodology.

8.7 Summary

This chapter has presented a methodology for producing a mathematical model of the heart based on logico-mathematical theory [33–35]. This model is the first computational model that considers the heart as an electrical conduction system. Given that a cardiac pacemaker interacts with the heart exactly at this level (i.e., electrical impulses), this model is a very promising "environmental model" to be used in parallel with a pacemaker model to form a closed-loop system. This model therefore has an immediate use in "the grand challenges in formal methods" where an industrial pacemaker specification has been elected as a benchmark. To formalise the heart system, we have used the Event-B modelling language [1, 38] to develop the proof-based formal model. Our approach involves formalising and reasoning about impulse propagation in the whole heart system through the conduction network (see Fig. 8.4(a)). More precisely, we would like to stress the original contribution of our work. We have proposed a method for modelling a human heart based on logico-mathematical theory. The main objectives of this proposed idea are as follows:

- To obtain a certification procedure for providing a higher safety integrity level.
- To verify the system in a patient model (in a formal representation).
- To analyse the biological environment (the heart) in a mathematical way.
- To analyse the interaction between the heart model and a cardiac pacemaker or ICD.

In summary, we have formalised the known characteristics and physiological behaviour of the heart. The formalisation highlights various aspects of the problem, making different assumptions about impulse propagation and establishing different properties related to the CA. We have outlined how an incremental refinement approach to the heart system enables a high degree of automatic proof using the Rodin tool. Our various developments reflect not only many facets of the problem, but also the learning process involved in understanding the problem and its ultimate possible solutions.

The consistency of our specification has been checked through reasoning, and validation experiments were performed using the ProB model checker with respect to safety conditions. As part of our reasoning, we have proved that the initialisation of the system is valid, and we have calculated the preconditions for operations. These have been executed to guarantee that our intention to have total operations has been fulfilled. At each stage of the refinement, we have introduced a new behaviour for the system and proved its *consistency* and *refinement checking*. We have introduced more general invariants at the refinement level, showing that the initialisation of the whole system is valid. Finally, we have validated the heart system using the ProB model checker as a validation tool and have verified the correctness of the exact behaviour of our heart system with the help of physiology and cardiology experts.

References

1. Abrial, J.-R. (2010). *Modeling in Event-B: System and software engineering* (1st ed.). New York: Cambridge University Press.
2. Adam, D. R. (1991). Propagation of depolarization and repolarization processes in the myocardium—an anisotropic model. *IEEE Transactions on Biomedical Engineering, 38*(2), 133–141.
3. Artigou, J. Y., & Monsuez, J. J. (2007). *Cardiologie et maladies vasculaires*. Paris: Elsevier Masson.
4. Back, R. J. R. (1981). On correct refinement of programs. *Journal of Computer and System Sciences, 23*(1), 49–68.
5. Barold, S. S., Stroobandt, R. X., & Sinnaeve, A. F. (2004). *Cardiac pacemakers step by step*. London: Futura. ISBN 1-4051-1647-1.

6. Bayes, B. V. N., de Luna, A., & Malik, M. (2006). The morphology of the electrocardiogram. In *The ESC textbook of cardiovascular medicine* (pp. 1–36). Oxford: Blackwell.

7. Bengtsson, J., Larsen, K., Larsson, F., Pettersson, P., & Yi, W. (1996). UPPAAL—a tool suite for automatic verification of real-time systems. In *Proceedings of the DIMACS/SYCON workshop on hybrid systems III: Verification and control* (pp. 232–243). Secaucus: Springer.

8. Berenfeld, O., & Abboud, S. (1996). Simulation of cardiac activity and the ECG using a heart model with a reaction-diffusion action potential. *Medical Engineering & Physics, 18*(8), 615–625.

9. Bowen, J., & Stavridou, V. (1993). Safety-critical systems, formal methods and standards. *Software Engineering Journal, 8*(4), 189–209.

10. CDRH (2006). Safety of marketed medical devices. Center for Devices and Radiological Health, US FDA.

11. Clarke, E. M., Grumberg, O., & Peled, D. (2001). *Model checking.* Cambridge: MIT Press.

12. Ellenbogen, K. A., & Wood, M. A. (2005). *Cardiac pacing and ICDs* (4th ed.). Oxford: Blackwell. ISBN 1-4051-0447-3.

13. Fitzgerald, J. (2007). The typed logic of partial functions and the Vienna development method. In D. Bjørner & M. C. Henson (Eds.), *EATCS textbook in computer science. Logics of specification languages* (pp. 431–465). Berlin: Springer.

14. Fitzgerald, J., Larsen, P. G., Pierce, K., Verhoef, M., & Wolff, S. (2010). Collaborative modelling and co-simulation in the development of dependable embedded systems. In *Lecture notes in computer science. Proceedings of the 8th international conference on integrated formal methods* (pp. 12–26). Berlin: Springer.

15. Harrild, D. M., & Henriquez, C. S. (2000). A computer model of normal conduction in the human atria. *Circulation Research, 87,* 25–36.

16. Hesselson, A. (2003). *Simplified interpretations of pacemaker ECGs.* Oxford: Blackwell. ISBN 978-1-4051-0372-5.

17. High Confidence Software and Systems Coordinating Group (2009). *High-confidence medical devices: Cyber-physical systems for 21st century health care* (Technical report). NITRD. http://www.nitrd.gov/About/MedDevice-FINAL1-web.pdf.

18. Jackson, D. (2002). Alloy: A lightweight object modelling notation. *ACM Transactions on Software Engineering and Methodology, 11*(2), 256–290.

19. Jee, E., Wang, S., Kim, J.-K., Lee, J., Sokolsky, O., & Lee, I. (2010). A safety-assured development approach for real-time software. In *16th IEEE international conference on embedded and real-time computing systems and applications,* RTCSA (pp. 133–142).

20. Jetley, R. P., Carlos, C., & Purushothaman Iyer, S. (2004). A case study on applying formal methods to medical devices: Computer-aided resuscitation algorithm. *International Journal on Software Tools for Technology Transfer, 5*(4), 320–330.

21. Jetley, R., Purushothaman Iyer, S., & Jones, P. (2006). A formal methods approach to medical device review. *Computer, 39*(4), 61–67.

22. Jiang, Z., Pajic, M., Connolly, A. T., Dixit, S., & Mangharam, R. (2010). Real-time heart model for implantable cardiac device validation and verification. In *22st Euromicro conference on real-time systems,* IEEE ECRTS'10, July 2010.

23. Keatley, K. L. (1999). A review of the FDA draft guidance document for software validation: Guidance for industry. *Quality Assurance, 7*(1), 49–55.

24. Khan, M. G. (2008). *Rapid ECG interpretation.* Clifton: Humana Press.

25. Lee, I., Pappas, G. J., Cleaveland, R., Hatcliff, J., Krogh, B. H., Lee, P., et al. (2006). High-confidence medical device software and systems. *Computer, 39*(4), 33–38.

26. Leuschel, M., & Butler, M. (2003). *Lecture notes in computer science. ProB: A model checker for B* (pp. 855–874). Berlin: Springer.

27. Love, C. J. (2006). *Cardiac pacemakers and defibrillators.* Georgetown: Landes Bioscience. ISBN 1-57059-691-3.

28. Maisel, W. H., Sweeney, M. O., Stevenson, W. G., Ellison, K. E., & Epstein, L. M. (2001). Recalls and safety alerts involving pacemakers and implantable cardioverter-defibrillator generators. *Journal of the American Medical Association, 286*(7), 793–799.

29. Makowiec, D. (2008). The heart pacemaker by cellular automata on complex networks. In *Proceedings of the 8th international conference on cellular automata for research and industry*, ACRI'08 (pp. 291–298). Berlin: Springer.

30. Malmivuo, J. (1995). *Bioelectromagnetism*. Oxford: Oxford University Press. ISBN 0-19-505823-2.

31. Méry, D., & Singh, N. K. (2010). Real-time animation for formal specification. In M. Aiguier, F. Bretaudeau, & D. Krob (Eds.), *Complex systems design & management* (pp. 49–60). Berlin: Springer.

32. Méry, D., & Singh, N. K. (2010). Trustable formal specification for software certification. In T. Margaria & B. Steffen (Eds.), *Lecture notes in computer science: Vol. 6416. Leveraging applications of formal methods, verification, and validation* (pp. 312–326). Berlin: Springer.

33. Méry, D., & Singh, N. K. (2011). Technical report on formalisation of the heart using analysis of conduction time and velocity of the electrocardiography and cellular-automata. MOSEL-LORIA-INRIA-CNRS: UMR7503-Université Henri Poincaré-Nancy I-Université Nancy II-Institut National Polytechnique de Lorraine. http://hal.inria.fr/inria-00600339/en/.

34. Méry, D., & Singh, N. K. (2012). Closed-loop modeling of cardiac pacemaker and heart. In *Foundations of health informatics engineering and systems*.

35. Méry, D., & Singh, N. K. (2012). Formalization of heart models based on the conduction of electrical impulses and cellular automata. In Z. Liu & A. Wassyng (Eds.), *Lecture notes in computer science: Vol. 7151. Foundations of health informatics engineering and systems* (pp. 140–159). Berlin: Springer.

36. Plonsey, R., & Barr, R. C. (1987). Mathematical modeling of electrical activity of the heart. *Journal of Electrocardiology, 20*(3), 219–226.

37. Seong, Y. R., Jun, K.-R., & Kim, T. G. (1994). A cellular automata model of activation process in ventricular muscle. In *SCSC'94* (pp. 769–774).

38. RODIN (2004). Rigorous open development environment for complex systems. http://rodin-b-sharp.sourceforge.net.

39. Vangheluwe, H., & Vansteenkiste, G. C. (2000). The cellular automata formalism and its relationship to DEVS. In *Proceedings of the 14th European simulation multiconference on simulation and modelling: Enablers for a better quality of life* (pp. 800–810). Ghent: SCS Europe.

40. von Neumann, J. (1966). *Theory of self-reproducing automata*. Chicago: University of Illinois Press. A. W. Burks (Ed.).

Chapter 9
The Cardiac Pacemaker

Abstract Building high quality and zero defects medical software-based devices is a critical task, and formal modelling techniques can effectively help to achieve this target at the certain level. Formal modelling of a high-confidence medical device, such as that is too much error prone in operating, is an international Grand Challenge in the area of Verified Software. Modelling a cardiac pacemaker is one of the proposed challenges, and we consider the complete description of pacemaker's functionalities using an incremental proof-based approach. To assess the effectiveness of our proposed development methodology and associated techniques and tools, we select this case study. This chapter presents the development of a cardiac pacemaker using our proposed development life-cycle methodology from requirement analysis to automatic code generation. In this development, we use formal verification to verify the correctness of the requirements for a simple and closed-loop model, model checking to verify the correctness of the system behaviours, real-time animator to check the system behaviours according to the domain experts (i.e. medical experts), and finally the code generation tool EB2ALL for generating the codes into several programming languages. The refinement charts are used to handle the complexity of the system, where it helps to organise the code structure according to the different operating modes. Formal models are expressed in the Event-B modelling language, which integrates conditions (called proof obligations) for checking their internal consistency with respect to the invariants and safety properties. The generated proof obligations of models are proved by the Rodin tool and desired behaviour of the system is validated by the ProB tool and real-time animator according to the medical experts.

9.1 Introduction

Development and production of medical device software and systems are common crucial issues [59] for ensuring safe advances in healthcare. The lack of uniform standard and formalism in the engineering of medical-device software leads many deficiencies in developing relatively low cost trustworthy software under a limit time frame. For decades, software failures have cost billions of dollars a year [60]. During

N.K. Singh, *Using Event-B for Critical Device Software Systems*,
DOI 10.1007/978-1-4471-5260-6_9, © Springer-Verlag London 2013

this period, software have been delivered with restricted warranties of failures and errors, resulting in the well-known software crisis. Due to software crisis, various formalisms and rigorous techniques (VDM, Z, Event-B, Alloy, etc.) have been used in the development process of safety-critical systems. These approaches provide a given level of reliability and confidence to develop the error-free systems. Formal methods and their tools have achieved some usability that could be applied even in industrial-scale applications allowing software developers to provide more meaningful guarantees to their projects.

Tony Hoare suggested Grand challenge for Computing Research [24] to integrate the research community to work together towards a common goal, agreed to be valuable and achievable by a team effort within a predicted time-scale. Verification Grand Challenge is one of them. From the Verification, Grand Challenges, many application areas were proposed by the Verified Software Initiative [25]. The pacemaker specification [7, 18] has been proposed by the software quality research laboratory at McMaster University as a pilot project for the Verified Software Initiative [38, 59]. The challenge is characterised by system aspects including hardware requirements and safety issues. Such a system demands high integrity to achieve safety requirements. The pacemaker device is highly sensitive, and lots of operating defects are coming day by day.

The contribution of this chapter is to give a complete idea of formal development of the cardiac pacemaker using our proposed framework and a set of techniques and tools. The cardiac pacemaker is a critical system, which is used here to show the usefulness of proposed approaches. Our approach is based on the Event-B modelling language which is supported by the Rodin platform integrating tools for proving models and refinements of models. Here, we present an incremental proof-based development to model and verify such interdisciplinary requirements in Event-B [1, 8]. Validation of the system is done by model checker as well as the real-time animator. The model checker, ProB tool [36] is used for validating and analysing the developed formal specifications. The cardiac pacemaker models must be validated to ensure that they meet requirements of the pacemaker. Hence, validation must be carried out by both formal modelling and domain experts. The real-time animator helps to the medical experts to verify the functional behaviour of the system. If medical experts are not agreed on the system behaviour, then the system specification is modified and again verify it. In addition, we have proposed the system integration approach using refinements charts to help a code designer to improve the code structure and code optimisation, and the code generation for synthesising and synchronising the software codes of the cardiac pacemaker. We have also used our proposed environment model of the heart to specify a closed-loop system of the heart and cardiac pacemaker. Finally, we have used our translator (EB2ALL) [13, 41, 45–47, 51] to generate the source code in multiple languages (C, C++, Java, C#). In the rest of the sections of this chapter, we describe step by step a development of the one- and two-electrode cardiac pacemaker.

9.1.1 Why Model-Checker?

Model checking [3] and theorem proving are both applicable in medical device development. This approach requires a model of the system under consideration together with a desired property and systematically checks whether the given model satisfies this property. The basic technique of model checking is a systematic, usually exhaustive, state-space search to check whether the property is satisfied in each state of the model, thereby using effective methods to combat the infamous state-space explosion problem. Using model checking with formal verification for medical device has several benefits:

- To understand the formal verification of any system is not an easy task. A group of non-formal people (doctors, engineering, coder and so on) cannot understand it due to lack of knowledge of formal mathematics. Non-formal people can understand the desirable system behaviour through model checker and can give the proper feedback.
- A model-checker is also useful for a model designer to improve the system. A model-checker may provide a counter-example showing under which circumstance the error can be generated. The counter-example provides evidence that the system is faulty and needs to be revised. This allows the user to locate the error and to repair the system before continuing. If no error is found, the user can refine the model description and can restart the verification process.

9.1.2 Related Work for the Cardiac Pacemaker

Macedo et al. [38] have developed a distributed real-time model of a cardiac pacemaker using a formal tool VDM [6], where they have modelled the subset of pacemaker functionalities. In another pacemaker case study, Manna et al. [34] have shown a simple pacemaker implementation. Gomes et al. [19] have presented a formal specification of a cardiac pacemaker using Z modelling language, and they have modelled the sequential model similar to Macedo et al. work [38]. A detailed formalisation of the one- and two electrode pacemaker is represented in [40, 43, 48]. The model has been developed in an incremental way using refinements in the Event-B modelling language. Tuan et al. [58] have proposed a formal model of the pacemaker based on its behaviour including the communication with the external environment. They have designed a real-time model of the pacemaker using timed extensions of CSP and used the model checker Process Analysis Toolkit (PAT) in order to verify the critical properties, such as deadlock freeness and heart rate limits. Recently, Gomes et al. [20] have presented the pacemaker case study by providing a means to execute the model using a translation of Z model into Perfect Developer [12]. They have used the existing tool Perfect Developer [12] to generate an executable code of Z model. In [30], authors have used dual chamber implantable pacemaker as a case study for modelling and verification of control algorithms for medical devices in UPPAAL.

Our models are superior to the sequential model of H.D. Macedo et al. [38] and Gomes et al. [19]. We have added the *threshold*, *hysteresis* and *rate adaptive* brady-cardia operating modes in our formal specification. We have developed the para-metric and functional incremental development of bradycardia operating modes. Incremental development is based on refinement approach and at every level of the development, we have proved all the required safety properties (*refinement* and *con-sistency checking*). Other specifications [19, 38] of the pacemaker developed as a one-shot model, means those are not based on the refinement and the correctness of a model is not checked by any model checker, for safely desired behaviour of the pacemaker system. We use the formal verification for consistency checking, and a model checker tool ProB is used to check the desired behaviour of the car-diac pacemaker. ProB animator helps to validate system behaviour according to the medical experts at each refinement level of the formal development. In this chapter, we present a complete system development of a cardiac pacemaker [48] from re-quirement analysis to source code generation in Event-B modelling language with several other techniques [13, 41, 46, 47].

9.1.3 Structure of This Chapter

The outline of the remaining chapter is as follows. We give a brief outline of the pacemaker and the heart system in Sect. 9.2. Section 9.3 presents patterns for mod-elling the cardiac pacemaker. Refinement structure of the cardiac pacemaker is given in Sect. 9.4. Section 9.5 presents development of the cardiac pacemaker using re-finement charts, and the control requirements of a cardiac pacemaker is given in Sect. 9.6. Sections 9.7 and 9.8 explore stepwise formal development of the one- and two-electrode cardiac pacemakers. Section 9.9 presents model validation using the ProB model checker. Section 9.10 presents a closed-loop formal model for the heart and cardiac pacemaker. Section 9.11 explores the requirements of the closed-loop modelling. Section 9.12 presents use of the real-time animator for validating the pacemaker models according to the domain experts. Section 9.13 presents code gen-eration process from formal specifications of the cardiac pacemaker using EB2ALL tool, and finally, Sects. 9.14 and 9.15 summarise this chapter with some discussions.

9.2 Basic Overview of Pacemaker System

The conventional pacemakers serve two major functions, namely *pacing* and *sensing*. The pacemaker actuator is pacing by the delivery of a short, intense elec-trical pulse into the heart. However, the pacemaker sensor uses the same electrode to detect the intrinsic activity of the heart. So, the pacemaker function of pacing and sensing activities are dependent on the behaviour of the heart. The sensing and pacing functions regulate the heart rhythm.

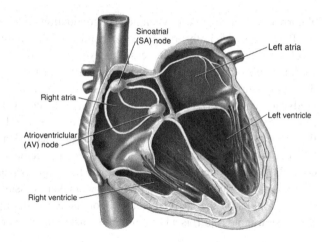

Fig. 9.1 Heart or natural pacemaker

The pacemaker system is a small electronic device that helps the heart to maintain the regular heart beat. In this study, the pacemaker is treated as an embedded system operating in an environment containing the heart. We first review the heart system that interact with the pacemaker (Sect. 9.2.1) and then consider elements of the pacemaker system itself (Sect. 9.2.2).

9.2.1 The Heart System

The human heart is wondrous in its ability to pump blood to the circulatory system continuously throughout a lifetime. The heart consists of four chambers: right atrial, right ventricle, left atrial and left ventricle, which contract and relax periodically. Atria form one unit and ventricles form another. The heart's mechanical system (the pump) requires at the very least impulses from the electrical system. An electrical stimulus is generated by the sinus node (see Fig. 9.1[1]), which is a small mass of specialised tissue located in the right atrium of the heart. This electrical stimulus travels down through the conduction pathways and causes the heart's lower chambers to contract and pump out blood. The right and left atrial are stimulated first and contract for a short period of time before the right and left ventricles. Each contraction of the ventricles represents one heartbeat. The atria contract for a fraction of a second before the ventricles, so their blood empties into the ventricles before the ventricles contract.

An artificial pacemaker is implanted to assist the heart in case of an arrhythmias condition to control the heart rate [39]. Arrhythmias are due to the cardiac problems producing abnormal heart rhythms. In general, arrhythmias reduce hemodynamic performance, including situations where the heart's natural pacemaker develops an

---

[1] Heart image is taken from http://media.summitmedicalgroup.com/media/db/relayhealth-images/nodes.jpg.

abnormal rate or rhythm or when normal conduction pathways are interrupted, and a different part of the heart takes over control of the rhythm. An arrhythmia can involve an abnormal rhythm increase (tachycardia; > 100 bpm) or decrease (brady-cardia; < 60 bpm), or may be characterised by an irregular cardiac rhythm, e.g. due to asynchrony of the cardiac chambers. The irregularity of the heartbeat, called bradycardia and tachycardia. The bradycardia indicates that the heart rate falls be-low the expected level while in tachycardia indicates that the heart rate goes above the expected level of the heart rate. An artificial pacemaker can restore synchrony between the atrial and ventricles. In an artificial pacemaker system, the firmware controls the hardware such that an adequate heart rate is maintained, which is nec-essary either because the heart's natural pacemaker is insufficiently fast or slow or there is a block in the heart's electrical conduction system [4, 14, 22, 35, 37, 39]. Beats per minute (bpm) is a basic unit to measure the rate of heart activity.

9.2.2 The Pacemaker System

The basic elements of the pacemaker system [4, 14] are:

1. *Leads*: One or more flexible coiled metal wires, normally two, that transmit elec-trical signals between the heart and the pacemaker. The same lead incorporate sensors, which are able to detect the intrinsic heart activity.
2. *The Pacemaker Generator*: This is both the power source and the brain of the artificial pacing and sensing systems. It contains an implanted battery and a con-troller.
3. *Device Controller-Monitor* (*DCM*) *or Programmer*: An external unit that inter-acts with the pacemaker device using a wireless connection. It consists of a hard-ware platform and the pacemaker application software.
4. *Accelerometer* (*Rate Modulation Sensor*): An electromechanical device inside the pacemaker that measures the body motion and acceleration of a body in or-der to allow modulated pacing. In the rate adaptive mode, a cardiac pacemaker automatically calculates the desire rate of the heart through the physical activities of the patient [31]. The rate modulation sensor is used to capture these physical activities and adjust the timing requirements for pacing.

The specification document [7] of our case study describes all possible operating modes that are controlled by the different programmable parameters of the pace-maker. All the programmable parameters are related to the real-time and action-reaction constraints that are used to regulate the heart rate.

Figure 9.2 depicts a basic block diagram of the cardiac pacemaker and shows the sensors and actuators that will be monitored and controlled in the design presented in the remainder of this chapter.

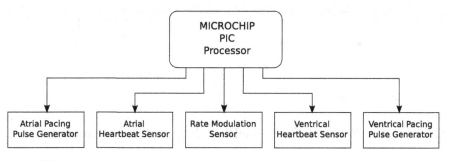

Fig. 9.2 Cardiac pacemaker sensors and actuators

Table 9.1 Bradycardia operating modes of pacemaker system

Category	Chambers paced	Chambers sensed	Response to sensing	Rate modulation
Letters	O—None	O—None	O—None	R—Rate modulation
	A—Atrium	A—Atrium	T—Triggered	
	V—Ventricle	V—Ventricle	I—Inhibited	
	D—Dual (A + V)	D—Dual (A + V)	D—Dual (T + I)	

9.2.3 Bradycardia Operating Modes

In order to understand the *language* of pacing, it is necessary to comprehend the coding system that produced by a combined working party of the North American Society of Pacing and Electrophysiology (NASPE) and the British Pacing and Electrophysiology Group (BPEG) known as NASPE/BPEG generic (NBG) pacemaker code [15]. This is a code of five letters of which the first three are most often used. The code provides a description of the pacemaker pacing and sensing functions. The sequence is referred to as *bradycardia operating modes* (see Table 9.1). In practice, only the first three or four-letter positions are commonly used to describe brady-cardia pacing functions. The first letter of the code indicates which chambers are being paced; the second letter indicates which chambers are being sensed; the third letter of the code indicates the response to sensing and the final letter, which is optional indicates the presence of rate modulation in response to the physical activity measured by the accelerometer. An accelerometer is an additional sensor in the pacemaker system that detects a physiological result of exercise or emotion, and increases the pacemaker rate on the basis of a programmable algorithm. "X" is a wildcard used to denote any letter (i.e. "O", "A", "V" or "D"). *Triggered (T)* refers to deliver a pacing stimulus and *Inhibited (I)* refers to an inhibition from further pacing after sensing of an intrinsic activity from the heart chambers.

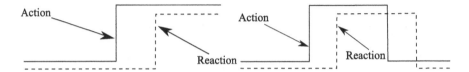

Fig. 9.3 Action-reaction patterns

9.3 Event-B Patterns for Modelling the Cardiac Pacemaker

Considering design patterns [17], the purpose is to capture structures and to make decisions within a design that are common to similar modelling and analysis tasks. They can be re-applied when undertaking similar tasks in order to reduce the duplication of effort. The design pattern approach is the possibility to reuse solutions from earlier developments in the current project. This will lead to a *correct refinement* in the chain of models, without producing proof obligations. Since the correctness (i.e. proof obligations are proved) of the pattern has been proved during its development, nothing is to be proved again when using this pattern.

Pacemaker systems are characterised by their functions, which can be expressed by analysing *action-reaction* and *real-time* patterns. Sequences of inputs are recognised, and outputs can be emitted in response within a fixed time interval. So, the most common elements in the pacemaker system are bounded time interval for every action, reaction and action-reaction pair. The action-reaction within a time limit can be viewed as an abstraction of the pacemaker system. We recognise the following two design patterns when modelling this kind of system according to the relationship between the action and corresponding reaction.

9.3.1 Action-Reaction Pattern

Under action-reaction chapter [1] two basic types of design patterns (see Fig. 9.3) are,

Action and Weak Reaction: Once an action emits, a reaction should start in response. For a quick instance, if an action stops, the reaction should follow. Sometimes reaction does not change immediately according to the action because the action moves too quickly (the continuance of an action is too short, or the interval between actions is too short). This is known as a pattern of action and weak reaction.

Action and Strong Reaction: When every reaction follows every action and there is proper synchronisation between action and corresponding reaction then this pattern is known as action and strong reaction.

9.3.2 Time-Based Pattern

The action-reaction events of a pacemaker system are based on the time constraint pattern in IEEE 1394 proposed by Cansell et al. and on the 2-Slots Simpson Al-

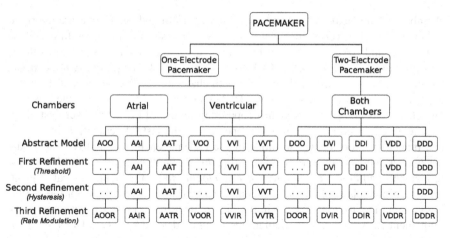

Fig. 9.4 Refinement structure of bradycardia operating modes of the pacemaker

gorithm case studies [9, 55]. This time pattern is fully based on a timed automaton. The timed automaton is a finite state machine that is useful to model the components of real-time systems. In a model, timed automata interacts with each other and defines a timed transition system. Besides ordinary action transitions that can represent input, output and internal actions. A timed transition system has time progress transitions. Such time progress transitions result in synchronous progress of all clock variables in the model. Here, we apply the time pattern in modelling to synchronise the sensing and pacing stimulus functions of the pacemaker system in continuous progressive time constraint. In the model, events are controlled under time constraints, which means action of any event activates only when time constraint satisfies on a specific time. The time progress is also an event, so there is no modification of the underlying Event-B language. It is only a modelling technique instead of a specialised formal system. The timed variable is in $\mathbb{N}$ (*natural numbers*), but time constraint can be written in terms involving unknown constants or expressions between different times. Finally, the timed event observations can be constrained by other events, which determine future activations.

9.4 Refinement Structure of a Cardiac Pacemaker

We present a block diagram (see Fig. 9.4) of a hierarchical tree structure of the possible bradycardia operating modes for a pacemaker. The hierarchical tree structure depicts a stepwise refinement from abstract to concrete models of the formal development for a pacemaker. Each level of refinement introduces new features of a pacemaker as functional and parametric requirements.

The root node indicates a cardiac pacemaker system. The next two branches show two classes of pacemaker: one-electrode pacemaker and two-electrode pacemaker. The one-electrode pacemaker branch is divided into two parts to indicate different chambers of the heart: atrium and ventricular. Atrium and ventricular are the right atrium and the right ventricular. The atrium chamber uses the three operating modes; AOO, AAI and AAT (see Table 9.1). Similarly, the ventricular chamber uses three operating modes: VOO, VVI and VVT (see Table 9.1). In the part of two-electrode pacemaker, there is only one branch for both chambers. Both chambers of the heart use the five operating modes: DOO, DVI, DDI, VDD and DDD. In the abstract model, we introduce the bradycardia operating modes of the pacemaker abstractly with required properties. From first refinement to the last refinement, there is only one branch in every operating mode of the pacemaker. In one and two-electrode pacemaker, there are three refinements: first *threshold* refinement; second *hysteresis* refinement; and third *rate adaptive or rate modulation* refinement. The subsequent refinement models introduce new features or functional requirements for the resulting system. The triple dots (. . .) in the hierarchical tree represents that there is no refinement at that level, in particular, operating modes (AOO, VOO, DOO, etc.). In the last refinement level, we have achieved the additional rate adaptive operating modes (i.e. AOOR, AAIR, VVTR, DOOR, DDDR, etc.). These operating modes are different from the previous levels of operating modes. This refinement structure is very helpful to model the functional requirements of the cardiac pacemaker.

9.5 Development of the Cardiac Pacemaker Using Refinement Chart

A formal specification serves as the central role of the development and evolution process. A refinement typically embodies a well-defined unit of programming knowledge. Figures 9.5 and 9.6 present the diagrams of the most abstract modal system for the one and two-electrode pacemaker system (A) and the resulting models of three successive refinement steps (B to D). The diagrams use a visual notation to represent the bradycardia operating modes of the pacemaker under functional and parametric requirements. An operating mode is represented by a box with a mode name; an operating mode transition is an arrow connecting two operating modes. The direction of an arrow indicates the previous and next operating modes in a transition. Refinement is expressed by nesting boxes [53].

A refined diagram of an abstract mode is equivalent to a concrete mode. These block wise refinements are similar to the hierarchical tree structure (see Fig. 9.4) of the bradycardia operating modes of the pacemaker. The nesting boxes in one- and two-electrode pacemakers (Figs. 9.5 and 9.6) represent equivalent to every refinement level of the hierarchical tree structure (see Fig. 9.4). Special initiating and terminating modes are *on* and *off* respectively of the pacemaker, which are omitted here in the refinement chart block diagram. At the most abstract level, we introduce *pacing* activity into single and both heart chambers. In Figs. 9.5(A) and 9.6(A), *pacing* is represented by transitions *Pace ON* and *Pace OFF* for single chamber or both chambers. It is the basic transitions for all bradycardia operating modes. During a pacing cycle, it is ensured that no other pacing activity has occurred. The model includes: the state of *pacing* (on/off) modelled by a boolean flag *Pacemaker_Actuator*;

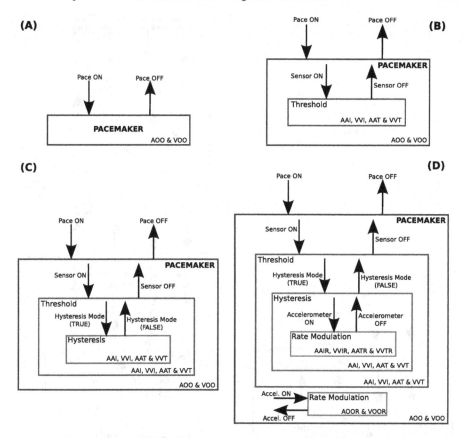

Fig. 9.5   Refinements of one-electrode pacemaker using the refinement chart

the current time control of the pacemaker, is stored in variable *tic*; a safe pacing interval is *Pace_Int* in which the pacemaker should not be paced.

In the next refinement (Figs. 9.5(B), 9.6(B)) step *pacing* is refined by *sensing*, corresponding to the activity of the heart, when sensing period is not under refractory period (RF^2). In the first refinement of two-electrode pacemaker, sensors are introduced in both chambers. In Fig. 9.5(B) of one-electrode, sensing is represented by transitions *Sensor ON* and *Sensor OFF*, while in Fig. 9.6(B) of two-electrode, sensing is represented by transitions *Sensor ON Atria*, *Sensor ON Ventricle*, *Sensor OFF Atria* and *Sensor OFF ventricle*. This refinement introduces: the state of pacemaker sensor (on/off), is modelled by a boolean flag *Pacemaker_Sensor*. The pacemaker's actuator and sensor are synchronising to each other under the real-time constraints. The block diagrams (Figs. 9.5(B), 9.6(B)) represent the *threshold* refinement, that is a measuring unit which measures a stimulation threshold voltage value of the heart and a pulse generator for delivering stimulation pulses to the heart. The

---

[2]RF: Atria Refractory Period (ARP) or Ventricular Refractory Period (VRP).

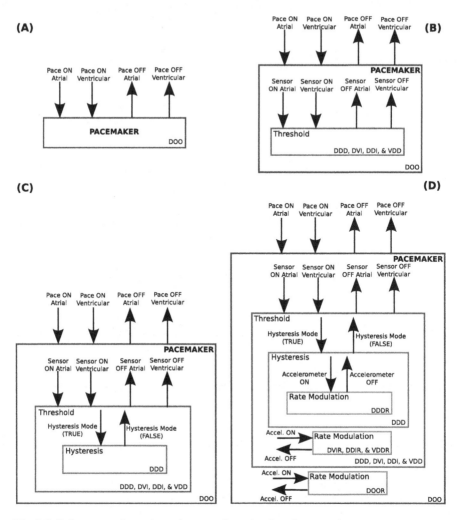

Fig. 9.6 Refinements of two-electrode pacemaker using the refinement chart

pacemaker's sensor starts sensing after the refractory period (*RF*) but pacemaker's actuator delivers a pacing stimulus when sensing value is greater than an equal to the standard threshold constant. Sensor-related transitions are available in all operating modes except AOO, VOO and DOO modes.

Third refinement step (Figs. 9.5(C), 9.6(C)) introduces different operating strategies under *hysteresis* interval: if the *hysteresis* mode is TRUE, then the pacemaker paces at a faster rate than the sensing rate to provide consistent pacing in one chamber (atrial or ventricle) or both chambers (atrial and ventricle), or prevents constant pacing in one chamber (atrial or ventricle) or both chambers (atrial and ventricle). In case of FALSE state of *hysteresis* mode of the pacemaker's sensor and actuator are working in normal state or does not try to maintain the consistent pacing. Hysteresis mode is represented by transitions *Hysteresis Mode TRUE* and *Hysteresis Mode FALSE*. The main objective of hysteresis is to allow the patient to have his or her own underlying rhythm as much as possible. The *hysteresis* operating mode is available in AAI, AAT, VVI, VVT and DDD modes.

According to the last refinement step (Figs. 9.5(D), 9.6(D)), it introduces the rate adapting pacing technique in the bradycardia operating modes of the pacemaker. The rate modulation mode is represented by transitions *Accel. ON* and *Accel. OFF*. The rate modulation operating modes are available in all pacemaker operating modes which are given under multiple refinements. The pacemaker uses the accelerometer sensors to sense the physiologic need of the heart and increase and decrease the pacing rate. The amount of rate increases is determined by the pacemaker based on maximum exertion is performed by the patient. This increased pacing rate is sometimes referred to as the "sensor indicated rate". When exertion has stopped the pacemaker will progressively decrease the pacing rate down to the lower rate.

The next section presents only selected parts of our formalisation and omit proof details. For instance, we have omitted the specification of refinement of every event from all operating modes. Only newly introduced event specifications are given in all refinements. To find more detailed information see the published papers and research reports [40, 43, 48].

9.6 Cardiac Pacemaker Control Requirements

There are several operating modes in the cardiac pacemaker, and DDD operating mode is one of the complex operating mode that contains the features of other operating modes. The data flow and pacing algorithm of DDD cover the functionality of the other operating modes. Therefore, this section presents only the control requirement of the DDD operating mode. As explained above, the DDD operating mode of the pacemaker is used, where the sensors sense intrinsic activities from both chambers and the actuators discharge electrical pulse in both chambers.

Figure 9.7 depicts the scenarios for sensing and pacing activities [4]. In Fig. 9.7, time goes left to right, and a flat line indicates no heart activity. A spike above the lines indicates intrinsic activity and a spike below the line indicates activity as a result of the action of the pacemaker. A rounded spike indicates activity in the atrial and a sharp spike indicates activity in the ventricle. The Ventriculoatrial Interval (VAI) is the maximum time the pacemaker should wait after sensing ventricle activity (either intrinsic or paced) for some indication of intrinsic activity in the atrium. If none is present, the pacemaker should pace in the atrial chamber. The Atrioventricular Interval (AVI) is the maximum time the pacemaker should wait after sensing atrial activity (either intrinsic or paced) for some indication of intrinsic activity in the ventricles. If none is present then the pacemaker should pace in the ventricle chamber. After every pace in the ventricle, there is some sensed activity in the atrial, but this is not true intrinsic heart activity and should be ignored. The Postventricular atrial refractory period (PVARP) indicates the length of time that such activity

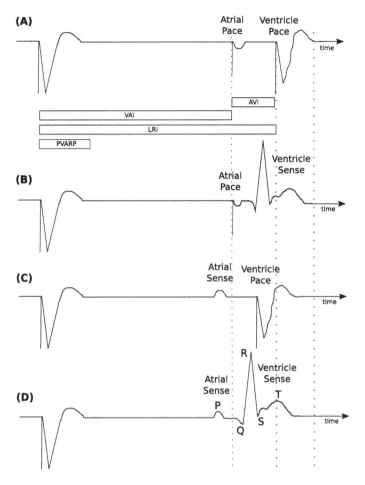

Fig. 9.7 The DDDR pacing scenarios

should be ignored. Sensed atrial activity is called a P wave, and sensed ventricular activity is called a QRS complex. A T wave follows a QRS complex and represents the recovery of the ventricles [57]. There are four possible scenarios for pacing and sensing activities, which are given in Fig. 9.7.

- Scenario A—shows a situation in which the pacemaker paces after a standard time interval in both chambers. This is the reaction when no intrinsic heart activity is detected.
- Scenario B—shows a situation in which the pacemaker paces in the atrial chamber after a standard interval, while the ventricular pacing is inhibited due to a sensing of intrinsic activity from the ventricle.
- Scenario C—shows a situation in which intrinsic atria activity is sensed, pacing inhibited in the atrial chamber but occurs in the ventricular chamber after AVI (due to a lack of intrinsic ventricular activity).

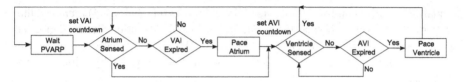

Fig. 9.8 The required DDDR pacing cycle

- Scenario D—represents the case where both pacing activities are inhibited due to a sensing of intrinsic activities in both chambers.

Figure 9.8 gives a flow chart for the basic required operations of the DDD mode. This gives an informal description of the requirements for the pacemaker operating in the DDDR mode. If a ventricle pulse has just been delivered, the pacemaker watches the atrial channel for a spontaneous P wave (intrinsic activity in the atrium). If the VAI times out, the pacer delivers a pacing pulse to the atrium; otherwise, the atrial output is inhibited. The pacemaker now watches the ventricle for a spontaneous QRS complex wave (indicating intrinsic activity in the ventricle). If it is detected, the ventricular pace is inhibited, otherwise the pacemaker delivers a pacing pulse. If the accelerometer detects a change in the patient's activity level, it changes the VAI timeout to compensate—thus speeding up or slowing down the heart beat [57].

9.7 Formal Development of the One-Electrode Cardiac Pacemaker

9.7.1 Context and Initial Model

Abstraction of AOO and VOO Modes

We begin by defining the Event-B context. The context uses sets and constants to define axioms and theorems. Axioms and theorems represent the logical theory of a system. The logical theory is the static properties and properties of the system. In the context, we define constants *LRL* and *URL* that relate to the lower rate limit (minimum number of pace pulses delivered per minute by pacemaker) and upper rate limit (how fast the pacemaker will allow the heart to be paced). These constants are extracted from the pacemaker specification document [7]. The lower rate limit (LRL) must be between 30 and 175 pulse per minute (ppm) and upper rate limit (URL) must be between 50 and 175 pulse per minute (ppm).

The two new constants *URI* and *LRI* represent the corresponding upper rate interval and lower rate interval, respectively. The pacemaker (or pacing) rate is programmed in milliseconds. To convert a heart rate from beats per minute (bpm) to milliseconds, 60,000 is divided by the heart rate. For example, a heart rate of 70 bpm equals 857 milliseconds. In the context, the axioms (*axm*3 and *axm*4) represent the upper rate interval (URI) and lower rate interval (LRI). Additionally, we define an enumerated set *status* of an electrode as ON or OFF states. Finally, we introduce some basic initial properties using defined constants of the system by axioms (*axm*6 and *axm*7).

$$
\begin{array}{l}
axm1 : LRL \in 30 .. 175 \\
axm2 : URL \in 50 .. 175 \\
axm3 : URI \in \mathbb{N}_1 \ \wedge \ URI = 60000/URL \\
axm4 : LRI \in \mathbb{N}_1 \ \wedge \ LRI = 60000/LRL \\
axm5 : status = \{ON, OFF\} \\
axm6 : LRL < URL \\
axm7 : URI < LRI
\end{array}
$$

In the one-electrode pacemaker system, the pacemaker delivers a pacing stimulus in the atrial or the ventricular chamber. In our initial model, we formalise the functional behaviours of the pacemaker system, where a new variable *Pace_Actu* is a pacemaker's actuator, represents the presence or absence of pulse. A variable *Pace_Int* is an interval between two paces, which is initialised by the system before starting the pacing process. A variable *sp* represents the current *clock counter* and a variable *last_sp* represents the last interval (in ms) between two paces. An invariant (*inv*5) states that the clock counter *sp* should be less than or equal to the lower rate interval (LRI). The next two invariants (*inv*6, *inv*7) introduce two variables *Pace_Int_flag* and *last_sp*. The variable *Pace_Int_flag* is defined as a boolean type to represent changing state of the pacing interval (*Pace_Int*), and the variable *last_sp* is used to store an interval between last two heart beats or paces. An invariant (*inv*8) represents safety properties: the pacemaker delivers a pacing stimulus into the heart chamber between upper rate interval (URI) and lower rate interval (LRI). Similarly, the next invariant (*inv*9) represents the states of the pacemaker's actuator under the heart environment as the safety properties, and state that it is never activated between two heart beats, means pacemaker's actuator is OFF during pace interval *Pace_Int*, and pace changing flag is FALSE. The last invariant (*inv*10) states that if pace changing flag is FALSE and the pacemaker's actuator is ON, then the current clock counter *sp* is equal to the pace interval *Pace_Int*.

$$
\begin{array}{l}
inv1 : Pace\_Actu \in status \\
inv2 : Pace\_Int \in URI .. LRI \\
inv3 : sp \in 1 .. \mathbb{N} \\
inv4 : last\_sp \in \mathbb{N} \\
inv5 : sp \leq LRI \\
inv6 : Pace\_Int\_flag \in BOOL \\
inv7 : last\_sp \in \mathbb{N} \\
inv8 : last\_sp \geq URI \ \wedge \ last\_sp \leq LRI \\
inv9 : Pace\_Int\_flag = FALSE \wedge sp < Pace\_Int \ \Rightarrow \ Pace\_Actu = OFF \\
inv10 : Pace\_Int\_flag = FALSE \wedge Pace\_Actu = ON \Rightarrow sp = Pace\_Int
\end{array}
$$

In our abstract specification, there are four events *Pace_ON* to start pacing, *Pace_OFF* to stop pacing, *tic* to increment the current clock counter under the time constraints and *Change_Pace_Int* to update the pace interval. The events *Pace_ON* and *Pace_OFF* start and stop the pulse stimulating into the heart chamber, respectively. The guards of these events synchronise ON and OFF states of the pacemaker system under the time constraints. The action part of event *Pace_ON* sets ON state of the pacemaker's actuator and assigns the value of current clock counter sp to a new variable *last_sp*. Similarly, an action part of the event *Pace_OFF* sets OFF state of the pacemaker's actuator and resets the current clock counter variable sp to 1.

```
EVENT Pace_ON
    WHEN
            grd1 : Pace_Actu = OFF
            grd2 : sp = Pace_Int
    THEN
            act1 : Pace_Actu := ON
            act2 : last_sp := sp
    END
```

```
EVENT Pace_OFF
    WHEN
            grd1 : Pace_Actu = ON
            grd2 : sp = Pace_Int
    THEN
            act1 : Pace_Actu := OFF
            act2 : sp := 1
    END
```

```
EVENT tic
    WHEN
            grd1 : sp < Pace_Int
    THEN
            act1 : sp := sp + 1
    END
```

The pacing and sensing events update a state every millisecond. We model this increment by the event *tic*, that increments time in 1 ms. The event *tic* progressively increases the current clock counter sp under pre-defined pace interval *Pace_Int*. The predicate in guard (*grd1*) of the event *tic* represents an upper bound time limit.

```
EVENT Change_Pace_Int
    WHEN
            grd1 : Pace_Int_flag = TRUE
    THEN
            act1 : Pace_Int :∈ URI .. LRI
    END
```

A new event *Change_Pace_Int* is introduced to update the current value of the pace interval. This event is defined abstractly, which is used in further refinement levels to modify the pace interval according to the introduction of different operating modes like *hysteresis* and *rate modulation*. This event represents that when the pace changing flag (*Pace_Int_flag*) is TRUE then the pace interval (*Pace_Int*) can be chosen from URI to LRI range.

Abstraction of AAI and VVI Modes

In the abstract model of AAI and VVI modes, all the constants, variables and events are common as the abstract model of AOO and VOO modes. In this section, we introduce only extra added new constants, variables and events. We introduce a new constant refractory period *RF* (*Atria Refractory Period* (*ARP*) *or Ventricular Refractory Period* (*VRP*)) that represents a period during which pacemaker timing in the heart chamber is not affected by events. Two new axioms (*axm*1, *axm*2) are introduced in this abstract level. The first axiom (*axm*1) represents a refractory period as a constant and the second axiom (*axm*2) represents a static property.

$$
\begin{array}{l}
axm1 : RF \in 150 \mathinner{\ldotp\ldotp} 500 \\
axm2 : URI > RF
\end{array}
$$

A new variable *Pace_Sensor* as a pacemaker's sensor, is defined as an enumerated type that represents the presence or absence of sensing pulse from the heart chamber and a variable *last_ss* represents the last interval (in ms) between two sensed pulses. Some new invariants are added here that are common to all other operating modes (except AOO and VOO) of the pacemaker system. An invariant (*inv*3) states that the interval between two sensed pulses is greater than or equal to the refractory period *RF* and less than or equal to the pace interval (*Pace_Int*). Invariants (*inv*4, *inv*5) state that the pacemaker's sensor and actuator are always in OFF state during the refractory period *RF*. These are the essential safety properties for the refractory period during which the pacemaker timing must not to be affected by any events that occur. The last invariant (*inv*6) states that when pace changing flag (*Pace_Int_flag*) is FALSE, current clock counter (*sp*) is greater than the refractory period (*RF*) and less than the pacing interval (*Pace_Int*), then the pacemaker's sensor should be ON, means the pacemaker's sensor is ON and continuously sensing the intrinsic activities from the heart chamber within an alert period (*Pace_Int* − *RF*).

$$
\begin{array}{l}
inv1 : Pace\_Sensor \in status \\
inv2 : last\_ss \in \mathbb{N} \\
inv3 : last\_ss \geq RF \wedge last\_ss \leq LRI \\
inv4 : sp < RF \Rightarrow Pace\_Sensor = OFF \\
inv5 : sp < RF \Rightarrow Pace\_Actu = OFF \\
inv6 : Pace\_Int\_flag = FALSE \wedge sp > RF \wedge sp \leq Pace\_Int \Rightarrow \\
\qquad Pace\_Sensor = ON
\end{array}
$$

We introduce extra events *Pace_OFF_with_Sensor* and *Sense_ON* in the abstraction model of the AAI and VVI modes. The guards of event *Pace_OFF_with_Sensor* state that, when the pacemaker's actuator is OFF, pacemaker's sensor is ON and current clock counter *sp* is greater than or equal to the refractory period *RF* then it stores the value of the current clock counter *sp* to the new variable *last_ss*, resets the current clock counter *sp* to 1 and sets OFF state of the pacemaker's sensor. It means that during the alert period (*Pace_Int* − *RF*), the pacemaker inhibits a pacing stimulus and resets the current clock counter whenever it senses an intrinsic activity from the heart chamber.

```
EVENT Pace_OFF_with_Sensor
   WHEN
            grd1 : Pace_Actu = OFF
            grd2 : Pace_Sensor = ON
            grd3 : sp ≥ RF
   THEN
            act1 : last_ss := sp
            act2 : sp := 1
            act3 : Pace_Sensor := OFF
   END
```

The event *Sense_ON* starts the sensing process of pacemaker's sensor when the sensor is OFF and the current clock counter *sp* is greater than or equal to the refractory period *RF* and lower than the pace interval *Pace_Int*. We have added some new guards in the events *Pace_OFF* of AAI and VVI operating modes to control the sensor under the current clock counter *sp*.

```
EVENT Sense_ON
   WHEN
            grd1 : Pace_Sensor = OFF
            grd2 : sp ≥ RF
            grd3 : sp < Pace_Int
   THEN
            act1 : Pace_Actu := ON
   END
```

We have added more real time constraints in the guard (*grd1*) of the event *tic* in all operating modes that control the progressive increment of the current clock counter *sp* as follows:

```
grd1 : (sp < RF ∧ Pace_Sensor = OFF ∧
         Pace_Actu = OFF)
         ∨
         (sp ≥ RF ∧ sp < Pace_Int ∧
         Pace_Sensor = ON ∧ Pace_Actu = OFF)
```

Abstraction of AAT and VVT Modes

The abstract model of AAT and VVT modes are similar to AAI and VVI modes. We introduce a new event *Pace_ON_with_Sensor* in place of event *Pace_OFF_with_Sensor* in this abstract model. The guards of this event state, when the pacemaker's actuator is OFF, the pacemaker's sensor is ON and the current clock counter *sp* is greater than or equal to the refractory period *RF* and less than or equal to pace interval *Pace_Int* then it stores the value of current clock counter *sp* to the variable *last_ss*, and the pacemaker's actuator sets ON under the sensing process. During the alert period (*Pace_Int* − *RF*), the pacemaker delivers a pacing stimulus whenever it senses an intrinsic activity from the heart chamber.

```
EVENT Pace_ON_with_Sensor
  WHEN
          grd1 : Pace_Actu = OFF
          grd2 : Pace_Sensor = ON
          grd3 : sp ≥ RF ∧ sp ≤ Pace_Int
  THEN
          act1 : Pace_Actu := ON
          act2 : last_ss := sp
  END
```

9.7.2 First Refinement: Threshold

The pacemaker control unit delivers stimulation to the heart chamber, on the basis of measured value under the safety margin. We define a new constant *THR* as *THR* ∈ $\mathbb{N}_1$ to hold standard threshold value, and we use the constant nominal threshold value for modelling that is different for the atria and the ventricular chambers.

The pacemaker's sensor starts sensing after the refractory period *RF* but pacemaker's actuator delivers a pacing stimulus when sensing value is greater than or equal to the standard threshold constant *THR*.[3] The first invariant is introduced in operating modes (AAI, VVI) that states that the pacemaker's actuator is OFF, when the pace changing flag (*Pace_Int_flag*) is FALSE, the pacemaker's sensor is ON; an obtained sensor value is greater than or equal to the standard threshold value, the current clock counter *sp* is within the alert period (*Pace_Int* − *RF*) and the state of threshold *thr_val_state* is TRUE. Similarly, the second invariant is introduced in the operating modes (AAT, VVT) that states that the pacemaker's actuator is ON, when the pace changing flag (*Pace_Int_flag*) is FALSE, the pacemaker's sensor is ON, an obtained sensor value is greater than or equal to the standard threshold constant *THR*, the current clock counter *sp* within the alert period (*Pace_Int* − *RF*), and the state of threshold *thr_val_state* is TRUE.

---

[3]Standard threshold constant values of atria and ventricular chambers are different.

$inv1 : Pace\_Int\_flag = FALSE \wedge Pace\_Sensor = ON \wedge thr \geq THR \wedge$
$\qquad sp > RF \wedge sp < Pace\_Int \wedge$
$\qquad thr\_val\_state = TRUE \Rightarrow$
$\qquad Pace\_Actu = OFF$

$inv2 : Pace\_Int\_flag = FALSE \wedge Pace\_Sensor = ON \wedge thr \geq THR \wedge$
$\qquad sp > RF \wedge sp < Pace\_Int \wedge$
$\qquad thr\_val\_state = TRUE \Rightarrow$
$\qquad Pace\_Actu = ON$

A new event *Thr_value* is introduced in all the operating modes (AAI, AAT, VVI and VVT) that obtains a measured value of the heart activities using the pacemaker's sensor. The guards of this event state that when the pacemaker's sensor is ON, the current clock counter *sp* is within the alert period (*Pace_Int* − *RF*) and the state of threshold value *thr_val_state* is TRUE then the sensed value *th* is assigned to the threshold variable *thr* and the state of threshold variable *thr_val_state* becomes FALSE.

EVENT Thr_value
   ANY
     th
   WHERE
        $grd1 : Pace\_Sensor = ON$
        $grd2 : sp \geq RF \ \wedge \ sp < Pace\_Int$
        $grd3 : thr\_val\_state = TRUE$
        $grd4 : th \in \mathbb{N}$
   THEN
        $act1 : thr := th$
        $act2 : thr\_val\_state := FALSE$
   END

In this refinement, we have added a new guard $thr \geq THR$ in the events (*Pace_OFF_with_Sensor* and *Pace_ON_with_Sensor*). Moreover, we modify the guard (*grd1*) of the event (*tic*) to synchronise the pacing-sensing events with a new threshold functional behaviour under the real-time constraints.

$grd1 : (sp < RF \wedge Pace\_Sensor = OFF \wedge$
$\qquad Pace\_Actu = OFF)$
$\qquad \vee$
$\qquad (sp \geq RF \wedge sp < Pace\_Int \wedge$
$\qquad Pace\_Sensor = ON \wedge Pace\_Actu = OFF \wedge$
$\qquad thr < THR \wedge thr\_val\_state = FALSE)$

9.7.3 Second Refinement: Hysteresis

Hysteresis is a programmed feature whereby the pacemaker paces at a faster rate than the sensing rate. For example, pacing at 80 pulses a minute with a hysteresis rate of 55 means that the pacemaker will be inhibited at all rates down to 55 beats per minute, having been activated at a rate below 55, the pacemaker then switches on and paces at 80 pulses a minute [22, 39]. The application of the hysteresis interval provides consistent pacing of the atrial or ventricle, or prevents constant pacing of the atrial or ventricle. The main purpose of hysteresis is to allow the patient to have his or her own underlying rhythm as much as possible. Two new variables (*Hyt_Pace_Int_flag*, *HYT_State*) are introduced to define the functional properties of the hysteresis operating modes. Both variables are defined as a boolean type. The hysteresis state *HYT_State* is used to set the hysteresis functional parameter as TRUE or FALSE, to apply the hysteresis operating modes.

$$\begin{array}{l} inv1 : Hyt\_Pace\_Int\_flag \in BOOL \\ inv2 : HYT\_State \in BOOL \end{array}$$

A new event *Hyt_Pace_Updating* is introduced to implement the functional properties of the hysteresis operating modes. In the hysteresis operating modes, the pacemaker tries to maintain own heart rhythm as much as possible. Hence, this event can change the pacing interval and set a pacing length longer than existing, which changes the pacing length of the cardiac pacemaker. This event is only used for updating the pacing interval (*Pace_Int*). Guards of this event state that the pace changing flag (*Pace_Int_flag*) is TRUE, the hysteresis pacing flag (*Hyt_Pace_Int_flag*) is TRUE and the hysteresis pace interval (*Hyt_Pace_Int*) should be within the range of the pace interval (*Pace_Int*) and lower rate interval (*LRI*). Actions of this event state that a new hysteresis pace interval (*Hyt_Pace_Int*) updates the pace interval *Pace_Int*, the hysteresis pacing flag (*Hyt_Pace_Int_flag*) sets to FALSE and the hysteresis state (*HYT_State*) becomes TRUE.

```
EVENT Hyt_Pace_Updating Refines Change_Pace_Int
   ANY
      Hyt_Pace_Int
   WHERE
         grd1 : Pace_Int_flag = TRUE
         grd2 : Hyt_Pace_Int_flag = TRUE
         grd3 : Hyt_Pace_Int ∈ Pace_Int .. LRI
   THEN
         act1 : Pace_Int := Hyt_Pace_Int
         act2 : Hyt_Pace_Int_flag := FALSE
         act3 : HYT_State := TRUE
   END
```

9.7.4 Third Refinement: Rate Modulation

Rate modulation term is used to describe the capacity of a pacing system to respond to physiologic needs by increasing and decreasing pacing rate. The rate modulation mode of the pacemaker can progressively pace faster than the lower rate, but no more than the upper sensor rate limit, when it determines that heart rate needs to increase. This typically occurs with exercise in patients who cannot increase their own heart rate. The amount of rate increases is determined by the pacemaker based on maximum exertion is performed by the patient. This increased pacing rate is sometimes referred to as the "sensor indicated rate". When exertion has stopped the pacemaker will progressively decrease the paced rate down to the lower rate.

In this last refinement, we introduce the rate modulation function and found some new operating modes (AOOR, VOOR, AAIR, VVIR, AATR and VVTR) of the pacemaker system. For modelling the rate modulation, we introduce some new constants maximum sensor rate MSR as $MSR \in 50 .. 175$ and acc_thr as $acc\_thr \in \mathbb{N}_1$ using axioms ($axm1$, $axm2$). The maximum sensor rate (MSR) is the maximum pacing rate allowed as a result of sensor control, and it must be between 50 and 175 pulse per minute (ppm). The constant acc_thr represents the activity threshold. Axiom ($axm3$) represents a static property for the rate modulation operating modes.

$$
\begin{array}{l}
axm1 : MSR \in 50 .. 175 \\
axm2 : acc\_thr \in \mathbb{N}_1 \\
axm3 : MSR = URL
\end{array}
$$

Two new variables $acler\_sensed$ and $acler\_sensed\_flag$ are defined as to store a measured value from the accelerometer and boolean type of the accelerometer sensor. Boolean type of the accelerometer sensor is used to synchronise with other functionalities of the system. The accelerometer is used to measure the physical activities of the body in the pacemaker system. Two new invariants ($inv3$, $inv4$) provide the safety margin and state that the heart rate never falls below the lower rate limit (LRL) and never exceeds the maximum sensor rate (MSR) limit.

$$
\begin{array}{l}
inv1 : acler\_sensed \in \mathbb{N} \\
inv2 : acler\_sensed\_flag \in BOOL \\
inv3 : HYT\_State = FALSE \wedge acler\_sensed < acc\_thr \wedge \\
\qquad acler\_sensed\_flag = TRUE \Rightarrow Pace\_Int = 60000/LRL \\
inv4 : HYT\_State = FALSE \wedge acler\_sensed => \geq acc\_thr \wedge \\
\qquad acler\_sensed\_flag = TRUE \Rightarrow Pace\_Int = 60000/MSR
\end{array}
$$

In this final refinement, we introduce two new events *Increase_Interval* and *Decrease_Interval*, which are the refinement of event *Change_Pace_Int*. These new events are used to control the pacing rate of the one-electrode pacemaker in the rate modulating operating modes. The new events *Increase_Interval* and *Decrease_Interval* control the value of the pace interval variable *Pace_Int*, whenever a measured value (*acler_sensed*) from the accelerometer sensor goes higher or lower than the activity threshold *acc_thr*.

```
EVENT Increase_Interval Refines Change_Pace_Int
   WHEN
          grd1 : Pace_Int_flag = TRUE
          grd1 : acler_sensed ≥ threshold
          grd1 : HYT_State = FALSE
   THEN
          act1 : Pace_Int := 60000/MSR
          act1 : acler_sensed_flag := TRUE
   END
```

```
EVENT Decrease_Interval Refines Change_Pace_Int
   WHEN
          grd1 : Pace_Int_flag = TRUE
          grd1 : acler_sensed < threshold
          grd1 : HYT_State = FALSE
   THEN
          act1 : Pace_Int := 60000/LRL
          act1 : acler_sensed_flag := TRUE
   END
```

A new event (*Acler_sensed*) is defined as to simulate the behaviour of accelerometer sensor. This event senses continue the motion of the body to increase or decrease the length of the pace interval (*Pace_Int*). In this event, the guards state that the accelerometer sensor flag is TRUE and the hysteresis state is FALSE. A new variable *acl_sen* is used to store the current sensing value. Actions of this event state that a local variable *acl_sen* updates accelerometer sensor (*acler_sensed*) and the accelerometer sensor flag (*acler_sensed_flag*) becomes FALSE.

```
EVENT Acler_sensed
   ANY
      acl_sen
   WHERE
          grd1 : acl_sen ∈ ℕ
          grd1 : acler_sensed_flag = TRUE
          grd1 : HYT_State = FALSE
   THEN
          act1 : acler_sensed := acl_sen
          act1 : acler_sensed_flag := FALSE
   END
```

In the next section, we explore the formal model of the two-electrode pacemaker system using incremental refinements.

9.8   Formal Development of the Two-Electrode Cardiac Pacemaker

9.8.1 Context and Abstract Model

In this section, we describe the formal development of initial modes of the two-electrode pacemaker system using the basic notion of action-reaction and real-time constraints, to focus on pacing and sensing activities of the pacemaker's actuator and sensor. The initial context of the two-electrode pacemaker is similar to the one-electrode pacemaker. We give here only newly defined constants and axioms. A new constant atrioventricular (AV) interval (FixedAV) is defined in *axm*8. Refractory period constants Atria Refractory Period (ARP), Ventricular Refractory Period (VRP) and Post Ventricular Atria Refractory Period (PVARP) are defined by axioms (*axm*9, *axm*10 and *axm*11). Another new constant *V_Blank* is defined as blanking period as an initial period of VRP. Finally, we introduce some basic initial properties using defined constants of the system by axioms (*axm*13, *axm*14 and *axm*15).

$$
\begin{aligned}
&axm8 : FixedAV \in 70 .. 300 \\
&axm9 : ARP \in 150 .. 500 \\
&axm10 : VRP \in 150 .. 500 \\
&axm11 : PVARP \in 150 .. 500 \\
&axm12 : V\_Blank \in 30 .. 60 \\
&axm13 : URI > PVARP \\
&axm14 : URI > VRP \\
&axm15 : VRP \geq PVARP
\end{aligned}
$$

Abstraction of DDD Mode

In the two-electrode pacemaker system, the pacemaker delivers a pacing stimulus in both atrial and ventricular chambers. In DDD operating mode, the first letter 'D' represents that the pacemaker paces in both atrial and ventricle chambers; second letter 'D' represents that the pacemaker senses intrinsic activities from both atrial and ventricle chambers and final letter 'D' represents two conditional meaning that depends on atrial and ventricular sensing; first is that atrial sensing inhibits atrial pacing and triggers ventricular pacing and second is that ventricular sensing inhibits ventricular and atrial pacing [22, 35].

Two new variables *PM_Actuator_A* and *PM_Actuator_V* are defined that represent ON or OFF state of the pacemaker's actuators for pacing in both atrial and ventricular chambers. Similarly next two variables *PM_Sensor_A* and *PM_Sensor_V* represent ON or OFF state of the pacemaker's sensor for sensing an intrinsic pulse from both atrial and ventricular chambers. An interval between two paces is defined by a new variable *Pace_Int* that must be between upper rate interval (URI) and lower rate interval (LRI), is represented by an invariant (*inv*5). A variable *sp* represents the current *clock counter*. A variable *last_sp* represents the last interval (in ms) between two paces, and a safety property in invariant (*inv*7) states that the last interval must be between PVARP and pace interval *Pace_Int*. Another new variable *AV_Count_STATE* is defined as a boolean type to control the atrioventricular (AV) interval state and the next variable *AV_Count* is defined as a natural number to count the atrioventricular (AV) interval. A variable (*Pace_Int_flag*) is defined as a boolean type to represent changing state of the pace interval (*Pace_Int*). Invariants (*inv*11, *inv*12 and *inv*13) represent the safety properties. The invariant *inv*11 states that, when the clock counter *sp* is less than VRP and atrioventricular (AV) counter state *AV_Count_State* is FALSE, then the pacemaker's actuators and sensors of both chambers are OFF. Similarly, the next invariants (*inv*12 and *inv*13) represent the conditions of ON state of the pacemaker's actuators in the both chambers.

$$
\begin{aligned}
&inv1 : PM\_Actuator\_A \in status \\
&inv2 : PM\_Actuator\_V \in status \\
&inv3 : PM\_Sensor\_A \in status \\
&inv4 : PM\_Sensor\_V \in status \\
&inv5 : Pace\_Int \in URI \mathinner{.\,.} LRI \\
&inv6 : sp \in 1 \mathinner{.\,.} Pace\_Int \\
&inv7 : last\_sp \geq PVARP \wedge last\_sp \leq Pace\_Int \\
&inv8 : AV\_Count\_STATE \in BOOL \\
&inv9 : AV\_Count \in \mathbb{N} \\
&inv10 : Pace\_Int\_flag \in BOOL \\
\\
&inv11 : sp < VRP \wedge AV\_Count\_STATE = FALSE \\
&\qquad\quad \Rightarrow \\
&\qquad\quad PM\_Actuator\_V = OFF \wedge \\
&\qquad\quad PM\_Sensor\_A = OFF \wedge \\
&\qquad\quad PM\_Sensor\_V = OFF \wedge \\
&\qquad\quad PM\_Actuator\_A = OFF \\
\\
&inv12 : Pace\_Int\_flag = FALSE \wedge PM\_Actuator\_V = ON \\
&\qquad\quad \Rightarrow \\
&\qquad\quad sp = Pace\_Int \vee (sp < Pace\_Int \wedge \\
&\qquad\quad AV\_Count > V\_Blank \wedge AV\_Count \geq FixedAV) \\
\\
&inv13 : Pace\_Int\_flag = FALSE \wedge PM\_Actuator\_A = ON \\
&\qquad\quad \Rightarrow \\
&\qquad\quad (sp \geq Pace\_Int - FixedAV)
\end{aligned}
$$

In the abstract specification of DDD operating mode, there are ten events *Actuator_ON_A* to start pacing in atrial, *Actuator_OFF_A* to stop pacing in atrial, *Actuator_ON_V* to start pacing in ventricular, *Actuator_OFF_V* to stop pacing in ventricular, *Sensor_ON_V* to start sensing in ventricular, *Sensor_OFF_V* to stop sensing in ventricular, *Sensor_ON_A* to star sensing in atrial, *Sensor_OFF_A* to stop sensing in atrial, *tic* to increment the current clock counter *sp* under the real time constraints and *tic_AV* to count the atrioventricular (AV) interval.

```
EVENT Actuator_ON_V
  WHEN
    grd1 : PM_Actuator_V = OFF
    grd2 : (sp = Pace_Int)
              ∨
           (sp < Pace_Int ∧ AV_Count > V_Blank ∧
            AV_Count ≥ FixedAV)
    grd3 : sp ≥ VRP ∧ sp ≥ PVARP
  THEN
    act1 : PM_Actuator_V := ON
    act2 : last_sp := sp
  END
```

The events *Actuator_ON_V* and *Actuator_OFF_V* are used to start and stop the pacemaker's actuator in the ventricular chamber under the real-time constraints. In the event (*Actuator_ON_V*), the first guard states that the pacemaker's actuator (*PM_Actuator_V*) of the ventricular is OFF, the next guard (*grd2*) states that the current clock counter *sp* is either equal to the pace interval *Pace_Int* or the clock counter *sp* is less than the pace interval *Pace_Int*, the atrioventricular counter is greater than the blanking period *V_Blank* and the atrioventricular counter is greater than the fixed atrioventricular interval *FixedAV*. The last guard (*grd3*) states that the clock counter *sp* is greater than or equal to the VRP and PVARP. The actions of this event show that when all guards are true then the pacemaker's actuator (*PM_Actuator_V*) of ventricular sets ON and assigns a value of the clock counter *sp* into other variable *last_sp*.

```
EVENT Actuator_OFF_V
  WHEN
    grd1 : PM_Actuator_V = ON
    grd2 : (sp = Pace_Int)
              ∨
           (sp < Pace_Int ∧ AV_Count > V_Blank ∧
            AV_Count ≥ FixedAV)
    grd3 : AV_Count_STATE = TRUE
    grd4 : PM_Actuator_A = OFF
    grd5 : PM_Sensor_A = OFF
  THEN
    act1 : PM_Actuator_V := OFF
    act2 : AV_Count := 0
    act3 : AV_Count_STATE := FALSE
    act4 : PM_Sensor_V := OFF
    act5 : sp := 1
  END
```

First two guards of the event (*Actuator_OFF_V*) state that the pacemaker's actuator (*PM_Actuator_V*) of ventricular is ON, and the clock counter (*sp*) is equal to the pace interval (*Pace_Int*), or less than the pace interval (*Pace_Int*), the atrioventricular (AV) counter (*AV_Count*) is greater than the blanking period (*V_Blank*) and the atrioventricular (AV) counter is greater than or equal to the atrioventricular (AV) interval (*FixedAV*). Third guard (*grd3*) states that the atrioventricular (AV) counter state (*AV_Count_STATE*) is TRUE, and the last two guards represent that the pacemaker's actuator and sensor (*PM_Actuator_A, PM_Sensor_A*) of atrial is OFF. In action's part, sets OFF state of the pacemaker's actuator (*PM_Actuator_V*) of ventricular, reassigns the value of variable (*AV_count*) as 0, sets FALSE state to the AV counter state (*AV_Count_STATE*), sets OFF state to the pacemaker's Sensor (*PM_Sensor_V*) of the ventricular chamber and finally assigns the value of the clock counter (*sp*) as 1.

EVENT Actuator_ON_A
  WHEN
    grd1 : $PM\_Sensor\_V = ON$
    grd2 : $sp \geq Pace\_Int - FixedAV \wedge$
            $sp \geq VRP \wedge sp \geq PVARP$
    grd3 : $PM\_Actuator\_A = OFF$
    grd4 : $PM\_Sensor\_A = ON$
  THEN
    act1 : $PM\_Actuator\_A := ON$
    act2 : $PM\_Sensor\_V := OFF$
    act3 : $PM\_Sensor\_A := OFF$
  END

A set of new events *Actuator_ON_A* and *Actuator_OFF_A* are introduced to start and stop the pacemaker's actuator in the atrial chamber. Actions (*act1–act3*) of the event (*Actuator_ON_A*) state that the pacemaker's actuator (*PM_Actuator_A*) of the atria sets ON and the pacemaker's sensors (*PM_Sensor_V, PM_Sensor_A*) of the ventricular and atrial set OFF when all the guards satisfy. The first guard of this event states that the pacemaker's sensor (*PM_Sensor_V*) of ventricular is ON, the next guard (*grd2*) states that the clock counter (*sp*) is greater than or equal to the ventriculoatrial (VA) interval, VRP and PVARP, the third guard shows that the pacemaker's actuator (*PM_Actuator_A*) of atrial is OFF and last guard states that the pacemaker's sensor (*PM_Sensor_A*) of atrial is ON.

EVENT Actuator_OFF_A
  WHEN
    grd1 : $PM\_Actuator\_A = ON$
    grd2 : $sp \geq Pace\_Int - FixedAV \wedge$
            $sp \geq VRP \wedge sp \geq PVARP$
    grd3 : $AV\_Count\_STATE = FALSE$
  THEN
    act1 : $PM\_Actuator\_A := OFF$
    act2 : $AV\_Count\_STATE := TRUE$
  END

First two actions (*act1, act2*) of the event (*Actuator_OFF_A*) state that the pacemaker's actuator (*PM_Actuator_A*) of atria is OFF and the atrioventricular (AV) counter state (*AV_Count_STATE*) is TRUE. The guards (*grd1*, *grd2*) of this event state that the acemaker's actuator (*PM_Actuator_A*) of the atria is ON, the current clock counter (*sp*) is greater than or equal to the ventriculoatrial (VA) interval, VRP and PVARP. The last guard presents that the atrioventricular (AV) counter state (*AV_Count_STATE*) is FALSE.

```
EVENT Sensor_ON_V
  WHEN
    grd1 : PM_Sensor_V = OFF
    grd2 : (sp ≥ VRP ∧ sp < Pace_Int − FixedAV∧
                PM_Sensor_A = ON)
            ∨
           (sp ≥ Pace_Int − FixedAV ∧
            AV_Count_STATE = TRUE)
    grd3 : PM_Actuator_A = OFF
  THEN
    act1 : PM_Sensor_V := ON
  END
```

The events (*Sensor_ON_V* and *Sensor_OFF_V*) are used to control the sensing activities from the ventricular chamber. The pacemaker's sensor (*PM_Sensor_V*) of ventricular chamber synchronises ON and OFF states under the real-time constraints. The pacemaker's sensor (*PM_Sensor_V*) of the ventricular is ON when all guards are satisfied. The event (*Sensor_OFF_V*) is used to set the pacemaker's sensor (*PM_Sensor_V*) of the ventricular as OFF and resets all other variables in the action part when all guards fulfil the required conditions. The guards represent the different states of the pacemaker's actuators and sensors under the real-time constraints with various time interval parameters (i.e. VRP, PVARP, *Pace_Int*, etc.).

```
EVENT Sensor_OFF_V
  WHEN
    grd1 : PM_Sensor_V = ON
    grd2 : sp ≥ VRP ∧ sp ≥ PVARP
    grd3 : (sp < Pace_Int − FixedAV)
            ∨
           (sp ≥ Pace_Int − FixedAV ∧
            sp < Pace_Int)
    grd4 : PM_Actuator_V = OFF
    grd5 : PM_Actuator_A = OFF
  THEN
    act1 : PM_Sensor_V := OFF
    act2 : AV_Count := 0
    act3 : AV_Count_STATE := FALSE
    act4 : last_sp := sp
    act5 : sp := 1
    act6 : PM_Sensor_A := OFF
  END
```

The event (*Sensor_OFF_V*) is used to set the pacemaker's sensor (*PM_Sensor_V*) of ventricular in OFF state. The guards (*grd*1, *grd*2) of this event represent that the pacemaker's sensor (*PM_Sensor_V*) of ventricular is ON, and the clock counter (*sp*) is greater than or equal to the VRP and PVARP. The next guard (*grd*3) represents that the clock counter *sp* is less than the ventriculoatrial (VA) interval, or greater than or equal to the ventriculoatrial (VA) interval and less than the pace interval (*Pace_Int*). The last two guards (*grd*4, *grd*5) state that the pacemaker's actuators (*PM_Actuator_V*, *PM_Actuator_A*) of the ventricular and atrial are OFF. The actions (*act*1–*act*6) of this event state that the pacemaker's sensor (*PM_Sensor_V*) of ventricular is OFF, assigns the value of variable (*AV_count*) as 0, the atrioventricular (AV) counter state (*AV_Count_STATE*) sets FALSE, assigns the value of the clock counter (*sp*) to new variable (*last_sp*), assigns the value of the clock counter (*sp*) as 1 and sets OFF state of the pacemaker's actuator (*PM_Actuator_A*) of atrial.

```
EVENT Sensor_ON_A
  WHEN
    grd1 : PM_Sensor_A = OFF
    grd2 : sp < Pace_Int − FixedAV ∧
                  sp ≥ VRP ∧ sp ≥ PVARP
    grd3 : PM_Sensor_V = OFF
  THEN
    act1 : PM_Sensor_A := ON
  END
```

The events (*Sensor_ON_A* and *Sensor_OFF_A*) are used to control the sensing activities of the atrial chamber. The pacemaker's sensor (*PM_Sensor_A*) of the atrial chamber synchronises ON and OFF states under the real time constraints. A guard (*grd*1) of the event (*Sensor_ON_A*) represents that if the pacemaker's sensor (*PM_Sensor_A*) of atrial is OFF and the second guard (*grd*2) represents that the clock counter (*sp*) is less than the ventriculoatrial (VA) interval and greater than or equal to the VRP and PVARP. The last guard (*grd*3) represents that the pacemaker's sensor (*PM_Sensor_V*) of ventricular is OFF. If all guards are true, then in action part of this event the pacemaker's sensor (*PM_Sensor_A*) of atrial sets ON.

```
EVENT Sensor_OFF_A
  WHEN
    grd1 : PM_Sensor_A = ON
    grd2 : sp < Pace_Int − FixedAV ∧
                sp ≥ VRP ∧ sp ≥ PVARP
  THEN
    act1 : PM_Sensor_A := OFF
    act2 : AV_Count_STATE := TRUE
  END
```

The event (*Sensor_OFF_A*) is used to set the pacemaker's sensor (*PM_Sensor_A*) of atrial in OFF state. The guards of this event represent that the pacemaker's sensor

(*PM_Sensor_A*) of atrial is ON, and the clock counter (*sp*) is less than the ventriculoatrial (VA) interval and greater than or equal to the VRP and PVARP. In actions of
this event state that the pacemaker's sensor (*PM_Sensor_A*) of atrial sets OFF and
the atrioventricular (AV) counter state (*AV_Count_STATE*) sets TRUE.

```
EVENT tic
  WHEN
    grd1 : (sp < VRP)
             ∨
           (sp ≥ VRP ∧ sp < Pace_Int − FixedAV ∧
            PM_Sensor_A = ON ∧ PM_Sensor_V = ON
  THEN
    act1 : sp := sp + 1
  END
```

The event (*tic*) of this abstraction progressively increases the current clock
counter *sp* under the pre-defined pace interval (*Pace_Int*). This event controls the
time line of pacing and sensing events. A guard (*grd1*) of this event provides the required conditions to increase the clock counter *sp* by 1 (ms). The last event (*tic_AV*)
of this abstraction progressively counts the atrioventricular (AV) interval and increases the current clock counter *sp* is represented by actions *act1* and *act2*, respectively.

```
EVENT tic_AV
  WHEN
    grd1 : AV_Count < FixedAV
    grd2 : AV_Count_STATE = TRUE
    grd3 : (sp ≥ VRP ∧ sp ≥ PVARP ∧
            sp < Pace_Int − FixedAV)
             ∨
           (sp ≥ Pace_Int − FixedAV ∧
            sp < Pace_Int)
  THEN
    act1 : AV_Count := AV_Count + 1
    act2 : sp := sp + 1
  END
```

A new event *Change_Pace_Int* is introduced to update the current value of the
pace interval. This event is defined abstractly, which is used in further refinement
levels to modify the pace interval according to the introduction of different operating
modes like hysteresis and rate modulation. This event represents that when pace
changing flag (*Pace_Int_flag*) is TRUE then the pace interval (*Pace_Int*) can be
chosen from URI to LRI ranges.

```
EVENT Change_Pace_Int
  WHEN
          grd1 : Pace_Int_flag = TRUE
  THEN
          act1 : Pace_Int :∈ URI .. LRI
  END
```

Abstraction of DVI Mode

In DVI operating mode of the two-electrode pacemaker system, the first letter 'D' represents that the pacemaker paces both atrial and ventricle; second letter 'V' represents that the pacemaker only senses the ventricle and final letter 'I' represents that the ventricular sensing inhibits atrial and ventricular pacing [22, 35].

In this subsection, we formalise the operating mode (DVI) of the two-electrode pacemaker system. Variables, constants and some invariants ($inv1$, $inv2$ and $inv4$–$inv10$) are similar to the previous operating mode; DDD. More invariants are introduced in this operating mode (DVI) as the safety properties. Invariant ($inv11$) states that, when the clock counter sp is less than VRP, then the pacemaker's actuator of both chambers and pacemaker's sensor of ventricular are OFF. Next two invariants ($inv12$ and $inv13$) state that, when the pacemaker's actuator ($PM\_Actuator\_A$) of atrial is ON, then the clock counter sp is greater than or equal to the ventriculoatrial (VA) interval $Pace\_Int$-$FixedAV$ and when the pacemaker's actuator ($PM\_Actuator\_V$) of ventricular is ON, then the clock counter sp is equal to the pace interval $Pace\_Int$, respectively.

$$inv11 : sp < VRP \Rightarrow PM\_Actuator\_A = OFF \wedge$$
$$PM\_Actuator\_V = OFF \wedge$$
$$PM\_Sensor\_V = OFF$$
$$inv12 : Pace\_Int\_flag = FALSE \wedge PM\_Actuator\_A = ON \Rightarrow$$
$$sp \geq Pace\_Int - FixedAV$$
$$inv13 : Pace\_Int\_flag = FALSE \wedge PM\_Actuator\_V = ON \Rightarrow sp = Pace\_Int$$

In the abstract specification of DVI operating mode, there are eight events $Actuator\_ON\_A$ to start pacing in atrial, $Actuator\_OFF\_A$ to stop pacing in atrial, $Actuator\_ON\_V$ to start pacing in ventricular, $Actuator\_OFF\_V$ to stop pacing in ventricular, $Sensor\_ON\_V$ to start sensing in ventricular, $Sensor\_OFF\_V$ to stop sensing in ventricular, tic to increment the current clock counter sp under the real time constraints and tic_AV to count the atrioventricular (AV) interval. All these events are similar to the DDD operating modes, which are already described. The guards of events are not exactly similar to the DDD operating modes. The guards and actions are changed according to the requirements of the DVI operating mode.

Abstraction of DDI Mode

In DDI operating mode of the two-electrode pacemaker system, the first letter 'D' represents that the pacemaker paces both atrial and ventricle; second letter 'D' represents that the pacemaker senses both atrial and ventricle and final letter 'I' represents two conditional meaning that depends on atrial and ventricular sensing; first, atrial sensing inhibits atrial pacing and does not trigger ventricular pacing and second, ventricular sensing inhibits ventricular and atrial pacing [22, 35].

We formalise the operating mode DDI of the two-electrode pacemaker system. Variables, constants and some invariants ($inv1$–$inv10$) are similar to the previous operating mode; DDD. Invariant ($inv11$) states that, when the clock counter sp is less than the VRP, and the atrioventricular (AV) counter state (AV_Count_STATE) is TRUE, then the pacemaker's actuators and sensors of both chambers are OFF. The next invariant ($inv12$) represents that, when the pacemaker's actuator of ventricular is ON, then the clock counter sp is equal to the pace interval $Pace\_Int$.

$$
\begin{aligned}
&inv11 : sp < VRP \wedge AV\_Count\_STATE = FALSE \Rightarrow \\
&\qquad PM\_Actuator\_A = OFF \wedge \\
&\qquad PM\_Actuator\_V = OFF \wedge \\
&\qquad PM\_Sensor\_A = OFF \wedge \\
&\qquad PM\_Sensor\_V = OFF \\
&inv12 : Pace\_Int\_flag = FALSE \wedge PM\_Actuator\_V = ON \Rightarrow sp = Pace\_Int
\end{aligned}
$$

In the abstract specification of the DDI operating mode, there are ten events exactly similar to the DDD operating mode, which are already described. The guards and actions of the events are changed according to the DDI operating mode requirements.

Abstraction of VDD Mode

In VDD operating mode of the two-electrode pacemaker system, the first letter 'V' represents that the pacemaker only paces ventricle; second letter 'D' represents that the pacemaker senses both atrial and ventricle and final letter 'D' represents two conditional meanings that depend on atrial and ventricular sensing; first, atrial sensing triggers ventricular pacing and second, ventricular sensing inhibits ventricular pacing [22, 35].

In this model, we formalise the functional behaviours of the pacemaker system in VDD operating mode, where all variables, constants and invariants ($inv2$–$inv10$) are similar to the previously described DDD operating mode. Here, a new invariant ($inv11$) states that, when the clock counter sp is less than VRP and the atrioventricular (AV) counter state (AV_Count_STATE) is FALSE, then the pacemaker's actuator ($PM\_Actuator\_V$) of the ventricular is OFF, and the pacemaker's sensors of both chambers are OFF. Next invariant ($inv12$) represents that, when the pacemaker's actuator ($PM\_Actuator\_V$) of ventricular is ON, then the clock counter sp is either equal to the pace interval $Pace\_Int$ or the clock counter sp is less than the pace interval $Pace\_Int$ and the atrioventricular (AV) counter (AV_Count) is greater than the

blanking period (*V_Blank*), and greater than or equal to the fixed atrioventricular
(AV) period (*FixedAV*).

$$inv11 : sp < VRP \wedge AV\_Count\_STATE = FALSE \Rightarrow$$
$$PM\_Actuator\_V = OFF \wedge$$
$$PM\_Sensor\_A = OFF \wedge$$
$$PM\_Sensor\_V = OFF$$
$$inv12 : Pace\_Int\_flag = FALSE \wedge PM\_Actuator\_V = ON \Rightarrow$$
$$(sp = Pace\_Int$$
$$\vee$$
$$(sp < Pace\_Int \wedge$$
$$AV\_Count > V\_Blank \wedge$$
$$AV\_Count \geq FixedAV))$$

In the abstract specification of VDD operating mode, there are eight events *Actuator_ON_V* to start pacing in ventricular, *Actuator_OFF_V* to stop pacing in ventricular, *Sensor_ON_V* to start sensing in ventricular, *Sensor_OFF_V* to stop sensing in ventricular, *Sensor_ON_A* to star sensing in atrial, *Sensor_OFF_A* to stop sensing in atrial, *tic* to increment the current clock counter *sp* under the real time constraints and *tic_AV* to count the atrioventricular (AV) interval. All these events are similar to the DDD operating modes, which are already described.

Abstraction of DOO Mode

In DOO operating mode of the two-electrode pacemaker system, the first letter 'D' represents that the pacemaker paces both atrial and ventricle, second letter 'O' represents that the pacemaker does not sense the atrial and ventricular chambers and final letter 'O' represents that there is no any inhibits or triggers modes in both chambers [22, 35].

In this model, we formalise the functional behaviours of the pacemaker system of DOO operating mode, where all variables, constants and invariants (*inv1*, *inv2* and *inv5–inv10*) are similar to the previous operating mode; DDD. New invariant (*inv11*) states that the pacemaker's actuator of the atrial and ventricular chambers are OFF, when the clock counter *sp* is less than the ventriculoatrial (VA) interval, and the atrial state (*Atria_state*) is FALSE. The next invariant (*inv12*) states that the pacemaker's actuators of both chambers are OFF, when the clock counter *sp* is greater than the atrioventricular (AV) interval, and the atrial state (*Atria_state*) is TRUE. The last invariants (*inv13* and *inv14*) state that, when the pacemaker's actuator of atrial is ON, then the clock counter *sp* is greater than or equal to the ventriculoatrial (VA) interval (*Pace_Int-FixedAV*) and when the pacemaker's actuator of the ventricular is ON, then the clock counter *sp* is equal to the pace interval *Pace_Int*, respectively.

$$
\begin{aligned}
inv11 : &\ Pace\_Int\_flag = FALSE \wedge sp < (Pace\_Int - FixedAV) \wedge \\
        &\ Atria\_state = FALSE \Rightarrow \\
        &\ PM\_Actuator\_V = OFF \wedge \\
        &\ PM\_Actuator\_A = OFF \\
inv12 : &\ Pace\_Int\_flag = FALSE \wedge sp > (Pace\_Int - FixedAV) \wedge \\
        &\ sp < Pace\_Int \wedge \\
        &\ Atria\_state = TRUE \Rightarrow \\
        &\ PM\_Actuator\_A = OFF \wedge \\
        &\ PM\_Actuator\_V = OFF \\
inv13 : &\ Pace\_Int\_flag = FALSE \wedge PM\_Actuator\_A = ON \Rightarrow \\
        &\ sp = Pace\_Int - FixedAV \\
inv14 : &\ Pace\_Int\_flag = FALSE \wedge PM\_Actuator\_V = ON \Rightarrow sp = Pace\_Int
\end{aligned}
$$

In the abstract specification of DOO operating mode, there are five events *Pace_ON_A* to start pacing in atrial, *Pace_OFF_A* to stop pacing in atrial, *Pace_ON_V* to start pacing in ventricular, *Pace_OFF_V* to stop pacing in ventricular and *tic* to increment the current clock counter *sp* under the real time constraints. These events are similar to the previously described events but guards, and actions are changed according to the requirements of the DOO operating mode.

9.8.2 First Refinement: Threshold

The pacemaker control unit delivers stimulation to the heart chambers, on the basis of measured threshold value under the safety margin. We define two new constants *STA_THR_A* and *STA_THR_V* to hold the standard threshold value in axioms (*axm1* and *axm2*). The threshold constants are different for the atrial and the ventricular chambers.

$$
\begin{aligned}
axm1 : &\ STA\_THR\_A \in nat_1 \wedge STA\_THR\_A = 75 \\
axm1 : &\ STA\_THR\_V \in nat_1 \wedge STA\_THR\_V = 250
\end{aligned}
$$

The pacemaker's sensor starts sensing after the refractory period but the pacemaker's actuator delivers a pacing stimulus, when sensing value is greater than or equal to the standard threshold constants *STA_THR_A* or *STA_THR_V*. In the DOO operating mode only the pacemaker's actuators paces in the atrial and ventricular chambers under the automatic pace interval without using any pacemaker's sensors, so in this mode none of the refinement is given related to the threshold. Table 9.2 shows a list of invariants common in this refinement of other operating modes. First column shows the group of operating modes and second column shows corresponding common invariants.

First Refinement of DDD Mode

A pacemaker has a stimulation threshold measuring unit which measures a stimulation threshold voltage value of heart and a pulse generator for delivering stimulation pulses to the heart. The pulse generator is controlled by a control unit to deliver the stimulation pulses with respective amplitudes related to the measured threshold value under the safety margin. We introduce two new variables Thr_A and Thr_V to hold the sensing threshold value of the pacemaker's sensor from the atrial and ventricular chambers. Similarly, next two variables Thr_A_State and Thr_V_State represent boolean states as TRUE or FALSE of the pacemaker's sensor to sense the intrinsic activity from the atrial and ventricular chambers.

$$
\begin{array}{l}
inv1 : Thr\_A \in \mathbb{N}_1 \\
inv2 : Thr\_V \in \mathbb{N}_1 \\
inv3 : Thr\_A\_State \in BOOL \\
inv4 : Thr\_V\_State \in BOOL \\
inv5 : Pace\_Int\_flag = FALSE \wedge PM\_Actuator\_A = ON \Rightarrow \\
\qquad\qquad sp \geq Pace\_Int - FixedAV
\end{array}
$$

Invariants are given in Table 9.2. An additional invariant ($inv5$) is introduced and states that, when the pacemaker's actuator of the atrial chamber is ON, then the current clock counter sp is greater than or equal to the ventriculoatrial (VA) interval ($Pace\_Int - FixedAV$).

```
EVENT Thr_Value_V
  ANY    Thr_V_val
  WHERE
    grd1 : Thr_V_val ∈ ℕ
    grd2 : PM_Sensor_V = ON
    grd3 : Thr_V_State = TRUE
    grd4 : Thr_V < STA_THR_V
    grd5 : (sp ≥ VRP ∧ sp < Pace_Int − FixedAV)
             ∨
           (sp ≥ Pace_Int − FixedAV ∧ sp < Pace_Int)
    grd6 : (Thr_A_State = FALSE∧
            Thr_A < STA_THR_A)
             ∨
           (PM_Sensor_A = OFF∧
            AV_Count < FixedAV)
  THEN
    act1 : Thr_V := Thr_V_val
    act2 : Thr_V_State := FALSE
  END
```

In this refinement, we introduce two new events (Thr_Value_V and Thr_Value_A) for sensing the intrinsic activities from the ventricular and atrial chambers. These events are synchronised with all other events of the operating mode under all the

Table 9.2 Common invariants list

Modes	Common invariants
DDD VDD DDI DVI	1. $Pace\_Int\_flag = FALSE \wedge sp > Pace\_Int - FixedAV \wedge$ $sp < Pace\_Int \wedge AV\_Count\_STATE = TRUE \Rightarrow$ $PM\_Sensor\_V = ON$
DDD DVI	2. $Pace\_Int\_flag = FALSE \wedge sp > VRP \wedge$ $sp < Pace\_Int - FixedAV \Rightarrow PM\_Sensor\_V = ON$
DDD VDD	3. $Pace\_Int\_flag = FALSE \wedge PM\_Actuator\_V = ON \Rightarrow$ $(sp = Pace\_Int) \vee (sp < Pace\_Int \wedge AV\_Count > V\_Blank \wedge$ $AV\_Count \geq FixedAV)$
	4. $Pace\_Int\_flag = FALSE \wedge sp > Pace\_Int - FixedAV \wedge$ $sp < Pace\_Int \wedge AV\_Count\_STATE = TRUE \Rightarrow$ $PM\_Sensor\_A = OFF$
DDD DVI DDI	5. $Pace\_Int\_flag = FALSE \wedge sp > Pace\_Int - FixedAV \wedge$ $sp < Pace\_Int \wedge AV\_Count\_STATE = TRUE \Rightarrow$ $PM\_Actuator\_A = OFF$
DVI DDI	6. $Pace\_Int\_flag = FALSE \wedge sp > Pace\_Int - FixedAV \wedge$ $sp < Pace\_Int \wedge AV\_Count\_STATE = TRUE \Rightarrow$ $PM\_Actuator\_V = OFF$

safety properties and real time constraints. The guards of the event (Thr_Value_V) are introduced as to fulfil all the requirements of the sensing intrinsic activities from the ventricular chamber and actions ($act1$–$act2$) of this event state that the actual sensed value from a chamber is assigned to the variable Thr_V and sets FALSE state of the variable threshold ventricular state (Thr_V_State), respectively.

```
EVENT Thr_Value_A
   ANY   Thr_A_val
   WHERE
      grd1 : Thr_A_val ∈ ℕ
      grd2 : PM_Sensor_A = ON
      grd3 : Thr_A_State = TRUE
      grd4 : Thr_A < STA_THR_A
      grd5 : (sp ≥ VRP ∧ sp < Pace_Int − FixedAV)
   THEN
      act1 : Thr_A := Thr_A_val
      act2 : Thr_A_State := FALSE
   END
```

In the event Thr_Value_A, the guards ($grd2$–$grd4$) state that the pacemaker's sensor (PM_Sensor_A) of atrial chamber is ON; the threshold state (Thr_A_State)

of atrial chamber is TRUE and the sensed value (*Thr_A*) from the atrial chamber is less than the standard threshold (*STA_THR_A*) of atrial chamber. The last guard of this event states that the clock counter *sp* is greater than or equal to the VRP and less than the ventriculoatrial (VA) interval. Actions (*act1–act2*) of this event state that the actual sensed value (*Thr_A_val*) of atrial chamber is assigned to a variable (*Thr_A*) and sets FALSE state of a variable threshold atrial state (*Thr_A_State*).

EVENT Actuator_OFF_V
⊕   act6 : *Thr_A* := 0
⊕   act7 : *Thr_V* := 0
⊕   act8 : *Thr_A_State* := *FALSE*
⊕   act9 : *Thr_V_State* := *FALSE*

EVENT Sensor_ON_A
⊕   act2 : *Thr_A_State* := *TRUE*

EVENT Sensor_OFF_A
⊕   grd3 : *Thr_A* ≥ *STA_THR_A*

EVENT Sensor_OFF_V
⊕   grd6 : *Thr_V* ≥ *STA_THR_V*
⊕   act7 : *Thr_A* := 0
⊕   act8 : *Thr_V* := 0
⊕   act9 : *Thr_A_State* := *FALSE*
⊕   act10 : *Thr_V_State* := *FALSE*

We have introduced some new actions and guards in events (*Actuator_OFF_V*, *Sensor_ON_A*, *Sensor_OFF_A*, and *Sensor_OFF_V*) to synchronise the sensing activities using events (*Thr_Value_V* and *Thr_Value_A*) under the real time constraints. These events are already defined in the abstract model.[4]

EVENT tic
WHEN
    grd1 : (sp < VRP ∧ AV_Count_STATE = $FALSE$
            ∨
            (sp ≥ VRP ∧ sp < $Pace\_Int$ − $FixedAV$∧
            PM_Sensor_V = ON∧
            PM_Sensor_A = ON∧
            Thr_V_State = $FALSE$∧
            Thr_V < STA_THR_V))
    grd2 : AV_Count_STATE = $FALSE$
THEN
⊕   act2 : *Thr_A_State* := *TRUE*
⊕   act3 : *Thr_V_State* := *TRUE*
END

---

[4] ⊕: To add a new guard and an action in the model. ⊖: To remove a new guard and an action in the model.

The event (*tic*) of this refinement model progressively increases the current clock counter *sp*. We have strengthened the guard of this event to properly synchronise with new introduced threshold events, and the pacing and sensing activities of both chambers. Some new actions (*act2* and *act3*) are added in this event. The additional guards and actions handle the behaviour of the events (*Thr_Value_A* and *Thr_Value_V*) to sense the intrinsic activities from the atrial and ventricular chambers.

```
EVENT tic_AV
   WHEN
⊕       grd4 : PM_Sensor_V = ON
⊕       grd5 : Thr_V_State = FALSE
⊕       grd6 : Thr_V < STA_THR_V
⊕       grd7 : PM_Actuator_V = OFF
⊕       grd8 : PM_Sensor_A = OFF
⊕       grd9 : PM_Actuator_A = OFF
   THEN
⊕       act3 : Thr_V_State := TRUE
   END
```

We have introduced some new guards (*grd4–grd9*) and an action (*act3*) in the event (*tic_AV*) of this refinement. New guards provide more specific conditions and some specific states of the pacemaker's actuators and sensors to count the atrioventricular (AV) interval. An extra action (*act3*) sets TRUE state of the variable threshold state of ventricular (*Thr_V_State*).

First Refinement of DVI Mode

In this refinement, we introduce two new variables *Thr_V* and *Thr_V_State* to hold the sensing threshold value as similar to the DDD operating mode. We introduce few more invariants except some defined common invariants (see Table 9.2).

$$inv1 : Pace\_Int\_flag = FALSE \;\wedge\; PM\_Actuator\_V = ON \Rightarrow sp = Pace\_Int$$
$$inv2 : Pace\_Int\_flag = FALSE \;\wedge\; sp > VRP \wedge sp < Pace\_Int a \wedge$$
$$Thr\_V \geq STA\_THR\_V \;\wedge\;$$
$$Thr\_V\_State = TRUE \Rightarrow$$
$$PM\_Sensor\_V = OFF$$
$$inv3 : Pace\_Int\_flag = FALSE \;\wedge\; PM\_Actuator\_A = ON \Rightarrow$$
$$sp \geq Pace\_Int - FixedAV \wedge sp \geq VRP \wedge sp < Pace\_Int$$

The first invariant (*inv1*) states that when the pacemaker's actuator (*PM_Actuator_V*) of ventricular is ON, then the current clock counter *sp* is equal to the pace interval *Pace_Int*. Second invariant (*inv2*) represents that the pacemaker's sensor (*PM_Sensor_V*) of ventricular is OFF, when the clock counter *sp* is greater than the VRP, less than the pace interval (*Pace_Int*), the sensed value (*Thr_V*) is greater than or equal to the standard threshold (*STA_THR_V*) value of ventricular chamber and the threshold ventricular state (*Thr_V_State*) is TRUE. The last invariant (*inv3*) states that, when the pacemaker's actuator of atrial chambers is ON, then the current clock counter *sp* is within the ventriculoatrial (VA) interval (*Pace_Int* − *FixedAV*) and greater than or equal to the VRP and less than the pace interval *Pace_Int*.

In this refinement, we introduce a new event (*Thr_Value_V*) for sensing the intrinsic activities of the ventricular chamber, and it is similar to the first refinement of DDD operating mode. This event is synchronised with all other events of this operating mode under all the safety properties and real time constraints. The other events *tic* and *tic_AV* are also modified in this refinement to synchronise sensors and actuators behaviour.

First Refinement of DDI Mode

We introduce some new variables (*Thr_A*, *Thr_V*, *Thr_A_State* and *Thr_V_State*) as similar to the refinement of the DDD operating modes. In this refinement, we introduce some new invariants except some defined common invariants (see Table 9.2).

$$
\begin{array}{l}
inv1 : Pace\_Int\_flag = FALSE \ \wedge PM\_Actuator\_V = ON \Rightarrow sp = Pace\_Int \\
inv2 : Pace\_Int\_flag = FALSE \ \wedge sp > VRP \wedge sp < Pace\_Int - FixedAV \Rightarrow \\
\qquad PM\_Actuator\_A = OFF \\
inv3 : Pace\_Int\_flag = FALSE \ \wedge PM\_Actuator\_A = ON \Rightarrow \\
\qquad sp = Pace\_Int - FixedAV
\end{array}
$$

The first invariant states that when the pacemaker's actuator (*PM_Actuator_V*) of ventricular is ON, then the clock counter *sp* is equal to the pace interval *Pace_Int*. The next invariant (*inv2*) states that the pacemaker's actuator (*PM_Actuator_A*) of atrial is OFF, when the current clock counter *sp* is greater than the VRP and less than the ventriculoatrial (VA) interval. The last invariant states that, when the pacemaker's actuator of atrial chamber is ON, then the current clock counter *sp* is equal to ventriculoatrial (VA) interval (*Pace_Int* − *FixedAV*).

In this refinement, we introduce two new events (*Thr_Value_V* and *Thr_Value_A*) for sensing the intrinsic activities from the ventricular and atrial chambers that are similar to the first refinement of DDD operating mode. These events are synchronised with all other events of this operating mode under all the safety properties and real time constraints. Other events are also modified in this refinement to synchronise the sensors and actuators behaviour as similar to the DDD operating mode.

First Refinement of VDD Mode

We introduce four new variables (*Thr_A*, *Thr_V*, *Thr_A_State* and *Thr_V_State*) as similar to the refinement of the DDD operating mode. In this refinement, we introduce an extra invariant except some defined common invariants (see Table 9.2).

Invariant (*inv*1) states that the pacemaker's sensor (*PM_Sensor_A*) of atrial is ON, when the clock counter *sp* is greater than the VRP and less than the pace interval (*Pace_Int*) and the atrioventricular (AV) counter state (*AV_Count_STATE*) is FALSE.

$$inv1 : Pace\_Int\_flag = FALSE \ \wedge sp > VRP \wedge sp < Pace\_Int \wedge$$
$$AV\_Count\_STATE = FALSE \Rightarrow$$
$$PM\_Sensor\_A = ON$$

In this refinement, we introduce two new events (*Thr_Value_V* and *Thr_Value_A*) as similar to the DDD operating mode. These events are synchronised with all other events of this operating mode under all the safety properties and real time constraints. Some guards and actions are added in the old events as defined in the DDD operating mode.

9.8.3 Second Refinement of DDD Mode: Hysteresis

In the two electrode pacemaker, *hysteresis* mode is applicable only in the DDD operating mode. *Hysteresis* is a programmed feature whereby the pacemaker paces at a faster rate than the sensing rate. For example, pacing at 80 pulses a minute with a hysteresis rate of 55 means that the pacemaker will be inhibited at all rates down to 55 beats per minute, having been activated at a rate below 55, the pacemaker then switches on and paces at 80 pulses a minute [22, 39]. The application of the hysteresis interval provides consistent pacing of the atrial or ventricle, or prevents constant pacing of the atrial or ventricle. The main purpose of hysteresis is to allow a patient to have his or her own underlying rhythm as much as possible. Two new variables (*Hyt_Pace_Int_flag*, *HYT_State*) are introduced to define functional properties of the hysteresis operating modes. Both variables are defined as a boolean type. The hysteresis state *HYT_State* is used to set the hysteresis functional parameter as TRUE or FALSE, to apply the hysteresis operating modes.

$$inv1 : Hyt\_Pace\_Int\_flag \in BOOL$$
$$inv2 : HYT\_State \in BOOL$$

A new event *Hyt_Pace_Updating* is introduced to implement the functional properties of the hysteresis operating modes, which is a refinement of the event *Change_Pace_Int*. In the hysteresis operating modes, the pacemaker is trying to maintain own heart rhythm as much as possible. Hence, this event can change the pacing interval and sets pacing length longer than existing, which changes the pacing length of the cardiac pacemaker. This event is only used for updating the pacing interval (*Pace_Int*). Guards of this event state that the pace changing flag (*Pace_Int_flag*) is TRUE, the hysteresis pacing flag (*Hyt_Pace_Int_flag*) is TRUE and the hysteresis pace interval (*Hyt_Pace_Int*) should be lied between the pace interval (*Pace_Int*) and lower rate interval (*LRI*). The actions of this event state that a new hysteresis pace interval (*Hyt_Pace_Int*) updates the pace interval *Pace_Int*, the hysteresis pacing flag (*Hyt_Pace_Int_flag*) sets FALSE and hysteresis state (*HYT_State*) sets TRUE.

```
EVENT Hyt_Pace_Updating Refines Change_Pace_Int
  ANY
     Hyt_Pace_Int
  WHERE
        grd1 : Pace_Int_flag = TRUE
        grd2 : Hyt_Pace_Int_flag = TRUE
        grd3 : Hyt_Pace_Int ∈ Pace_Int .. LRI
  THEN
        act1 : Pace_Int := Hyt_Pace_Int
        act2 : Hyt_Pace_Int_flag := FALSE
        act3 : HYT_State := TRUE
  END
```

9.8.4 Third Refinement: Rate Modulation

Rate modulation is the final refinement of the two-electrode pacemaker. Rate modulation refers to the ability of the pacemaker to increase the rate of pacing on its own. The manner that the pacemaker does this is by having its own special sensor's measure such as things as vibration or minute ventilation (volume of air moved in 1 minute's time). The pacemaker uses these measurements as a determination of at least how fast heart rate should be. This rate is termed the "sensor indicated rate."

Rate modulation is typically used when a patient's heart does not appropriately increase its own rate with exertion or stress. This intrinsic inability to increase heart rate is called "chronotropic incompetence." Use of rate modulation also demands to set an upper limit on how fast the heart may be paced.

This refinement is similar to the one-electrode pacemaker and pacing rate control both chambers according to the required physiologic need. Here, we introduce the rate modulation function and found some new operating modes (DDDR, DVIR, AAIR, DDIR, VDDR and DOOR) of the two-electrode pacemaker system. For modelling the rate modulation, we introduce some new constants maximum sensor rate *MSR* as $MSR \in 50 .. 175$ and *acc_thr* as $acc\_thr \in \mathbb{N}_1$ using axioms (*axm*1, *axm*2). The maximum sensor rate (*MSR*) is the maximum pacing rate allowed as a result of sensor control, and it must be between 50 and 175 pulse per minute (ppm). The constant *acc_thr* represents the activity threshold. Axiom (*axm*3) represents a static property for the rate modulation operating modes.

$$axm1 : MSR \in 50..175$$
$$axm2 : acc\_thr \in \mathbb{N}_1$$
$$axm3 : MSR = URL$$

Two new variables *acler_sensed* and *acler_sensed_flag* are defined as to store the measured value from the accelerometer and boolean stats of the accelerometer sensor. Boolean state of the accelerometer sensor is used to synchronise with other functionalities of the system. The accelerometer is used to measure the physical activities of the body in the pacemaker system. Two invariants (*inv3*, *inv4*) provide the safety margin and state that the heart rate never falls below the lower rate limit (LRL) and never exceeds the maximum sensor rate (MSR) limit.

$$inv1 : acler\_sensed \in \mathbb{N}$$
$$inv2 : acler\_sensed\_flag \in BOOL$$
$$inv3 : HYT\_State = FALSE \ \wedge acler\_sensed < acc\_thr \wedge$$
$$acler\_sensed\_flag = TRUE \Rightarrow Pace\_Int = 60000/LRL$$
$$inv4 : HYT\_State = FALSE \ \wedge acler\_sensed => acc\_thr \wedge$$
$$acler\_sensed\_flag = TRUE \Rightarrow Pace\_Int = 60000/MSR$$

In this final refinement, we introduce two new events *Increase_Interval* and *Decrease_Interval*, which are the refinements of the event *Change_Pace_Int*. These new events are used to control the pacing rate of the one-electrode pacemaker in the rate modulating operating modes. The new events *Increase_Interval* and *Decrease_Interval* control the value of the pace interval variable *Pace_Int*, whenever a measured value (*acler_sensed*) from the accelerometer sensor goes higher or lower than the activity threshold *acc_thr*.

EVENT Increase_Interval Refines Change_Pace_Int
WHEN
   grd1 : $Pace\_Int\_flag = TRUE$
   grd1 : $acler\_sensed \geq threshold$
   grd1 : $HYT\_State = FALSE$
THEN
   act1 : $Pace\_Int := 60000/MSR$
   act1 : $acler\_sensed\_flag := TRUE$
END

EVENT Decrease_Interval Refines Change_Pace_Int
WHEN
   grd1 : $Pace\_Int\_flag = TRUE$
   grd1 : $acler\_sensed < threshold$
   grd1 : $HYT\_State = FALSE$
THEN
   act1 : $Pace\_Int := 60000/LRL$
   act1 : $acler\_sensed\_flag := TRUE$
END

A new event (*Acler_sensed*) is defined as to simulate the behaviour of the accelerometer sensor. This event is continued sensing the motion of the body to increase or decrease the length of the pace interval (*Pace_Int*). In this event, the guards state that the accelerometer sensor flag is TRUE and the hysteresis state is FALSE. A new variable *acl_sen* is used to store the current sensing value. The actions of this event state that the local variable *acl_sen* updates the accelerometer sensor (*acler_sensed*) and the accelerometer sensor flag (*acler_sensed_flag*) sets FALSE.

```
EVENT Acler_sensed
  ANY
    acl_sen
  WHERE
        grd1 : acl_sen ∈ ℕ
        grd1 : acler_sensed_flag = TRUE
        grd1 : HYT_State = FALSE
  THEN
        act1 : acler_sensed := acl_sen
        act1 : acler_sensed_flag := FALSE
  END
```

Finally, we have completed the formal specifications of the one- and two-electrode cardiac pacemaker. The next section describes the validation of the formal model using ProB animator.

9.9 Model Validation and Analysis

There are two main validation activities in Event-B, and both are complementary for designing a consistent system:

- *Consistency checking*, which is used to show that the events of a machine preserve the invariant, and *refinement checking*, which is used to show that one machine is a valid refinement of another. A list of automatically generated proof obligations should be discharged by the proof tool of the Rodin platform.
- *Model analysis*, which is done by the ProB tool and consists in exploring traces or scenarios of our consistent Event-B models. For instance, the ProB may discover possible deadlocks or hidden properties that are not expressed by generated proof obligations.

This section conveys the validity of the model by using ProB tool [36] and Proof Statistics. "Validation" refers to the activity of gaining confidence that the developed formal models are consistent with the requirements, which expressed in the requirements document [7]. We have used the ProB tool [36] that supports *automated consistency checking* of Event-B machines via model checking [10] and constraint-based checking [28]. Animation using ProB worked very well, and we have then used ProB to validate the Event-B machine. This tool assists us to find

Table 9.3 Proof statistics

Model	Total number of POs	Automatic proof	Interactive proof
One-electrode pacemaker			
Abstract model	203	199 (98 %)	4 (2 %)
First refinement	48	44 (91 %)	4 (9 %)
Second refinement	12	8 (66 %)	4 (34 %)
Third refinement	105	99 (94 %)	6 (6 %)
Two-electrode pacemaker			
Abstract model	204	195 (95 %)	9 (5 %)
First refinement	234	223 (95 %)	11 (5 %)
Second refinement	3	3 (100 %)	0 (0 %)
Third refinement	83	74 (89 %)	9 (11 %)
Total	892	845 (94 %)	47 (6 %)

potential problems, to improve invariant's expressions in our Event-B models, for instance, by generating counter-examples when it discovers an invariant violation. ProB may help in improving invariant expression by suggesting hints for strengthening the invariant and each time an invariant is modified; new proof obligations are generated by the Rodin platform. It is the complementary use of both techniques to develop formal models of critical systems, where high safety and security are required. More errors are corrected during the elaboration of the specifications while discharging the proof obligations and careful cross-reading than during the animations. We have validated all operating modes of the pacemaker in each refinement of models. The pacemaker specification is developed and formally proved by the Rodin tool.

ProB was very useful in the development of the pacemaker specification, and was able to animate all of our models and able to prove the absence of error (no counter example exist). The ProB model checker also discovered several invariant violations, e.g., related to incorrect responses or unordered pacing and sensing activities. It was also able to discover a deadlock in two of the models, which was due to the fact that "clock counter" were not properly recycled, meaning that after a while no pacing or sensing activities occur into the system. Such kind of errors would have been more difficult to uncover with the prover of Rodin tool.

Table 9.3 is expressing proof statistics for the formal development of the pacemaker using the Rodin platform. These statistics measure the size of the model, the proof obligations generated and discharged by the Rodin prover, and those are interactively proved. The complete development of the pacemaker system results in 892 (100 %) proof obligations, in which 845 (94 %) are proved automatically by the Rodin tool. The remaining 47 (6 %) proof obligations are proved interactively using the Rodin tool. In the Event-B models, many proof obligations are generated due to the introduction of new functional behaviours and their parameters (threshold, hysteresis and rate modulation) under the real-time constraints. In order to guarantee the correctness of these functional behaviours, we have established various invariants in the stepwise refinements. As it can be seen, the abstract model in one electrode required by far the largest number of proofs: it is due to the large number of invariants (57), together with the number of events (26) which shows a size of the model. Similarly, large numbers of proofs are in the abstract model and the first refinement of two electrodes, where a large number of invariants (36 (abstract), 30 (refinement 1)), together with the number of events (41 (abstract), 43 (refinement 1)). It should be noted that the manual proofs were not difficult. Proofs are quite simple, and have been achieved with the help of *do case* operation. Guards of some events are very complex, so for proving invariants and theorems; we simplify guards using *do case*. The stepwise refinement of the pacemaker system helps to achieve a high degree of automatic proofs.

9.10 Closed-Loop Model of Heart and Cardiac Pacemaker

A detailed description of the heart model based on electrocardiography analysis [5, 21, 33] and cellular automata is given in Chap. 8. The heart model is based on logico-mathematical theory. The logico-mathematical based heart model is developed using refinement approach in Event-B modelling language [1, 56]. In this investigation, we present a methodology for modelling a heart model, to extract a set of biological nodes (i.e. SA node, AV node, etc.), impulse propagation speed between nodes, impulse propagation time between nodes and cellular automata for propagating impulses at the cellular level. A main key feature of this heart model is a representation of all the possible morphological states of the electrocardiogram (ECG) [2, 5]. The morphological states represent the normal and abnormal states of the electrocardiogram (ECG). The morphological representation generates any kind of heart model (patients model or normal heart model using ECG). This model can observe a failure of the impulse generation and a failure of the impulse propagation. This model is also verified through electro-physiologist and cardiac experts.

Formal specification of the cardiac pacemaker is expressed in this chapter. But this cardiac pacemaker is modelled without any biological environment like the heart system. This section describes a closed-loop formal model of a cardiac pacemaker and the heart system, where the cardiac pacemaker responses according to the functional behaviour of the heart [49, 50, 52]. The main objective of this model is to verify the complex properties of the cardiac pacemaker under the virtual environment. Figure 9.9 represents a block diagram of the cardiac pacemaker and the heart system, where the cardiac pacemaker responses when it senses intrinsic activities from the heart. In this system specification, the heart model simulates the functional behaviour of the normal and abnormal heart. The heart model activities are always monitored by the cardiac pacemaker and it responses according to the user needs.

This section presents a closed-loop model of the cardiac pacemaker, where the heart is used as an environment. For developing this closed-loop model [50], we

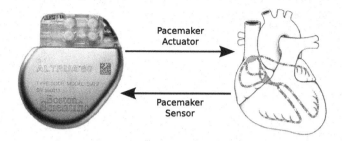

Fig. 9.9   Closed-loop model

borrow formal specifications from the previously developed and verified formal models of the cardiac pacemaker [48] and heart system [52]. However, to develop the closed-loop model, we have done substantial changes in the existing models to specify the desired behaviour of the system. Moreover, we develop the whole system from the scratch using progressive refinement. Each refinement level introduces both cardiac pacemaker and heart system behaviours. To check the correctness of the closed-loop system we have introduced many safety properties using invariants, and discharged all the generated proof obligations at each refinement level.

The closed-loop model of the cardiac pacemaker is also based on *action-reaction* and *time patterns*. We apply the action-reaction and time patterns in modelling to synchronise the sensing and pacing stimulus functions of the pacemaker system in a continuous progressive time constraint. We present here only summary informations about each refinement of one- and two-electrode pacemakers and omit detailed formalisation and proof details. The following outline is given about every refinement level to understand the basic formalism structure of the closed-loop model of the cardiac pacemaker. We have combined the model of the heart and the cardiac pacemaker to formalise the closed-loop model. To know more about detailed formalism see individual model of the heart system and the cardiac pacemaker. We have described here only summary informations about each refinement in form of very basic description of the heart modelling and the cardiac pacemaker modelling incremental refinement-based approach and omit detailed formalisation of events and proof details due to repetition of the formalism. To find more detailed information about developed formal model of the cardiac pacemaker and the heart model, see the published papers and research reports [40, 43, 48, 49].

9.10.1 The Context and Initial Model

To formalise the heart behaviour, we capture the electrical features. We identify a set of landmark nodes from the conduction network (see Fig. 9.10(a)) of the heart. These landmark nodes are also known as the electrical impulse propagation nodes *ConductionNode*, which enable expression of the normal and abnormal behaviours of the heart system. We find the direct connections among the impulse propagation

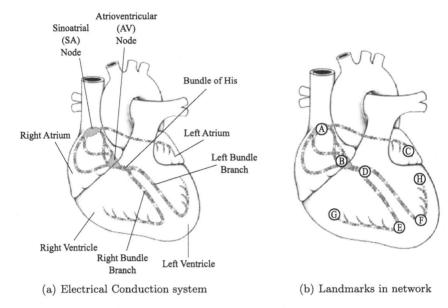

(a) Electrical Conduction system   (b) Landmarks in network

Fig. 9.10 The electrical conduction and landmarks of the heart system

nodes, which constitute the impulse propagation path. The impulse propagation time
and impulse propagation velocity for each pair of nodes vary due to different types
of muscles in the heart. To formalise the heart system, we define three constants impulse propagation time *ConductionTime*, impulse propagation path *ConductionPath*
and impulse propagation velocity *ConductionSpeed*. All these constants are initial
components, which are defined through a set of axioms (*axm1–axm4*).

To formalise the cardiac pacemaker, we define a set of constants (*LRL, URL,
ARP, VRP, PVARP*, etc.), which expresses timing intervals. These timing intervals
are used as a set of configuration parameters. To model boolean behaviour of the
sensor and actuator, we define an enumerated set *status*. A set of axioms for the
cardiac pacemaker is defined in *axm5* and *axm6*. All these constants and axioms
have been extracted from the technical specification [7], which are validated by the
cardiologist and the physiologist.

$axm1 : partition(ConductionNode, \{A\}, \{B\}, \{C\}, \{D\}, \{E\}, \{F\}, \{G\}, \{H\})$
$axm2 : ConductionTime \in ConductionNode \rightarrow \mathbb{P}(0..230)$
$axm3 : ConductionPath \subseteq ConductionNode \times ConductionNode$
$axm4 : ConductionSpeed \in ConductionPath \rightarrow \mathbb{P}(5..400)$
$axm5 : LRL \in 30..175 \wedge URL \in 50..175 \wedge PVARP \in 150..500$
$axm6 : ARP \in 150..500 \wedge VRP \in 150..500 \wedge status = \{ON, OFF\}$

To define an abstract model of the closed-loop system, we develop the combined
model of the cardiac pacemaker and heart, where the cardiac pacemaker acts according to the heart behaviour. The environment model of the heart behaves according

to observations of the impulse propagation in the conduction nodes. We define a set of variables to model the heart and pacemaker models, where four variables (*ConductionNodeState*, *CConductionTime*, *CConductionSpeed* and *HeartState*) are used to model the heart behaviour, and six variables (*PM_Actuator_A*, *PM_Actuator_V*, *PM_Sensor_A*, *PM_Sensor_V*, *Pace_Int* and *sp*) are used to express the cardiac pacemaker behaviour. All these variables are defined using a set of invariants (*inv*1–*inv*7). The cardiac pacemaker variables are introduced for modelling actuators, sensors and timing intervals. A group of invariants (*inv*8, *inv*9 and *inv*10) presents safety properties. The invariant *inv*8 states that, when the clock counter *sp* is less than the VRP and the atrioventricular (AV) counter state *AV_Count_State* is FALSE, then the pacemaker's actuators and sensors of both chambers are OFF. Similarly, the next invariants (*inv*9 and *inv*10) represent required properties of ON state of the pacemaker's actuators in both chambers.

$$
\begin{aligned}
&inv1 : ConductionNodeState \in ConductionNode \rightarrow BOOL \\
&inv2 : CConductionTime \in ConductionNode \rightarrow 0 .. 300 \\
&inv3 : CConductionSpeed \in ConductionPath \rightarrow 0 .. 500 \\
&inv4 : HeartState \in BOOL \\
&inv5 : PM\_Actuator\_A \in status \wedge PM\_Actuator\_V \in status \\
&inv6 : PM\_Sensor\_A \in status \wedge PM\_Sensor\_V \in status \\
&inv7 : Pace\_Int \in URI .. LRI \wedge sp \in 1 .. Pace\_Int \\
&inv8 : sp < VRP \wedge AV\_Count\_STATE = FALSE \Rightarrow \\
&\qquad\qquad PM\_Actuator\_V = OFF \wedge PM\_Sensor\_A = OFF \wedge \\
&\qquad\qquad PM\_Sensor\_V = OFF \wedge PM\_Actuator\_A = OFF \\
&inv9 : PM\_Actuator\_V = ON \Rightarrow sp = Pace\_Int \vee (sp < Pace\_Int \wedge \\
&\qquad\qquad AV\_Count > V\_Blank \wedge AV\_Count \geq FixedAV) \\
&inv10 : PM\_Actuator\_A = ON \Rightarrow (sp \geq Pace\_Int - FixedAV)
\end{aligned}
$$

The abstract specification of the closed-loop model contains several events related to the cardiac pacemaker and heart system. There are many events, namely *HeartOK* to represent a normal state of the heart, *HeartKO* to express an abnormal state of the heart, *HeartConduction* to trace the current updated value of each landmark node in the conduction network, *Actuator_ON_V*, *Actuator_OFF_V*, *Actuator_ON_A* and *Actuator_OFF_A* to represent ON and OFF states of pacemaker's actuators for both chambers, *Sensor_ON_A*, *Sensor_OFF_A*, *Sensor_ON_V*, and *Sensor_OFF_V* to represent ON and OFF states of pacemaker's sensors for both chambers, and *tic* to represent the clock counter.

The event *HeartOK* expresses desired behaviour of the normal heart, where a set of guards formulates the required conditions. The first guard (*grd*1) states that all the landmark nodes must be visited for one cycle during impulse propagation using conduction network. The second guard specifies that the current impulse propagation time for each landmark node should be lie in the pre-specified ranges (Chap. 8, Property 1). Similarly, the last guard states that the current impulse propagation velocity of each path should lie between pre-defined impulse propagation velocities (Chap. 8, Property 2). The action predicate (*act*1) denotes the normal state of the heart, when all these set of guards are satisfied.

```
EVENT HeartOK
  WHEN
    grd1 : ∀i · i ∈ ConductionNode ⇒ ConductionNodeState(i) = TRUE
    grd2 : ∀i · i ∈ ConductionNode ⇒
           CConductionTime(i) ∈ ConductionTime(i)
    grd3 : ∀i, j · i ↦ j ∈ ConductionPath ⇒
           CConductionSpeed(i ↦ j) ∈ ConductionSpeed(i ↦ j)
  THEN
    act1 : HeartState := TRUE
  END
```

In the two electrode pacemaker, we use two sensors and two actuators for capturing the required behaviour of the cardiac pacemaker. In this section, we consider to show only actuator and sensor events of the ventricle chamber. Moreover, other events related to the sensor and actuator of the atrial chamber are same. The events *Actuator_ON_V* and *Sensor_ON_V* excerpt from the abstract model to describe *ON* state of the actuator and sensor of the cardiac pacemaker. A set of guards of both events enables to set *ON* state of both actuator and sensor, which allows to pace and sense in the ventricular chamber under the desired conditions using real-time constraints.

```
EVENT Actuator_ON_V
  WHEN
    grd1 : PM_Actuator_V = OFF
    grd2 : (sp = Pace_Int)∨
           (sp < Pace_Int∧
           AV_Count > V_Blank ∧
           AV_Count ≥ FixedAV)
    grd3 : sp ≥ VRP ∧ sp ≥ PVARP
           ∧sp ≥ URI
  THEN
    act1 : PM_Actuator_V := ON
    act2 : last_sp := sp
  END
```

```
EVENT Sensor_ON_V
  WHEN
    grd1 : PM_Sensor_V = OFF
    grd2 : (sp ≥ VRP ∧ sp < Pace_Int − FixedAV∧
           PM_Sensor_A = ON)
           ∨
           (sp ≥ Pace_Int − FixedAV ∧
           AV_Count_STATE = TRUE)
    grd3 : PM_Actuator_A = OFF
  THEN
    act1 : PM_Sensor_V := ON
  END
```

In our previous models of the cardiac pacemaker and the heart system, we use the *tic* event to model a clock, separately. However, in the closed-loop model, we use a *single* event *tic* to specify a common clock for both cardiac pacemaker and heart environment models. The event (*tic*) models the clock behaviour, where time is progressively increased using the current clock counter *sp*. This event controls the time line of pacing and sensing events. A guard (*grd1*) of this event provides the required conditions to increase the clock counter *sp* by 1 (ms).

```
EVENT tic
   WHEN
      grd1 : (sp < VRP)
              ∨
              (sp ≥ VRP ∧ sp < Pace_Int − FixedAV ∧
              PM_Sensor_A = ON ∧ PM_Sensor_V = ON
   THEN
      act1 : sp := sp + 1
   END
```

9.10.2 Chain of Refinements

So far, we have described our abstract model of the closed-loop model [50]. Each refinement level is used to introduce a new set of functional properties for modelling normal and abnormal behaviours of the heart and pacemaker. Rather than presenting the chain of refinement stages in great detail, we will just give an overview of the remaining refinement stages, sufficient to explain the rationale of each refinement stage in formalising the system.

Refinement 1: *Introducing* threshold *in cardiac pacemaker and impulse propagation in the heart system.* This refinement step is known as a conduction model, which introduces the impulse propagation in the conduction network of the heart. The impulse propagation originates from the SA node and pass through all the landmark nodes and reached at the Purkinje fibres of the ventricles. Formalising the conduction model, we introduce a set of events, which supports piecewise development of the impulse propagation. The electrical impulse passes through several intermediate landmark nodes and finally sink to the terminal nodes (C, G, H). The conduction model uses the clock counter to model the real-time system to satisfy the required temporal properties for the impulse propagation. A set of new events simulates the desired behaviour of the impulse propagation into the heart conduction network, where each new refined event formalises impulse flow between two landmark nodes; for instance, the electrical impulse moves from SA node (A) to AV node (B).

In the refinement of the closed-loop system, the cardiac pacemaker development introduces sensors behaviour for both atrial and ventricular chambers, which models to capture the sensing activities using some standard threshold values. The threshold values are different for both atria and ventricle chambers. The heart conduction behaviour is continue monitored by the cardiac pacemaker model. The monitored value is compared with the standard threshold value under required timing intervals to allow or inhibit to pace into the heart chamber to control the desired behaviours of the heart.

Refinement 2: *Introduction of hysteresis for cardiac pacemaker model and perturbation the conduction for the heart model.* This refinement step introduces an abnormal behaviour in the closed-loop model through introduction of the blocking activities, and *hysteresis* operating mode in the cardiac pacemaker model. The blocking behaviour in the heart network is known as perturbation model, which specifies perturbation in the heart conduction system and helps to discover exact block into the heart conduction network. We introduce a set of events through progressive refinement to simulate the desired blocking behaviour. The blocking behaviour generates trouble into electrical impulse propagation. Different types of heart blocks are presented through the partition of the landmark nodes in the conduction network.

The cardiac pacemaker model uses refinement to introduce a new feature related to the operating modes. This new feature is know as *hysteresis* operating mode, which prevents the constant pacing and allows a patient to have his or her own underlying rhythm as much as possible. The *hysteresis* is a programmed feature whereby the pacemaker paces at a faster rate than the sensing rate. This refinement introduces a new event, which allows to set *hysteresis* mode, and the cardiac pacemaker operates according to the desired rate.

Refinement 3: *Introduction of rate modulation for the cardiac pacemaker model and a cellular model for the heart system.* This is the final refinement of the closed-loop system, which introduces cellular level modelling for the heart system and rate modulation for the cardiac pacemaker. The final refinement of the heart system provides simulation model, which introduces the impulse propagation at the cellular level using cellular automata. The electrical impulse propagates at the cells level. A set of constants and mathematical properties are introduced using axioms, and a set of events are used to formalise the desired behaviour of the heart using cellular automata, which are described in [52].

In the final model of the cardiac pacemaker, we describe a rate adapting pacing technique. The rate adapting pacing technique gives freedom to select automatically desired pacing rate according to the physiologic needs. Automatic selection of the desired pacing rate helps to increase or decrease the pacing rate and assists a patient for controlling the heart rate according to the different day to day activities. In the rate modulation mode, the pacemaker operates faster than the lower rate, but no more than the upper sensor rate limit, when it determines that the heart rate needs to increase. For instance, when a patient does exercise and the heart rate cannot increase automatically to fulfil the required pupping rate. The rate modulation sensor is used to determine the maximum exertion performed by the patient. This increased pacing rate refers to the *sensor indicated rate*. Reducing the physical activities helps to progressively decrease the pacing rate down to the lower rate. A set of new refined events models increasing and decreasing pacing rate of the cardiac pacemaker [50].

Table 9.4 Proof statistics

Model	Total number of POs	Automatic proof	Interactive proof
Closed-loop model of one-electrode pacemaker			
Abstract model	304	258 (85 %)	46 (15 %)
First refinement	1015	730 (72 %)	285 (28 %)
Second refinement	72	8 (11 %)	64 (89 %)
Third refinement	153	79 (52 %)	74 (48 %)
Closed-loop model of two-electrode pacemaker			
Abstract model	291	244 (84 %)	47 (16 %)
First refinement	1039	766 (74 %)	273 (26 %)
Second refinement	53	2 (4 %)	51 (96 %)
Third refinement	122	60 (49 %)	62 (51 %)
Total	3049	2147 (70 %)	902 (30 %)

9.10.3 Proof Statistics

Table 9.4 expresses the proof statistics of the development of the closed-loop model of the cardiac pacemaker with the heart system. These statistics measure the size of the model, the proof obligations (POs) generated and discharged by the Rodin prover and those that are interactively proved. The complete development of the heart model results in 3049 (100 %) POs, within which 2147 (70 %) are proved automatically by the Rodin tool. The remaining 902 (30 %) POs are proved interactively using the Rodin tool. Integration of the heart model and the cardiac pacemaker model generates lots of extra POs. The main reason of these new POs is to use shared variables in both models to link between the heart and pacemaker models. A set of invariants corresponding to the shared variables generates new POs. For example, the current clock counter variable (sp) is shared, which has been used in events of the heart and pacemaker models. The combined invariants of the heart and pacemaker models generate new POs corresponding to the current clock counter variable (sp). The whole system represents functional properties of the cardiac pacemaker operating modes under the biological environment in the heart. The heart model represents normal and abnormal states of the heart, which is estimated by the physiological analysis. To guarantee the correctness of these functional behaviours, we have established various invariants in the incremental refinements.

The use of model checker helps to discover some unexpected behaviours, and assists to verify all the operating modes of the cardiac pacemaker in the heart environment model. A tool ProB [36] is used to animate the closed-loop model and able to prove the absence of errors.

9.11 Closed-Loop Modelling Requirements

This section presents a set of requirements for modelling the closed-loop system to guarantee the safety properties [29]. These requirements are useful for verifying the closed-loop system.

9.11.1 Patient Safety in Closed-Loop

The closed-loop system must hold a set of requirements related to the physiological needs. Few properties are constant and others are conditional. The heart indicates the patient condition, which presents conditional properties. In the closed-loop system the heart states are connected to the heart model parameters, which are not affected by pacemaker therapy. The integration of the heart model and pacemaker model allow us to evaluate whether the pacemaker provides an appropriate therapy for any arrhythmias.

9.11.2 Behavioural Requirements

The closed-loop system exposes several conditions for normal and abnormal heart, which are represented through node automata (Fig. 9.10(b)) using ranges of impulse propagation speed and impulse propagation time. Condition is a boolean value for whether the heart state is true. The cardiac pacemaker presents pacing and sensing activities under specified conditions. Some behaviour requirements are given as follows: (1) Atria and ventricular pace should not occur during atrial and ventricle refractory period, respectively. This requirement is an important safety properties, which is verified in the closed-loop model. Any pacing during the refractory period creates derangements in timing for the atria and ventricle. (2) Intrinsic activities of the atrial and ventricles should be sensed by different leads. The intrinsic activities are essential input for the pacemaker. The pacemaker should ensure that the intrinsic activities are sensed accurately. (3) Natural pacing in the atria and ventricle, and artificial pacing and sensing activities of the pacemaker must be coordinated to ensure efficient pumping for maintaining the heart rhythm.

9.11.3 Clinical Requirements with Closed-Loop

Clinical requirements are depended on the patient needs such as normal sinus rhythm, bradycardia, heart block and tachycardia. These requirements are common critical conditions, which can vary for each patient because of different physiological needs.

In this section, the heart model is presented as abstract as possible to capture all possible scenarios of the heart, which is completely based on the conduction speed and conduction time. Whenever these two parameters change or lie out of the range, then the ECG signal deforms and we cannot obtain the desired ECG signal, which represents an abnormal heart state. Moreover, we have introduced heart blocking behaviour using stepwise refinement. Rather than considering any particular behaviour of the heart, we have formalised the heart abstractly. For instance, we have not done any special treatment in our model to capture the retrograde conduction (travel backward). We have considered the perfect heart condition (see HeartOK, we have only forward conduction network). The retrograde conduction results in many symptoms, primarily those symptoms result from the delayed, non-physiologic timing of atrial contraction in relation to ventricular contraction. According to our model, if the retrograde conduction affects the timing cycle or conduction speed, then the heart presents an abnormal state. Normal state of the closed-loop model is presented according to the timing and speed of the conduction requirements. In case of abnormal state of the heart, the cardiac pacemaker does pacing and sensing according to the patient needs. In this closed-loop system, the cardiac pacemaker can take effect when the heart presents an abnormal state, which helps to maintain the patient heart rhythm. We have considered heart state (*OK* or *KO*) for each cycle. If the cycle has any abnormality, heart will be in abnormal state and pacemaker takes over to maintain heart rhythm. However, this closed-loop model helps to identify the pacemaker requirements according to the heart behaviour.

9.11.4 *To Discover Essential Safety Properties*

The closed-loop model provides higher insurance for safety and security. The number of POs of the closed-loop model of the cardiac pacemaker are higher than the simple model of the cardiac pacemaker model (see Tables 9.3 and 9.4). In the closed-loop model invariants are stronger than the plain model. The closed model generates more than 70 % extra POs.

9.12 Real-Time Animation Using Pacemaker Case Study

This section shows an applicability of the real-time animator [42] through animation of formal models of the pacemaker using real-time data sets. Figure 9.11 represents an implementation of the given architecture for the formal model of a cardiac pacemaker case study. We have mainly used this case study to experiment on our proposed architecture, which enables the animation of a proved specification with real-time data set without generating the source code in any programming language. According to the proposed architecture (see Fig. 9.11) for this experiment, we have not used any data-acquisition device to collect the ECG (electrocardiogram) signal.

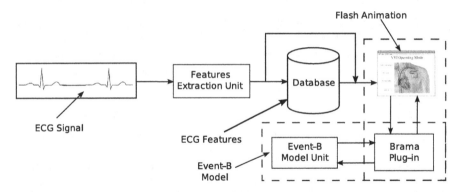

Fig. 9.11 Real-time animation of cardiac pacemaker

We have done this experiment in off-line mode, means we have used our architecture to test the real-time data set of ECG signal that is already collected. ECG signal collection and features extraction in on-line mode is too expensive due to complex data-acquisition process and limitation of feature extracting algorithms. So, we have used the ECG signal and feature extraction algorithms for our experiment from the MIT-BIH Database Distribution [54].

We have downloaded the ECG signal from ECG data bank [54]. The ECG signals are freely available for academic experiments. We have applied some algorithms to extract the features (P, QRS, PR, etc.) from the ECG signal and stored it into a database. We have written down some Macromedia Flash scripts to interface between Flash tool and Brama component, to pass the real data set as a parameter from a database to the Event-B model. No any tool is available to interface between database and the Event-B model. Extra Macromedia Flash script coding and the Brama animation tool help to test the Event-B formal model of the cardiac pacemaker on the real-time data set. We have designed an animated graphic of heart and pacemaker in Macromedia Flash, where this animated model represents the pacing activity in the right ventricular chamber. This animated model simulates the behaviour of heart according to the bradycardia operating modes and animates the graphic model. The animation of the model is fully based on the Event-B model. Event-B model is executing all events according to the parametric value. These parametric values are the extracted features from the ECG signal, which are passing into the Event-B model.

Figure 9.11 represents an implementation of proposed architecture on the formal model of a cardiac pacemaker case study. According to the architecture, data acquisition unit collects the ECG signal and features extractions are done by the feature extraction or parameter estimation unit. The extracting features are stored in the database XML file format. Macromedia Flash tool helps to design the animated graphics of the heart and pacemaker. Brama plug-in helps to communicate between animated graphics and Event-B formal model of the single electrode cardiac pacemaker. Finally, we have tested a real-time data set in the formal models without generating the source code.

One- and two-electrode Pacemaker's pacing and sensing behaviours are validated through cardiologist experts using real-time data; ECG signal. We have found some unexpected behaviours of the formal model according to the cardiologist experts in visualisation. We have modified the pacemaker formal model according to cardiologist experts and verify through the real-time animation tool. So, we consider that the real-time animation tool has a very important role in the area of development of the formal methods, and it can help to obtain a trust-able formal model, which can be helpful to obtain the certification assurances [11, 16, 23, 26, 27, 44].

9.13 Code Generation Using EB2ALL Tool

We have presented a proof-based an incremental formal development of a cardiac pacemaker in [40, 43, 48, 53] using our proposed tool and techniques. This section presents an automatic code generation from developed and proved formal specification of a cardiac pacemaker. We now illustrate the use of EB2C, EB2C++, EB2J and EB2C# tools [13, 41, 46, 47] by means of the automatic generation of C, C++, Java and C# codes for the cardiac pacemaker system described with EVENT B in [45, 51]. This tool has a technique of automatic support of safety assurance of a generated code. To achieve a verified source code of the cardiac pacemaker, we have done further refinement of the concrete models of the cardiac pacemaker using a new context, which has some data ranges (see Table 7.1) corresponding to the programming languages. The context file provides deterministic ranges for all kinds of data types. This refinement makes the model deterministic and generates some proof obligations due to defining the fixed data ranges of all constants and variables of the cardiac pacemaker model. The generated proof obligations are discharged by automatic as well as manual, and all these proofs are necessary to verify the specification in order to guarantee the consistency and correctness of the system. We have discharged all the generated proof obligations before generating the source code. This level of refinement complies system specification abstractly. Now, we move to the next level of code translation methodology as to pass the concrete model for continuing translation process.

The code translation from Event-B formal specification into any programming language using EB2ALL is straightforward using a set of plug-ins (EB2C, EB2C++, EB2J and EB2C#) [13, 41, 46, 47]. The main idea is to translate an Event-B model into any programming language code using the last concrete model. The EB2ALL tool generates programming language files corresponding to the concrete models. A generated source file using EB2ALL tool has a basic structure: a set of constants, variables and functions. A set of constants and variables are extracted from the context and machines sections of the Event-B model of the cardiac pacemaker, respectively. Data type of constant is defined as an axiom in Event-B model. Similarly, data type of variable is extracted from the invariant section of the model. Initial value of the constants and variables are initialised, if their initial values are declared. A set of constants and variables are given as follows, which are excerpted from the translated 'C' codes of the cardiac pacemaker model.

```
enum status {ON, OFF}; /* Enumerated  definition */
const int FixedAV=90; /* Integer in range 70-300 */
const int LRL=60; /* Integer in range 30-175 */
const int ARP=200; /* Integer in range 50-175 */
const int URL=120; /* Integer in range 50-175 */
const int VRP=250;
const int PVARP=150;
const int V_Blank=50;
. . .
enum status PM_Actuator_V; /* Enumerated  type variable */
enum status PM_Sensor_V; /* Enumerated  type variable */
unsigned long int Thr_V; /* Integer in range undefined */
unsigned long int AV_Count; /* Integer in range undefined */
BOOL AV_Count_STATE;
unsigned long last_sp;
unsigned long int sp;
unsigned long int Pace_Int;
. . .
```

A set of functions are extracted equivalent to a set of events of the pacemaker formal model. All the events of Event-B are translated into equivalent programming language functions. An event INITIALISATION is a programming language function, which initialise default values of all the variables. An event of Event-B model has fixed organisation of the internal components; local variables, guards (pre-conditions) and actions. An event may contain some local variables. The global constants and variables are declared on the top of the programming language source file, while local variables are declared within the function body. All events of a formal model is translated as a set of programming language functions. This function has the similar structure as an event. During the translation of the events, the guards are translated into equivalent to 'if' statement using logical conjunction, disjunction, implication and equivalence. Each guard represents into a separate 'if' statement like nested 'if' structure. All these guards represent a set of preconditions, which are required to satisfy for executing the action predicates. All action predicates of a formal model event are directly translatable equivalent into programming language assignment expressions. The EB2ALL tool is capable to analyse the syntax of Event-B guards and actions predicate. In the cardiac pacemaker formal model, their predicates are simple, which are obtained through several refinements. All preconditions or guards are required to be TRUE for executing all actions. However, despite being a complex system, the pacemaker pre-conditions are fairly simple to calculate. If all the guards are true, then the action's predicates execute and return TRUE for successful execution of the function. If any 'if' condition false, then the function returns FALSE and action's part of the function does not execute.

```
. . .
BOOL Actuator_ON_V ( void )
{
    /* Guards No.  1 */
```

```
if (PM_Actuator_V == OFF){
/* Guards No. 2*/
if ((sp == Pace_Int) || ((sp < Pace_Int) &&
(AV_Count > V_Blank) && (AV_Count >= FixedAV))){
/* Guards No. 3*/
if ((sp >= VRP)&&(sp >= PVARP) && (sp >= URI)){
/* Actions */
PM_Actuator_V = ON;
last_sp = sp;
return TRUE;
}}}
  return FALSE;
}
...
```

To make the generated code executable, the EB2ALL tool generates an *Iterate*
function that contains a list of all functions as in form of a function call. Another
function is a main body of the program like *main*() in 'C', which calls *Iterate* function. These two extra functions are used to compile and execute the generated code.

```
...
BOOL Iterate(void)
{
    if ( Actuator_ON_V ()==TRUE ) return TRUE;
    if ( Actuator_OFF_V ()==TRUE ) return TRUE;
    if ( Actuator_ON_A ()==TRUE ) return TRUE;
    if ( Actuator_OFF_A ()==TRUE ) return TRUE;
    if ( Sensor_ON_A ()==TRUE ) return TRUE;
    if ( Sensor_OFF_A ()==TRUE ) return TRUE;
    if ( Sensor_ON_V ()==TRUE ) return TRUE;
    if ( Sensor_OFF_V ()==TRUE ) return TRUE;
    if ( tic ()==TRUE ) return TRUE;
    if ( tic_AV ()==TRUE ) return TRUE;
    if ( Thr_Value_A ()==TRUE ) return TRUE;
    if ( Thr_Value_V ()==TRUE ) return TRUE;
    if ( Hyt_Pace_Updating ()==TRUE ) return TRUE;
    if ( Increase_Interval ()==TRUE ) return TRUE;
    if ( Decrease_Interval ()==TRUE ) return TRUE;
    if ( Acler_sensed ()==TRUE ) return TRUE;

    /* Signal deadlock */
    return FALSE;
}
...
```

The source code is automatically generated in any programming language (C,
C++, Java and C#) from the verified specification in less than five seconds. The
generated code resulted in over 5000 lines in all operating modes. Here, we have
presented a brief overview of the translation from the Event-B specification of the

cardiac pacemaker formal model into 'C' using EB2C tool. Based on this translation, we were able to automatically generate 'C' code and execute a simulation of
the pacemaker.

9.14   Discussion

New development methodology is successfully applied for developing the cardiac
pacemaker from requirement analysis to code implementation. The whole system
development life-cycle is based on formal techniques. The complete system is designed using different kinds of tools related to the formal techniques. The Event-B
modelling language is used for formalising the pacemaker system using refinement
techniques. Each level of refinements is validated through the ProB model checker
and the real-time animator for verifying the correctness of the system behaviours
against requirements and according to the medical experts, respectively. If any error is discovered during verification, validation or domain experts reviews, then the
pacemaker specification is modified and again follow the verification, validation and
domain experts reviews. This process is continued applied in a loop until not find
the correct proved formal specification of the cardiac pacemaker. The verification,
validation and domains experts reviews are applied on each refinement level for
modelling the whole system. To handle the complexity of a system according to the
refinements, we have used the refinement chart to model the cardiac pacemaker system. The refinement charts of the pacemaker present integration architecture of the
system in form of all possible operating modes. Some operating modes are an extension of the existing operating modes, it is clearly expressible from the refinement
charts. This technique is not only for code integration, but also it helps for analysing
the operating modes and code structuring of the system. Finally, we have used the
tool EB2ALL for generating the source code into multiple languages (C, C++, C#,
and Java) from the formal specifications. In this development process, we have not
considered the safety assessment approach.

According to the existing development life cycle, we use formal methods only on
the selected part of the system for verifying the correctness of the system against requirement. No formal methods are likely to be suitable for describing and analysing
every aspect of a complex system; a practical approach is to use different methods in combination. In this book, we have provided some possible solutions for
emerging problems in area of software engineering related to the development of
critical systems, where we have proposed a development life-cycle and associated
a set of techniques and tools to develop the highly critical systems using formal
techniques from requirements analysis to automatic source code generation. There
is not a set of supporting tools, which can be used for system development using
only formal techniques. We have developed a set of new tools, which support a rigorous framework for the system development and finally; we have applied this new
development life-cycle methodology and associated tools for developing the cardiac pacemaker system for assessing the usability of our proposed approach. This

methodology uses only refinement approach to build the complete system and each refinement level is verified using different techniques. Last level of the system is the concrete model, which has been used for producing the source code. The code generation tool EB2ALL is very simple in use, which can generate the optimised codes for future use. The process for system development is user friendly, but a developer has required the strong knowledge of formalisation and refinement techniques to build the correct system using this new system development methodology and associated techniques and tools.

9.15 Summary

In this chapter, we have presented the pacemaker specification, one of the challenges proposed by the Verified Software Initiative [25]. We have developed the formal model of the pacemaker system in Event-B and discovered the exact functional behaviour of the pacing and sensing events. Our approach for formalising and reasoning about action-reaction is based on real-time as a pacemaker system. The pacemaker case study suggests that such an approach can yield a viable model that can be subjected to useful validation against system-level properties at the early stage of the development process. The proposed techniques based on development patterns intend to assist in the design process of the system where correctness and safety are important issues.

A series of high confidence medical devices of increasing scope and complexity will follow the pacemaker system. Main advantage of proposed development methodology and a set of associated techniques and tools is the ability to develop the whole system from requirement analysis to code generation. Proposed methodology exploits the advance capabilities of the combined approach of formal verification and model validation using a model-checker, use of real time animation to test system behaviour and, finally automatic source code generation from a verified formal model in order to achieve the considerable advantages for a critical system design.

The proposed approach has also involved the use of the real-time animator for executing formal specification to validate the actual requirements. The main objectives of this real-time animator [42] are to promote the use of such kinds of tool to bridge a gap between software engineers and stakeholders to build quality system and to discover all the ambiguous information from the requirements. Moreover, this tool helps to verify the correctness of behaviour of the system according to the stakeholders requirements. The combined approach of the formal verification and real-time animation allows the systematic development of a clear, concise, precise and unambiguous specification of a software system and enables to the software engineers to animate the formal specification at the early stage of the development. The formal specification animation is supported by both software engineers and stakeholders. Our case study on cardiac pacemaker illustrates the potential value which is a formal specification, and its subsequent animation can bring to the comprehension and clarification of the informal requirements.

System integration methodology using refinements charts (see Figs. 9.5, 9.6) are also used for system development, which helps a code designer to improve the code structure and code optimisation, and the code generation for synthesising and synchronising the software codes of a critical system like the cardiac pacemaker. In the pacemaker case study, each operating mode (see Table 9.1) have different kinds of functional requirements, and all the operating modes are decomposed in the refinement chart using multiple refinements. The refinement chart and formal specifications support more systematic and error-free designing and implementation rather than other traditional approaches of system designing and implementation. Here, the refinement chart is tightly coupled with the formal specifications. A set of requirements are formally represented in the specifications. The complexity of formal specifications is the amounts of proof obligations (see Tables 9.3 and 9.4). Therefore use of the refinement chart, and formal specifications states the correctness of the system design and implementation.

The refinement chart specially covers component-based design frameworks and decomposition, integration of the critical infrastructure and device integration. We can see from our pacemaker case study that all these claims help to design error-free system and different phase of the pacemaker has been shown by refinements in form of formal development as well as refinement charts. We have presented evidence that such an analysis is fruitful for both formal and non-formal group of people. The second observation from our experiments is that the development of multiple models helped us not only find errors in the requirement documents but also gave us an opportunity to better understand intricate requirements such as the control algorithm of a medical system. Moreover, we believe that the effort needed is commensurate with the benefits we derive from developing the multiple models. An ideal critical system has the following characteristics:

- Embedded real-time system's design.
- To obtain the certification for providing the higher safety integrity level.
- Helps to domain experts to analyse work process guidelines.
- Sufficient complexity that traditional methods, such as testing and code reviews, are inadequate to establish its correctness.
- Model-based development and component-based design frameworks.
- Animator assists to regulatory agencies and helps to meet ISO/IEC and IEEE standards.
- Ability to monitor a real-time environment using animator at animation time and analyse the requirements, violations of goals, expectations on the environments, and domain properties.
- Real-time animation of a specification supplements inspection and reasoning as means for validation. This is especially important for the validation of non-functional behaviour.
- Real-time animation technique is available in early phase of the system development life-cycle, which can be used to correct validation errors immediately, without incurring costly redevelopment.
- Infrastructure for critical system integration and inter-operation.
- System integration of critical infrastructure.

- Possibility of annotating models for different purposes (e.g., directing synthesis or hooking to verification tools).
- To discover the complex situation using refinement approach.
- Decomposition of the complex system into different independent subsystems.
- To reduce the gap between software engineers and stakeholders requirements using real-time animator and easy to explain model behaviour to domain experts as well stakeholders.
- Ambiguous and incomplete requirements can be clarified and completed by hands-on experience with the specifications using our approach.

Code generation is a process, which is used to transform a formal specification into any programming language like C, C++, C#, Java, etc. Code generation from the verified formal model is our main objective. For generating the source code into different kinds of programming languages (C, C++, Java and C#), we have used a tool EB2ALL [13, 41, 46, 47]. We have developed a set of plug-ins tools [13, 41, 46, 47], which provides fully automatic code generation from Event-B formal specification into programming languages. The adaptations of the translation rules are required more complete experiments, especially with the large formal models for checking the impact on the execution time for some specific platforms. Finally, we have shown a satisfactory result and demonstrate the ability to generate automatically source code from EVENT B specification of the cardiac pacemaker in C, C++, Java and C# languages, which are comparable to a code written by hand with ordinary programming languages. The gains rely then on the guarantees provided using formal methods and on the certification level which can be obtained by this way. As far as we know, only few formal methods support code generation, which is as time/space efficient as handwritten code.

This chapter also presents an approach for modelling the closed-loop system of the cardiac pacemaker. The prime objective of this approach is to provide a new modelling technique, which helps to combine the formal models of a critical system and related environment. For example, the cardiac pacemaker operates in the biological heart system. The closed-loop modelling is an effective approach, which guarantees the correctness of the operating behaviour of the critical system. Moreover, this approach can be viable to obtain the certification standards for the developing system. To build a closed-loop model using both environment and device modelling is considered as a standard approach for validation, given that designing an environment model is a challenging problem in the real world. Industry has long sought such an approach to validating system models in a biological environment.

Proposed development methodology and associated techniques and tools enable us to design a new environment for medical device modelling and simulating and offers to obtain that challenge of complying with FDA's QSR and ISO's 13485 quality system directives [23, 32].

In order to assess the overall utility of our approach, a selection of the results of the formalisation and verification steps have been presented to a group of pacemaker developers (French-Italian based pacemaker company). The developers are satisfied by the results of pacemaker development using all proposed approaches in sense of incremental development, real-time animation of formal model, integration of hardware and software and automatically code generation approach from verified formal specifications. They are really agreed on the refinement charts for showing operating mode relation and their mode transitions. Based on the experiment described above and our conclusions we are convinced of the usefulness on certain areas, and therefore, we are considering to use all these tools and methodology, which are very helpful to design not even in a medical domain but also for other industrial domains, such as avionic and automotive domains.

References

1. Abrial, J.-R. (2010). *Modeling in Event-B: System and software engineering* (1st ed.). New York: Cambridge University Press.
2. Artigou, J. Y., & Monsuez, J. J. (2007). *Cardiologie et maladies vasculaires*. Paris: Elsevier Masson.
3. Baier, C., & Katoen, J.-P. (2008). *Principles of model checking (representation and mind series)*. Cambridge: MIT Press.
4. Barold, S. S., Stroobandt, R. X., & Sinnaeve, A. F. (2004). *Cardiac pacemakers step by step*. London: Futura. ISBN 1-4051-1647-1.
5. Bayes, B. V. N., de Luna, A., & Malik, M. (2006). The morphology of the electrocardiogram. In *The ESC textbook of cardiovascular medicine* (pp. 1–36). Oxford: Blackwell.
6. Bjørner, D., & Jones, C. B. (Eds.) (1978). *The Vienna development method: The metalanguage*. London: Springer.
7. Boston Scientific (2007). *Pacemaker system specification* (Technical report). http://www.cas.mcmaster.ca/sqrl/~SQRLDocuments/PACEMAKER.pdf.
8. Cansell, D., & Méry, D. (2008). The Event-B modelling method: Concepts and case studies. In D. Bjørner & M. C. Henson (Eds.), *Monographs in theoretical computer science. Logics of specification languages* (pp. 47–152). Berlin: Springer.
9. Cansell, D., Méry, D., & Rehm, J. (2006). Time constraint patterns for Event B development. In J. Julliand & O. Kouchnarenko (Eds.), *Lecture notes in computer science: Vol. 4355. B 2007: Formal specification and development in B* (pp. 140–154). Berlin: Springer.
10. Clarke, E. M., Grumberg, O., & Peled, D. (2001). *Model checking*. Cambridge: MIT Press.
11. CC. Common criteria. http://www.commoncriteriaportal.org/.
12. Crocker, D. (2003). Perfect developer: A tool for object-oriented formal specification and refinement. Tools exhibition notes at formal methods Europe. In *Tools exhibition notes at formal methods Europe* (p. 2003).
13. EB2ALL (2011). Automatic code generation from Event-B to many programming languages. http://eb2all.loria.fr/.
14. Ellenbogen, K. A., & Wood, M. A. (2005). *Cardiac pacing and ICDs* (4th ed.). Oxford: Blackwell. ISBN 1-4051-0447-3.
15. Epstein, A. E., DiMarco, J. P., Ellenbogen, K. A., Estes, N. A. M., III, Freedman, R. A., Gettes, L. S., et al. (2008). ACC/AHA/HRS 2008 guidelines for device-based therapy of cardiac rhythm abnormalities: A report of the American College of Cardiology/American Heart Association task force on practice guidelines (writing committee to revise the ACC/AHA/NASPE 2002 guideline update for implantation of cardiac pacemakers and antiarrhythmia devices) developed in collaboration with the American Association for Thoracic Surgery and Society of Thoracic Surgeons. *Journal of the American College of Cardiology, 51*(21), e1–e62.
16. FDA. Food and Drug Administration. http://www.fda.gov/.

17. Gamma, E., Helm, R., Johnson, R., Vlissides, R., & Gamma, P. (1994). *Design patterns: Elements of reusable object-oriented software design patterns*. Reading: Addison-Wesley Professional.
18. Goldman, B. S., Noble, E. J., Heller, J. G., & Covvey, D. (1974). The pacemaker challenge. *CMAJ. Canadian Medical Association Journal, 110*(1), 28–31.
19. Gomes, A., & Oliveira, M. (2009). Formal specification of a cardiac pacing system. In A. Cavalcanti & D. Dams (Eds.), *Lecture notes in computer science: Vol. 5850. FM 2009: Formal methods* (pp. 692–707). Berlin: Springer.
20. Gomes, A. O., & Oliveira, M. V. M. (2010). Formal development of a cardiac pacemaker: From specification to code. In *Lecture notes in computer science. SBFM 2010* (pp. 213–228).
21. Harrild, D. M., & Henriquez, C. S. (2000). A computer model of normal conduction in the human atria. *Circulation Research, 87*, 25–36.
22. Hesselson, A. (2003). *Simplified interpretations of pacemaker ECGs*. Oxford: Blackwell. ISBN 978-1-4051-0372-5.
23. High Confidence Software and Systems Coordinating Group (2009). *High-confidence medical devices: Cyber-physical systems for 21st century health care* (Technical report). NITRD. http://www.nitrd.gov/About/MedDevice-FINAL1-web.pdf.
24. Hoare, C. A. R. (2003). The verifying compiler: A grand challenge for computing research. In H. Kosch, L. Böszörményi, & H. Hellwagner (Eds.), *Lecture notes in computer science: Vol. 2790. Euro-Par 2003 parallel processing* (p. 1). Berlin: Springer.
25. Hoare, C. A. R., Misra, J., Leavens, G. T., & Shankar, N. (2009). The verified software initiative: A manifesto. *ACM Computing Surveys, 41*(4), 22:1–22:8.
26. IEEE-SA. IEEE Standards Association. http://standards.ieee.org/.
27. ISO. International Organization for Standardization. http://www.iso.org/.
28. Jackson, D. (2002). Alloy: A lightweight object modelling notation. *ACM Transactions on Software Engineering and Methodology, 11*(2), 256–290.
29. Jiang, Z., Pajic, M., & Mangharam, R. (2011). Model-based closed-loop testing of implantable pacemakers. In *2011 IEEE/ACM international conference on cyber-physical systems*, ICCPS (pp. 131–140).
30. Jiang, Z., Pajic, M., Moarref, S., Alur, R., & Mangharam, R. (2012). Modeling and verification of a dual chamber implantable pacemaker. In C. Flanagan & B. König (Eds.), *Lecture notes in computer science: Vol. 7214. Tools and algorithms for the construction and analysis of systems* (pp. 188–203). Berlin: Springer.
31. Kantharia, B. K., & Kutalek, S. P. (1999). Optimal programming of rate modulation functions. *Cardiac Electrophysiology Review, 3*, 53–55. doi:10.1023/A:1009935600754.
32. Keatley, K. L. (1999). A review of the FDA draft guidance document for software validation: Guidance for industry. *Quality Assurance, 7*(1), 49–55.
33. Khan, M. G. (2008). *Rapid ECG interpretation*. Clifton: Humana Press.
34. La Manna, V. P., Bonanno, A. T., & Motta, A. (2009). Poster on a simple pacemaker implementation. New York: ACM.
35. Lee, I., Pappas, G. J., Cleaveland, R., Hatcliff, J., Krogh, B. H., Lee, P., et al. (2006). High-confidence medical device software and systems. *Computer, 39*(4), 33–38.
36. Leuschel, M., & Butler, M. (2003). *Lecture notes in computer science. ProB: A model checker for B* (pp. 855–874). Berlin: Springer.
37. Love, C. J. (2006). *Cardiac pacemakers and defibrillators*. Georgetown: Landes Bioscience. ISBN 1-57059-691-3.
38. Macedo, H. D., Larsen, P. G., & Fitzgerald, J. (2008). Incremental development of a distributed real-time model of a cardiac pacing system using VDM. In *Lecture notes in computer science. Proceedings of the 15th international symposium on formal methods*, FM'08 (pp. 181–197). Berlin: Springer.
39. Malmivuo, J. (1995). *Bioelectromagnetism*. Oxford: Oxford University Press. ISBN 0-19-505823-2.
40. Méry, D., & Singh, N. K. (2009). *Pacemaker's functional behaviors in Event-B* (Research report). MOSEL-LORIA-INRIA-CNRS: UMR7503-Université Henri Poincaré-

Nancy I-Université Nancy II-Institut National Polytechnique de Lorraine. http://hal.inria.fr/inria-00419973/en/.

41. Méry, D., & Singh, N. K. (2010). *EB2C: A tool for Event-B to C conversion support*. Poster and tool demo submission, published in a CNR technical report in SEFM.

42. Méry, D., & Singh, N. K. (2010). Real-time animation for formal specification. In M. Aiguier, F. Bretaudeau, & D. Krob (Eds.), *Complex systems design & management* (pp. 49–60). Berlin: Springer.

43. Méry, D., & Singh, N. K. (2010). Technical report on formal development of two-electrode cardiac pacing system. MOSEL-LORIA-INRIA-CNRS: UMR7503-Université Henri Poincaré-Nancy I-Université Nancy II-Institut National Polytechnique de Lorraine. http://hal.archives-ouvertes.fr/inria-00465061/en/.

44. Méry, D., & Singh, N. K. (2010). Trustable formal specification for software certification. In T. Margaria & B. Steffen (Eds.), *Lecture notes in computer science: Vol. 6416. Leveraging applications of formal methods, verification, and validation* (pp. 312–326). Berlin: Springer.

45. Méry, D., & Singh, N. (2011). A generic framework: From modeling to code. In *Innovations in systems and software engineering* (pp. 1–9).

46. Méry, D., & Singh, N. K. (2011). Automatic code generation from Event-B models. In *Proceedings of the second symposium on information and communication technology*, SoICT'11 (pp. 179–188). New York: ACM.

47. Méry, D., & Singh, N. K. (2011). *EB2J: Code generation from Event-B to Java*. Short paper presented at the 14th Brazilian symposium on formal methods, SBMF'11.

48. Méry, D., & Singh, N. K. (2011). Functional behavior of a cardiac pacing system. *International Journal of Discrete Event Control Systems*, *1*(2), 129–149.

49. Méry, D., & Singh, N. K. (2011). Technical report on formalisation of the heart using analysis of conduction time and velocity of the electrocardiography and cellular-automata. MOSEL-LORIA-INRIA-CNRS: UMR7503-Université Henri Poincaré-Nancy I-Université Nancy II-Institut National Polytechnique de Lorraine. http://hal.inria.fr/inria-00600339/en/.

50. Méry, D., & Singh, N. K. (2012). Closed-loop modeling of cardiac pacemaker and heart. In *Foundations of health informatics engineering and systems*.

51. Méry, D., & Singh, N. K. (2012). *Formal development and automatic code generation: Cardiac pacemaker*. New York: ASME Press.

52. Méry, D., & Singh, N. K. (2012). Formalization of heart models based on the conduction of electrical impulses and cellular automata. In Z. Liu & A. Wassyng (Eds.), *Lecture notes in computer science: Vol. 7151. Foundations of health informatics engineering and systems* (pp. 140–159). Berlin: Springer.

53. Méry, D., & Singh, N. K. (2013). Formal specification of medical systems by proof-based refinement. *ACM Transactions on Embedded Computing Systems*, *12*(1), 15:1–15:25.

54. MIT-BIH. MIT-BIH database distribution and software. http://ecg.mit.edu/index.html.

55. Rehm, J. (2010). Proved development of the real-time properties of the IEEE 1394 Root Contention Protocol with the Event-B method. *International Journal on Software Tools for Technology Transfer*, *12*(1), 39–51.

56. RODIN (2004). Rigorous open development environment for complex systems. http://rodin-b-sharp.sourceforge.net.

57. Singh, N. K., Wellings, A., & Cavalcanti, A. (2012). The cardiac pacemaker case study and its implementation in safety-critical Java and Ravenscar Ada. In *Proceedings of the 10th international workshop on Java technologies for real-time and embedded systems*, JTRES'12 (pp. 62–71). New York: ACM.

58. Tuan, L. A., Zheng, M. C., & Tho, Q. T. (2010). Modeling and verification of safety critical systems: A case study on pacemaker. In *Secure system integration and reliability improvement* (pp. 23–32).

59. Woodcock, J. (2006). First steps in the verified software grand challenge. *Computer*, *39*(10), 57–64.

60. Woodcock, J., & Banach, R. (2007). The verification grand challenge. *Journal of Universal Computer Science*, *13*(5), 661–668.

Chapter 10
Formalisation of Electrocardiogram (ECG)

Abstract Today, an evidence-based medicine has given number of medical practice clinical guidelines and protocols. Clinical guidelines systematically assist practitioners with providing appropriate health care for specific clinical circumstances. However, a significant number of guidelines and protocols are lacking in quality. Indeed, ambiguity and incompleteness are more likely anomalies in medical practices. From last few years, many researchers have tried to address the problem of protocol improvement in clinical guidelines, but results are not sufficient since they believe on informal processes and notations. Our objective is to find anomalies and to improve the quality of medical protocols using well known formal techniques, such as Event-B. In this chapter; we use a modelling language to capture the guidelines for their validation. We have established a classification of the possible properties to be verified in a guideline. Our approach is illustrated with a guideline which published by the National Guideline Clearing House (NGC) and AHA/ACC Society. Our main contribution is to evaluate the real-life medical protocols using refinement based formal methods for improving quality of the protocols. Refinement based formalisation is very easy to handle any complex medical protocols. For this evaluation, we have selected a real-life reference protocol (ECG Interpretation), which covers a wide variety of protocol characteristics related to the several heart diseases. We formalise the given reference protocol, verify a set of interesting properties of the protocol and finally determine anomalies. Our main results are: to formalise an ECG interpretation protocol for diagnosing the ECG signal in an optimal way; to discover a hierarchical structure for the ECG interpretation efficiently using incremental refinement approach; a set of properties which should be satisfied by the medical protocol; verification proofs for the protocol and properties according to the medical experts; and perspectives of the potentials of this approach. Finally, we have shown the feasibility of our approach for analysing the medical protocols.

10.1 Introduction

A promising and challenging application area for the application of formal methods is a clinical decision making, as it is vital that the clinical decisions are sound. In fact, ensuring safety is the primary preoccupation of medical regulatory agencies. Medical guidelines are "systematically developed statements to assist

N.K. Singh, *Using Event-B for Critical Device Software Systems*,
DOI 10.1007/978-1-4471-5260-6_10, © Springer-Verlag London 2013

practitioners and patient decisions about appropriate health care for specific circumstances" [11, 36]. Based on updated empirical evidence; the medical protocols to provide clinicians with health-care testimonial and facilitate the spreading of high-standard practices. In fact, this way represents that adherence to protocol may reduce the costs of care up to 25 % [36]. In order to reach their potential benefits, protocols must fulfil strong quality requirements. Medical bodies worldwide have made efforts in this direction, e.g. elaborating appraisal documents that take into account a variety of aspects, of both protocols and their development process. However, these initiatives are not sufficient since they rely on informal methods and notations. The informal methods and notations have not any mathematical foundation.

We are concerned with a different approach, namely the quality improvement of medical protocols through formal methods. In this chapter, we report on our experiences in the formalisation and verification of a medical protocol for diagnosis of the Electrocardiogram (ECG) [21, 22]. The ECG signals are too complex for diagnosis. All kinds of diseases related to the heart are predictable using 12-lead ECG signals. A high number of medical guidelines for the ECG interpretation has been published in the literature and on the Internet, making them more accessible. Currently, protocols are described using a combination of different formats, e.g. text, flow diagrams and tables. These approaches are used in form of informal processes and notations for analysing the medical protocols, which are not sufficient for medical practices. As a result, the ECG interpretation guidelines and protocols[1] still contain ambiguous, incomplete or even inconsistent elements.

The idea of our work is translating the informal descriptions of the ECG interpretation into a more formal language, with the aim of analysing a set of properties of the ECG protocol. In addition to the advantages of such a kind of formal verification, making these descriptions more formal can serve to expose problematic parts in the protocols.

Formal methods have well structured representation language with clear and well-defined semantics, which can be used for taxonomy verification of clinical the guidelines and medical protocols. The representation language represents guidelines and protocols explicitly and in a non-ambiguous way. The process of verification using formal semantic representation of guidelines and protocols to allow the determination of consistency and correctness.

Formal modelling and verification of medical protocol to have been carried out as a case study to assess the feasibility of this approach. Throughout our case study, we have shown formal specification and verification of medical protocols. The ECG interpretation protocol is very complex, ambiguous, incomplete and inconsistent.

The contribution of this chapter is to give a complete idea of formal development of the ECG interpretation protocol, and we have discovered a hierarchical structure for the ECG interpretation efficiently using incremental refinement approach [21, 22]. Same approach can be also applied for developing a formal model of the protocol of any other disease. Our approach is based on the Event-B [1, 7]

---

[1]Guideline and protocol are different terms. The term protocol is used to represent a specialised version of a guideline. In this chapter, we use them indistinctively.

modelling language which is supported by the Rodin platform integrating tools for proving models and refinements of the models. Here, we present an incremental proof-based development to model and verify such interdisciplinary requirements in the Event-B [1, 7]. The ECG interpretation models must be validated to ensure that they meet requirements of the ECG protocols. Hence, validation must be carried out by both formal modelling and medical domain experts.

We have used a general formal modelling tool like Event-B [1] for modelling a complex medical protocol related to diagnoses of the ECG signal. To apply a refinement based technique to model a medical protocol is our main objective. The Event-B supports refinement technique. The refinement supported by the Rodin [29] platform guarantees the preservation of safety properties. The safety properties are detection of an actual disease under the certain conditions. The behaviour of the final system is preserved by an abstract model as well as in the correctly refined models. This technique is used to model a medical protocol more rigorously based on formal mathematics, which helps to find the anomalies and provide the consistency and correctness of the medical protocol. The current work intends to explore those problems related to the modelling of the ECG protocols. The formalisation of the ECG protocol is based on the original protocol, and all the safety properties and related assumptions are verified with the medical experts. Moreover, an incremental development of the ECG interpretation protocol model helps to discover the ambiguous, incomplete or even inconsistent elements in current the ECG interpretation protocol.

10.1.1　Structure of This Chapter

The outline of the remaining chapter is as follows. Section 10.2 contains related work. Section 10.3 presents selection of medical protocol for formalisation. We give a brief outline of the ECG in Sect. 10.4. In Sect. 10.5, we explore the incremental proof-based formal development of the ECG interpretation protocol. The verification results are discussed in Sect. 10.6. Finally, Sect. 10.7 summarises the chapter.

10.2　Related Work

Section 10.2 currently presents ongoing research work related to computer-based medical guidelines and protocols for clinical purposes. From past few years many languages have been developed for representing medical guidelines and protocols using various levels of formality based on expert's requirements. Although we have used the Event-B modelling language for guidelines and protocol representation in our case study. Various kinds of protocol representation languages like Asbru [33, 36], EON [26], PROforma [12] and others [27, 38] are used to represent a formal semantics of guidelines and medical protocols.

Clinical guidelines are useful tools to provide some standardisation and helps for improving the protocols. A survey paper [15] presents benefits and comparison through an analysis of different kinds of systems, which are used by clinical guidelines. This paper covers a wide scope of clinical guidelines related literatures and tools, which are collected from the medical informatics area.

An approach for improving guidelines and protocols is by evaluating the physician. Evaluation process involves the scenario and evidence based testing, which compares the actions. The actions are performed by physicians to handle particular patient case using testimonials that are prescribed by the guidelines [24]. When results of the actions deviate, evaluation process can be either focused on the explanation alternatively provide some valuable feedback for improving the guidelines and protocols [20]. An intention based evaluation process are deduced by the physicians from both the patient data and the performed actions. These are then verified against the intentions reported in the guidelines.

Automated quality assessment of clinical actions and patient outcomes is another area of related work, which is used to derive structured quality indicators from formal specifications of guidelines. This technique is used in decision support [2]. Such kinds of indicators is used as formal properties in our work that guideline must comply with.

Decision-table based techniques for the verification and simplification of guidelines are presented by Shiffman et al. [34, 35]. The basic idea behind this approach is to describe guidelines as condition/action statements: *If the antecedent circumstances exist, then one should perform the recommended actions* [34]. Completeness and consistency are two main properties for verification, when guidelines and protocols are expressed in terms of decision-table. Again, these properties are internal coherence properties, whereas we are focused on domain-specific properties.

Formal development of the guidelines and protocols using clinical logic may be incomplete or inconsistent. This problem is tackled by Miller et al. [25]. *If "if-then" rules are used as representation language for guidelines, incompleteness means that there are combinations of clinically meaningful conditions to which the system (guideline) is not able to respond* [25]. The verification of rule-based clinical guidelines using semantic constraints is supported by the commander tool. This tool is able to identify clinical conditions where the rules are incomplete. Miller et al. [25] were able to find a number of missing rules in various case studies of the guidelines and protocols.

Guidelines enhancement is represented through adoption of an advanced Artificial Intelligence techniques [6]. This paper has proposed an approach for verification of the guidelines, which is based on the integration of a computerised guidelines management system with a model-checker. They have used SPIN model checker [8, 14] for executing and verifying medical protocols or guidelines. A framework for authoring and verification of clinical guidelines is provided by Beatriz et al. [28]. The verification process of guidelines is based on combined approach of Model Driven Development (MDD) and Model Checking [8] to verify guidelines against semantic errors and inconsistencies. UML [30, 39] tool is used for modelling the guidelines, and a generated formal model is used as the input model for a model checker.

Jonathan et al. [31] have proposed a way to apply formal methods, namely interactive verification to improve the quality of medical protocols or guidelines. They have applied this technique for the management of jaundice in newborns based on guidelines of American Academy of Pediatrics. This paper includes formalisation of the jaundice protocol and verifies some interesting properties. Simon et al. [5] have used the same protocol for improvement purpose using a modelling language Asbru, temporal logic for expressing the quality requirements, and model checking for proof and error detection.

Applying a formal approach for improving medical protocol is one major area of research, which helps to the medical practitioners for improve the quality of patient care. A project Protocure [37] is a European project, which is carried out by five different institutions. The main objective of this project is for improving medical protocol through integration of formal methods. The main motivation of this project is to identify anomalies like ambiguity and incompleteness in the medical guidelines and protocols. Presently, all medical protocols and guidelines are in text, flow diagrams and tables formats, which are easily understandable by the medical practitioners. But these are incomplete and ambiguous due to lack of formal semantics. The idea of using formal methods is to uncover these ambiguous, incomplete or even inconsistent parts of the protocols, by defining all the different descriptions more precisely using a formal language and to enable verification. Mainly, the researchers have used Asbru [36] language for protocol description and KIV for interactive verification system [3].

Asbru [36] is a main modelling language for describing medical protocol and formal proof of the medical protocol is possible through KIV interactive theorem prover [3]. Guideline Markup Tool (GMT) [17] is an editor who helps to translate guidelines into Asbru. An additional functionality of the tool is to define relations between the original protocol and its Asbru translation with a link macro [17]. Asbru language is used for protocol description and Asbru formalisations are translated into KIV. Asbru is considered as a semi-formal language to support the tasks necessary for protocol-based care. It is called a semi-formal language because of its semantics, although more precise than in other protocol representation languages, are not defined in a formal way. This semi-formal quality makes Asbru suitable for an initial analysis but not for systematic verification of protocols [23].

According to our literatures survey, existing medical protocol tools are based on semi-formal techniques. Existing techniques [6, 25, 36] based on formal techniques are failed to scale the complexity of the protocol. They have not given any proper idea to model the medical protocols only using formal techniques due to complex nature of the medical protocol. To tackle the complexity of the protocol in formal methods is only a solution to use the refinement approach to model the whole protocol from abstract level to a final concrete model. In this chapter, we have provided sufficient detailed information about modelling a complex protocol using any formal method technique. In this study, we have tried to model a medical protocol, completely based on formal semantics and to check various anomalies. To overcome from the existing problems [23, 32] in the area of development of medical protocols, we have used the general formal modelling tool like Event-B [1] for specifying a complex medical protocol related to the diagnoses of ECG signal. The main objective to use Event-B modelling language is to model medical protocols using the refinement approach. The medical protocols are very complex and to model a complex protocol, a refinement approach is very helpful, which introduces peculiarity of the protocols in an incremental way. This technique is used to model a medical protocol more rigorously based on formal mathematics, which helps to find the anomalies and provide the consistency and correctness of the medical protocol.

10.3 Selection of Medical Protocol

Concerning the protocols that is the object of our study, we have selected the ECG interpretation that covers a wide range of protocol characteristics related to the heart diseases. All kinds of medical guidelines and protocols to differ from each others along several dimensions, which can be referred to the contents of the protocols or to its form. General practitioners (GPs), nurses and a large group of people related to this domain[2] are the *most important target users* of the guidelines and protocols, and the main aspects of clinical practice are to cover *diagnosis* as well as help in treatments. The medical guidelines and protocols, which are used by general practitioners and nurses, are also characterised by time dimensions; short time-span protocols; long-time span protocols. The form of guidelines and protocols are related to the textual descriptions. Sometimes it is also represented in the textual form as well as the combination with *tables* and *flowcharts*.

The ECG interpretation protocol [4, 16] aims at cardiologist as well as GPs and covers both diagnosis and treatment over a long period of time. The ECG interpretation protocol can be considered more precisely: one is in daily use by cardiologist, and the other is included in the repository of the National Guideline Clearinghouse (NGC), American College of Cardiology/American Heart Association (ACC/AHA). The basic standard for inclusion in the NGC and ACC/AHA are that the guidelines and protocols to contain well structured meaningful informations and systematically developed statements. The contents are produced under the supervision of medical specialty associations. It should be also based on literatures, reviewed and revised within the last 5 years. Furthermore, the ECG interpretation protocol has been published in a peer-reviewed scientific journal. In summary, the chosen protocol covers different aspects while fulfilling high-quality standards, which are the good criteria for selection of our case study.

In the following sections, we will use the ECG interpretation protocol as the main example in our explanations, and we therefore give a brief description of this protocol. The Electrocardiogram (ECG or EKG) interpretation is a common technique to trace abnormalities in the heart system and various levels of tracing help to find severe diseases. The guideline is more than 100 pages document, which contains knowledge in various notations: the main text; a list of factors to be considered

---

[2]http://www.guideline.gov/.

when assessing an abnormality in the ECG signal and a flowchart describing the steps in the ECG interpretation protocol. The protocol consists of an evaluation (or diagnosis) part and a treatment part, to be performed in the successive way. During the application of guidelines and protocols, as soon as the possibility of a more serious disease is uncovered, the recommendation is to leave the protocol without any further actions.

10.4 Basic Overview of Electrocardiogram (ECG)

The electrocardiogram (ECG or EKG) [13, 16] is a diagnostic tool that measures and records the electrical activity of the heart precisely in the form of signals. Clinicians can evaluate the conditions of a patient's heart from the ECG and perform further diagnosis. Analysis of these signals can be used for interpreting diagnosis of a wide range of the heart conditions and to predict the related diseases. The ECG records are obtained by sampling the bioelectric currents sensed by several electrodes, known as leads. A typical one-cycle ECG tracing is shown in Fig. 10.1. Electrocardiogram term is introduced by Willem Einthoven in 1893 at the meeting of Dutch Medical Society. In 1924, Einthoven received the Nobel Prize for his life's work in developing the ECG [4, 9, 10, 13, 16, 18, 19].

The normal electrocardiogram (ECG or EKG) is depicted in Fig. 10.1. All kinds of segments and intervals are represented in this ECG diagram. The depolarisation and repolarisation of the ventricular and atrial chambers are presented by deflection of the ECG signal. All these deflections are denoted by alphabetic order (P-QRS-T). Letter P indicates the atrial depolarisation, and the ventricular depolarisation is represented by QRS complex. The ventricular repolarisation is represented by T-wave. The atrial repolarisation appears during the QRS complex and generates a very low amplitude signal which cannot be uncovered from a normal ECG signal.

10.4.1 Differentiating the P-, QRS- and T-waves

Sequential activation, depolarisation, and repolarisation are deflected distinctly in the ECG due to anatomical difference of the atria and ventricles. Even all sequences are easily distinguishable when they are not in a correct sequence: P-QRS-T. The QRS-complex is easily identifiable between P- and T-waves because it has characteristic waveform and dominating amplitude. This amplitude is about 1000 µm in a normal heart and can be much greater in the ventricular hypertrophy. Normal duration of the QRS-complex is 80–90 ms. In case of non-existence of the atrial hypertrophy; an amplitude and duration of the P-wave are about 100 µm and 100 ms, respectively. The T-wave has about twice of the amplitude and duration of the P-wave. The T-wave can be differentiated from the P-wave by observing that the T-wave follows the QRS-complex after about 200 ms. In the ECG signal several parameters are used to evaluate the conditions of a patient's heart from the ECG. The

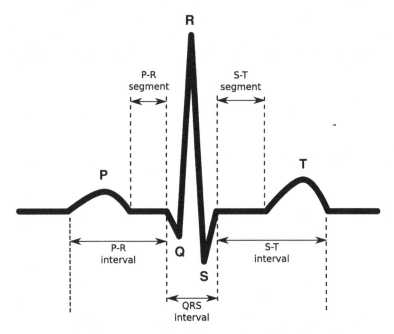

Fig. 10.1 A typical one-cycle ECG tracing

parameters are: PR-interval, P-wave, QRS duration, Q-wave, R-wave, ST-segment, T-wave, Axis, QT-interval. All these parameters have several characteristics that are used for diagnosis.

10.5 Formal Development of the ECG Interpretation

10.5.1 Abstract Model: Assessing Rhythm and Rate

We begin by defining the Event-B context. The context uses sets and constants to define axioms and theorems. Axioms and theorems represent the logical theory of a system. The logical theory is the static properties and properties of the target system. In the context, we define constants *LEADS*, *HState* and *YesNoState* that are related to an enumerated set of the ECG leads, normal and abnormal states of the heart and yes-no states, respectively. These constants are extracted from the ECG interpretation protocol [9, 10, 13, 16]. The standard 12-lead electrocardiogram is a representation of the heart's electrical activity recorded from electrodes on the body surface. A set of leads is represented as $LEADS = \{I, II, III, aVR, aVL, aVF, V1, V2, V3, V4, V5, V6\}$. Normal and abnormal states of the heart are represented by $HState = \{OK, KO\}$ and yes-no states are represented by $YesNoState = \{Yes, No\}$. Figure 10.2 depicts an incremental formal development

Fig. 10.2 ECG interpretation
protocols refinements

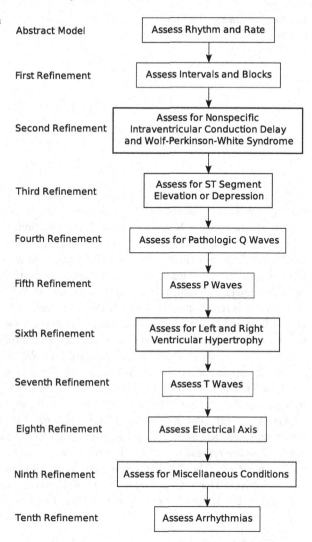

of the ECG interpretation protocol. In our development process, some refinements
are decomposed into several refinements for the simplicity. Every refinement level
introduces a *diagnosis* criteria for different components of the ECG signal, and each
new criteria helps to analyse a particular set of diseases. A particular set of diseases
is introduced in the multiple context related to each refinement.

Figure 10.3 shows an abstract representation of a *diagnostic-based* system development, where a root node (top circle in Fig. 10.3) represents a set of conditions for
testing any particular disease abstractly. The possible abstract outcomes of a diagnosis criterion are in form of *OK* and *KO*, which are represented by two branches.
The *KO* represents that the diagnosis criteria have found some conditions for further testing, while the *OK* represents the absence of any disease. The dash line of

Fig. 10.3 Abstract
representation

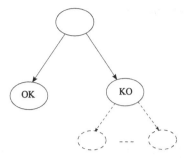

circles and arrows represent the next level of refinement for further analysing of any
particular diseases according to the guidelines and protocol.

Our abstract Event-B model of the ECG interpretation protocol assesses the
rhythm and *heart rate* to distinguish between normal and abnormal heart. Figure 10.4 presents a basic diagram of the ECG analysis at an abstract level according
to the standard procedure of the ECG protocol analysis. The specification consists
of just three-state variables (*inv1–int3*) *Sinus*, *Heart_Rate* and *Heart_State*. The *Sinus* variable is represented by *YesNoState* as enumerated sets. The last two variables
Heart_Rate and *Heart_State* are introduced as to show the heart rate limit and heart
states. One possible approach is to introduce a set of variables (*RR_Int_equidistant*,
PP_Int_equidistant, *P_Positive*, *PP_Interval* and *RR_Interval*) representing total
functions mapping leads (LEADS) to a standard data type (*BOOL*, $\mathbb{N}$) in invariants
(*inv4–inv8*). The RR and PP equidistant intervals in the ECG signal are represented
by variables *RR_Int_equidistant* and *PP_Int_equidistant* as the total functions from
LEADS to *BOOL*. The *RR_Int_equidistant* and *PP_Int_equidistant* are functions,
which represent RR and PP equidistant interval's states in a boolean form. A variable *P_Positive* represents a positive wave of the signal also as a total function from
LEADS to *BOOL*. The *P_Positive* function is used to show the positive visualisation
of the P-waves. The next variables PP and RR intervals in the ECG signal are represented by the variables *PP_Interval* and *RR_Interval* as the total functions from

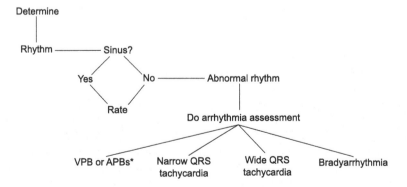

Fig. 10.4 Basic diagram of assessing rhythm and rate (adapted from [16])

LEADS to $\mathbb{N}$. The *PP_Interval* and *RR_Interval* functions are used to calculate the PP and RR-intervals.

$inv1 : Sinus \in YesNoState$

$inv2 : Heart\_Rate \in 1..300$

$inv3 : Heart\_State \in HState$

$inv4 : RR\_Int\_equidistant \in LEADS \rightarrow BOOL$

$inv5 : PP\_Int\_equidistant \in LEADS \rightarrow BOOL$

$inv6 : P\_Positive \in LEADS \rightarrow BOOL$

$inv7 : PP\_Interval \in LEADS \rightarrow \mathbb{N}$

$inv8 : RR\_Interval \in LEADS \rightarrow \mathbb{N}$

$inv9 : P\_Positive(II) = FALSE \Rightarrow Sinus = No$

$inv10 : ((\forall l \cdot l \in \{II, V1, V2\}$
$\qquad\qquad \Rightarrow$
$\qquad\qquad PP\_Int\_equidistant(l) = FALSE \lor$
$\qquad\qquad RR\_Int\_equidistant(l) = FALSE \lor$
$\qquad\qquad RR\_Interval(l) \neq PP\_Interval(l))$
$\qquad\qquad \lor$
$\qquad\qquad P\_Positive(II) = FALSE) \Rightarrow Sinus = No$

$inv11 : Sinus = Yes \Rightarrow ((\exists l \cdot l \in \{II, V1, V2\} \land$
$\qquad\qquad PP\_Int\_equidistant(l) = TRUE \land$
$\qquad\qquad RR\_Int\_equidistant(l) = TRUE \land$
$\qquad\qquad RR\_Interval(l) = PP\_Interval(l))$
$\qquad\qquad \land$
$\qquad\qquad P\_Positive(II) = TRUE)$

$inv12 : Heart\_Rate \in 60..100 \land Sinus = Yes$
$\qquad\qquad \Rightarrow$
$\qquad\qquad Heart\_State = OK$

$inv13 : Heart\_Rate \in 1..300 \setminus 60..100 \land Sinus = Yes$
$\qquad\qquad \Rightarrow$
$\qquad\qquad Heart\_State = KO$

$inv14 : Heart\_Rate \in 60..100 \land Sinus = No$
$\qquad\qquad \Rightarrow$
$\qquad\qquad Heart\_State = KO$

A set of invariants (*inv9–inv14*) represents the safety properties, and these are used to verify the required conditions for the ECG interpretation protocol using all possible behaviour of the heart system and analysis of the signal features, which are collected from the ECG signals. All these safety properties are designed under the supervision of cardiologist experts to verify the correctness of the formal model. These invariants in form of safety properties are extracted from the original protocol.

The invariant (*inv9*) states that if positive visualisation of the P-wave is *FALSE*, then there is no sinus rhythm. According to the clinical document, lead II is best for visualisation of the P-waves to determine the presence of sinus rhythm. The next invariant (*inv10*) is stronger invariant to identify the non-existence of the sinus rhythm. This invariant states that if the PP intervals (*PP_Int_equidistant*) or

RR intervals (*RR_Int_equidistant*) is not equidistant (*FALSE*), or the RR intervals (*RR_Interval*) and PP intervals (*PP_Interval*) are not equivalent, in all leads (II, V1, V2), or positive visualisation of the P-wave in lead II is *FALSE*, then there is no sinus rhythm. Similarly, next invariant (*inv*11) confirms, if the rhythm is sinus, then the PP intervals (*PP_Int_equidistant*) and RR intervals (*RR_Int_equidistant*) are equidistant, and the RR intervals (*RR_Interval*) and PP intervals (*PP_Interval*) are equal, exist in any leads (II, V1, V2), and the P-wave is positive in lead II. The invariant (*inv*12) represents that if the heart rate (*Heart_Rate*) is belonging between 60–100 bpm and the sinus rhythm is *Yes*, then the *Heart_State* is *OK*. The next two invariants (*inv*13–*inv*14) represent *KO* state of the Heart, mean the heart has any disease. The invariant (*inv*13) states that if the heart rate (*Heart_Rate*) is belonging between less than 60 bpm and greater than 100 bpm but less than 300 bpm, and the sinus rhythm is *Yes*, then the heart state (*Heart_State*) is *KO*. Similarly, the last invariant (*inv*14) represents that if the heart rate (*Heart_Rate*) is in between 60–100 bpm and the sinus rhythm is *No*, then the *Heart_State* is *KO*, means heart has any disease.

Three significant events *Rhythm_test_TRUE*, *Rhythm_test_FALSE* and *Rhythm_test_TRUE_abRate* are introduced in the abstract model. The *Rhythm_test_TRUE* represents successful ECG testing and found the sinus rhythm *Yes* and the heart state is *OK*. The next event *Rhythm_test_FALSE* represents successful ECG testing and found the sinus rhythm is *No* and the heart state is *KO*. Third event *Rhythm_test_TRUE_abRate* represents successful ECG testing and found the sinus rhythm is *Yes* and the heart state is *KO* due to abnormal heart rate. These events are the abstract events, which are equivalent to the first step of diagnosis of the ECG signal of the original protocol. We have taken some assumptions for modelling the medical protocol. These assumptions are extracted from the original protocol. In our formal model, all invariants and assumptions are verified with the medical experts. Our developed formal models are always complied with existing original protocols.

Mostly, events are used to test the criteria of possible disease using the ECG features. The criteria for testing the sinus rhythm is to focus on leads V1, V2, and II. The leads V1 and II are best for visualisation of the P-waves to determine the presence of the sinus rhythm or an arrhythmia, and the V1 and V2 are best to observe for the bundle branch block. If the P-waves are not clearly visible in V1, assess them in lead II, which usually shows well-formed P-waves [16]. Identification of the P-wave and then the RR intervals allow the interpreter to discover immediately whether the rhythm is sinus or other and to take the following steps:

- Confirm, if the rhythm is sinus, that the RR intervals are equidistant, that the P-wave is positive in lead II, and that the PP intervals are equidistant and equal to the RR interval.
- Do an arrhythmia assessment if the rhythm is abnormal.
- Determine the heart rate.

EVENT Rhythm_test_TRUE
  ANY *rate*
  WHERE
    grd1 : $(\exists l \cdot l \in \{II, V1, V2\} \wedge PP\_Int\_equidistant(l) = TRUE \wedge$
           $RR\_Int\_equidistant(l) = TRUE \wedge$
           $RR\_Interval(l) = PP\_Interval(l)) \wedge$
           $P\_Positive(II) = TRUE$
    grd2 : $rate \in 60 .. 100$
  THEN
    act1 : $Sinus := Yes$
    act2 : $Heart\_Rate := rate$
    act3 : $Heart\_State := OK$
END

EVENT Rhythm_test_FALSE
  ANY *rate*
  WHERE
    grd1 : $(\forall l \cdot l \in \{II, V1, V2\} \Rightarrow PP\_Int\_equidistant(l) = FALSE$
          $\vee RR\_Int\_equidistant(l) = FALSE \vee$
          $RR\_Interval(l) \neq PP\_Interval(l)) \vee$
          $P\_Positive(II) = FALSE$
    grd2 : $rate \in 1 .. 300$
  THEN
    act1 : $Sinus := No$
    act2 : $Heart\_Rate := rate$
    act3 : $Heart\_State := KO$
END

EVENT Rhythm_test_TRUE_abRate
  ANY *rate*
  WHERE
    grd1 : $(\exists l \cdot l \in \{II, V1, V2\} \wedge PP\_Int\_equidistant(l) = TRUE \wedge$
           $RR\_Int\_equidistant(l) = TRUE \wedge$
           $RR\_Interval(l) = PP\_Interval(l)) \wedge$
           $P\_Positive(II) = TRUE$
    grd2 : $rate \in 1 .. 300 \setminus 60 .. 100$
  THEN
    act1 : $Sinus := Yes$
    act2 : $Heart\_Rate := rate$
    act3 : $Heart\_State := KO$
END

In the abstract model, we have seen that the sinus rhythm and heart rate are introduced for the ECG interpretation in a single atomic step. This provides for a clear and simple specification of the essence of the basic ECG interpretation protocol and predicts the heart state (*OK* or *KO*). However, in the real protocol, the ECG interpretation and heart state prediction is not atomic. Instead, the ECG interpretation and prediction are also encountered lots of diagnosis to find the various kinds of heart diseases.

This section describes the abstract model of the ECG interpretation protocol. Every level of refinement introduces new context file for adding static properties of the system and list of heart diseases after introducing certain protocol of the ECG interpretation. Every refinement level is used to introduce a new set of diagnosis criteria to test the ECG signals. The following sections presents a sufficient detail information of the remaining refinement stages helping a reader to understand the rational of each refinement stage for formalising the ECG interpretation protocol.

10.5.2 First Refinement: Assess Intervals and Blocks

In an abnormal ECG signal, all the ECG features are varying according to the symptoms of heart diseases. We formalise the ECG interpretation protocol using an incremental approach, where we determine all features of the ECG signal. This level of refinement determines the PR- and QRS-intervals for the ECG interpretation. These intervals classify different kinds of the heart diseases.

Invariants (*inv*1–*inv*3) represent a set of new introduced variables in the refinement for expressing formalisation of the ECG interpretation protocol. These variables are *PR_Int*, *Disease_step2*, *QRS_Int*. Other variables (*M_Shape_Complex*, *Slurred_S*, *Notched_R*, *Small_R_QS* and *Slurred_S_duration*) are introduced as total functions in invariants (*inv*4–*inv*8) where total functions are mapping from leads (LEADS) to *BOOL* and $\mathbb{N}_1$, respectively. The function *M_Shape_Complex* returns existence of M-shape complex from the ECG signals in form of *TRUE* or *FALSE*. The function *Slurred_S* represents Slurred S-wave, the function *Notched_R* represents notched R-wave and the function *Small_R_QS* represents small R- or QS-waves, in boolean type. The function *Slurred_S_duration* is used to calculate Slurred-S duration.

A set of invariants (*inv*9–*inv*14) presents safety properties to validate formal representation of the ECG interpretation protocol. All these properties are derived from the original protocol to verify the correctness and consistency of the system. These properties are formulated through logic experts as well as cardiologist experts according to the original protocol. The main advantage of this technique is that if any property does not hold by the model, then it helps to find anomalies or to find missing parts of the model such as required conditions and parameters.

Invariants (*inv*9–*inv*13) represent an abnormal state of the heart (*KO*) to identify any disease and unsatisfying condition for features of the ECG signal, in the formal diagnosis process. While the last invariant (*inv*14) presents all the required properties for a normal heart. It states that if the heart rate is in between 60 to 100 bpm, the sinus rhythm is *Yes*, the PR interval is less than or equal to 200 ms and the QRS interval is less than 120 ms, then the heart state is *OK*.

$inv1 : PR\_Int \in 120 .. 250$

$inv2 : Disease\_step2 \in Disease\_Codes\_Step2$

$inv3 : QRS\_Int \in 50 .. 150$

$inv4 : M\_Shape\_Complex \in LEADS \rightarrow BOOL$

$inv5 : Slurred\_S \in LEADS \rightarrow BOOL$

$inv6 : Notched\_R \in LEADS \rightarrow BOOL$

$inv7 : Small\_R\_QS \in LEADS \rightarrow BOOL$

$inv8 : Slurred\_S\_duration \in LEADS \rightarrow \mathbb{N}_1$

$inv9 : Sinus = Yes \wedge PR\_Int > 200 \wedge Disease\_step2 = First\_degree\_AV\_Block$
$$\Rightarrow$$
$Heart\_State = KO$

$inv10 : Sinus = Yes \wedge QRS\_Int \geq 120 \wedge Disease\_step2 \in \{LBBB, RBBB\}$
$$\Rightarrow$$
$Heart\_State = KO$

$inv11 : Sinus = Yes \wedge Disease\_step2 = First\_degree\_AV\_Block$
$$\Rightarrow$$
$Heart\_State = KO$

$inv12 : Sinus = Yes \wedge Disease\_step2 = LBBB$
$$\Rightarrow$$
$Heart\_State = KO$

$inv13 : Sinus = Yes \wedge Disease\_step2 = RBBB$
$$\Rightarrow$$
$Heart\_State = KO$

$inv14 : Heart\_Rate \in 60 .. 100 \wedge Sinus = Yes \wedge PR\_Int \leq 200 \wedge QRS\_Int < 120$
$$\Rightarrow$$
$Heart\_State = OK$

To express formal logic for a new set of diagnoses for the ECG signal, we introduce three events *PR_Test*, *QRS_Test_LBBB* and *QRS_Test_RBBB*. The *PR_Test* interval represents, if the PR intervals are abnormal (>200 ms), then consider the first-degree atrioventricular (AV) block. The next two events *QRS_Test_LBBB* and *QRS_Test_RBBB* are used to assess the QRS duration for the bundle branch block and states that, if the QRS interval is ≥120 ms, the bundle branch block is present. Understanding the genesis of the QRS complex is an essential step and clarifies the ECG manifestations of bundle branch blocks [16]. We formalise the basic criteria to distinguish between RBBB and LBBB in the diagnosis process.

Left Bundle Branch Block (LBBB)

- QRS duration ≥ 120 ms.
- A small R- or QS-wave in V1 and V2.
- A notched R-wave in leads I, V5, and V6.

Right Bundle Branch Block (RBBB)

- QRS duration ≥ 120 ms.
- M-shaped complex in V1 and V2.
- Slurred S-wave in leads 1, V5, V6; and an S-wave that is of greater amplitude (length) than the preceding R-wave.

Right Bundle Branch Block (RBBB)

- QRS duration ≥120 ms.
- M-shaped complex in V1 and V2.
- Slurred S-wave in leads I, V5, V6; and an S-wave that is of greater amplitude (length) than the preceding R-wave.

The event PR_Test is used to capture the PR interval in the ECG signal, and to assess the first degree AV block. A set of guards of this event states that the current PR interval is within the range of 120 ms to 220 ms, and it is greater than 200 ms, sinus rhythm is *Yes*, and the heart is in abnormal state.

```
EVENT PR_Test
    ANY pr
    WHERE
        grd1 : pr ∈ 120 .. 220
        grd2 : pr > 200
        grd3 : Sinus = Yes
        grd4 : Heart_State = KO
    THEN
        act1 : PR_Int := pr
        act2 : Disease_step2 := First_degree_AV_Block
END
```

The event QRS_Test_LBBB is used to diagnose left bundle branch block through testing of QRS-wave. This event refines QRS_Test. The guards of this event state that the current QRS interval is within the range of 50 ms to 150 ms, and it is greater than or equal to 120 ms, sinus rhythm is *Yes*, the heart is in abnormal state, notched R-wave is TRUE in leads (I, V5, and V6), and small R- or QS-wave is TRUE in leads V1 and V2.

```
EVENT QRS_Test_LBBB Refines QRS_Test
    ANY qrs
    WHERE
        grd1 : qrs ∈ 50 .. 150
        grd2 : qrs ≥ 120
        grd3 : Sinus = Yes
        grd4 : Heart_State = KO
        grd5 : Notched_R(I) = TRUE ∧ Notched_R(V5) = TRUE ∧
               Notched_R(V6) = TRUE
        grd6 : Small_R_QS(V1) = TRUE ∧ Small_R_QS(V2) = TRUE
    THEN
        act1 : QRS_Int := qrs
        act2 : Disease_step2 := LBBB
END
```

The event QRS_Test_RBBB refines QRS_Test that is used to diagnose right bundle branch block through the testing of QRS-wave. The guards of this event state that the current QRS interval is within the range of 50 ms to 150 ms, and it is greater than or equal to 120 ms, sinus rhythm is *Yes*, the heart is in abnormal state, M-shaped complex is TRUE in leads (V1 and V2), slurred S-wave is TRUE in leads I, V5 and V6, and slurred S-wave duration is greater than 40 ms in leads I, V5, and V6.

```
EVENT QRS_Test_RBBB Refines QRS_Test
   ANY qrs
   WHERE
      grd1 : qrs ∈ 50 .. 150
      grd2 : qrs ≥ 120
      grd3 : Sinus = Yes
      grd4 : Heart_State = KO
      grd5 : M_Shape_Complex(V1) = TRUE ∧
             M_Shape_Complex(V2) = TRUE
      grd6 : Slurred_S(I) = TRUE ∧ Slurred_S(V5) = TRUE ∧
             Slurred_S(V6) = TRUE∧
      grd7 : Slurred_S_duration(I) > 40 ∧ Slurred_S_duration(V5) > 40 ∧
             Slurred_S_duration(V6) > 40
   THEN
      act1 : QRS_Int := qrs
      act2 : Disvease_step2 := RBBB
   END
```

10.5.3 Second Refinement: Assess for Nonspecific Intraventricular Conduction Delay and Wolff-Parkinson-White Syndrome

This level of refinement of the ECG interpretation assesses for nonspecific intraventricular conduction delay (IVCD) and Wolff-Parkinson-White (WPW) syndrome. The WPW syndrome may mimic an inferior MI (see in further refinements). If the WPW syndrome, RBBB, or LBBB is not present, interpret as nonspecific intraventricular conduction delay (IVCD) and assess for the presence of electronic pacing [16]. Some new variables (*Delta_Wave* and *Disease_step3*) are introduced in this refinement to assess atypical right bundle branch block using ECG signal. Two invariants (*inv3–inv4*) are used to declare new variables in form of the total functions mapping leads (LEADS) to *BOOL*. These functions are used to calculate the ST-segment elevation and epsilon wave, respectively. Invariants (*inv5–inv8*) represent an abnormal state of the heart (*KO*) when the sinus rhythm is *Yes* and any new particular disease is found in this refinement. All these properties are derived from the original protocol to verify the correctness and consistency of the system according to the cardiologist.

$inv1 : Delta\_Wave \in \mathbb{N}$
$inv2 : Disease\_step3 \in Disease\_Codes\_Step3$
$inv3 : ST\_elevation \in LEADS \rightarrow BOOL$
$inv4 : Epsilon\_Wave \in LEADS \rightarrow BOOL$
$inv5 : Sinus = Yes \wedge Disease\_step3 = WPW\_Syndrome$
$\qquad \Rightarrow$
$\qquad Heart\_State = KO$
$inv6 : Sinus = Yes \wedge Disease\_step3 = Brugada\_Syndrome$
$\qquad \Rightarrow$
$\qquad Heart\_State = KO$
$inv7 : Sinus = Yes \wedge Disease\_step3 = RV\_Dysplasia$
$\qquad \Rightarrow$
$\qquad Heart\_State = KO$
$inv8 : Sinus = Yes \wedge Disease\_step3 = IVCD$
$\qquad \Rightarrow$
$\qquad Heart\_State = KO$

We have introduced four events *QRS_Test_Atypical_RLBBB_WPW_Syndrome*, *QRS_Test_Atypical_RBBB_Brugada_Syndrome*, *QRS_Test_Atypical_RBBB_RV_ Dysplasia* and *QRS_Test_Atypical_RBBB_IVCD* to interpret atypical right bundle branch block using QRS interval. The basic rules for assessing the ECG signal in this refinement are given as follows:

- If the QRS duration is prolonged ≥ 110 ms and bundle branch block appears to be present but is atypical, consider WPW syndrome, particularly if there is a tall R-wave in leads V1 and V2.
- Assess for a short PR interval ≤ 120 ms and for a delta wave.

The event *QRS_Test_Atypical_RLBBB_WPW_Syndrome* is used to identify a disease WPM Syndrome, where a set of required conditions for diagnosis purpose is given in form of guard predicates. The guards of this event state that the QRS interval is greater than or equal to 110 ms, already symptoms of RBBB or LBBB is identified, summation of delta wave and PR interval is less than or equal to 120 ms, and the heart is in abnormal state (*KO*).

EVENT QRS_Test_Atypical_RLBBB_WPW_Syndrome
  ANY *sympt, d_wave*
  WHERE
    $grd1 : QRS\_Int \geq 110$
    $grd2 : sympt = A\_RBBB \vee sympt = A\_LBBB$
    $grd3 : d\_wave \in \mathbb{N}$
    $grd4 : (d\_wave + PR\_Int) \leq 120$
    $grd5 : Heart\_State = KO$
  THEN
    $act1 : Delta\_Wave := d\_wave$
    $act2 : Disease\_step3 := WPW\_Syndrome$
  END

The next event *QRS_Test_Atypical_RBBB_Brugada_Syndrome* is used to trace the symptoms of Brugada Syndrome. The guards of this event presents that the heart is in state of Atypical RBBB, QRS interval is greater than or equal to 110 ms, slurred S-wave is FALSE in leads V5 and V6, the heart has not the symptoms of WPW syndrome and the possibility of any other diseases, ST elevation is TRUE in leads V1 and V2, and the sinus rhythm is *Yes*.

EVENT QRS_Test_Atypical_RBBB_Brugada_Syndrome
  ANY *sympt, dis*
  WHERE
    grd1 : *sympt = A_RBBB*
    grd2 : $QRS\_Int \geq 110$
    grd3 : $Slurred\_S(V5) = FALSE \wedge Slurred\_S(V6) = FALSE$
    grd4 : $dis \in Disease\_Codes\_Step3 \setminus \{WPW\_Syndrome, NDS3\}$
    grd5 : $ST\_elevation(V1) = TRUE \wedge ST\_elevation(V2) = TRUE$
    grd6 : *Sinus = Yes*
  THEN
    act1 : $Disease\_step3 := Brugada\_Syndrome$
END

The event *QRS_Test_Atypical_RBBB_RV_Dysplasia* captures the diagnosis process for Right Ventricular Dysplasia (RV Dysplasia), where a set of guards explores the required symptoms using predicates. These predicates express that the heart is in state of Atypical RBBB, QRS interval is greater than or equal to 110 ms, the heart has not the symptoms of WPW syndrome, Brugada Syndrome and the possibility of any other diseases, and epsilon wave is TRUE in leads V1 and V3.

EVENT QRS_Test_Atypical_RBBB_RV_Dysplasia
  ANY *sympt, dis*
  WHERE
    grd1 : *sympt = A_RBBB*
    grd2 : $QRS\_Int \geq 110$
    grd3 : $dis \in Disease\_Codes\_Step3 \setminus \{WPW\_Syndrome,$
          $Brugada\_Syndrome, NDS3\}$
    grd4 : $Epsilon\_Wave(V1) = TRUE \wedge Epsilon\_Wave(V3) = TRUE$
  THEN
    act1 : $Disease\_step3 := RV\_Dysplasia$
END

The event *QRS_Test_Atypical_RBBB_IVCD* captures the essential conditions to determine the IVCD. A set of guards of this event describes that QRS interval is greater than or equal to 110 ms, the heart has not the symptoms of WPW syndrome, Brugada Syndrome, RV Dysplasia, and the possibility of any other disease.

EVENT QRS_Test_Atypical_RBBB_IVCD
  ANY *dis*
  WHERE
    grd1 : $QRS\_Int \geq 110$
    grd2 : $dis \in Disease\_Codes\_Step3 \setminus \{WPW\_Syndrome,$
                $Brugada\_Syndrome, RV\_Dysplasia, NDS3\}$
  THEN
    act1 : $Disease\_step3 := IVCD$
END

10.5.4 Third Refinement: Assess for ST-segment Elevation or Depression

This refinement provides a criterion for the ST-segments assessment by introducing some new variables (*ST_seg_ele* and *ST_depression*) in form of total functions mapping leads (LEADS) to $\mathbb{N}$ in invariants (*inv2–inv3*). The ST-segment for elevation and ST depression features are calculated by the *ST_seg_ele* and *ST_depression* functions. Invariants (*inv4–inv8*) are introduced for representing the safety properties to confirm an abnormal state of the heart (*KO*) when sinus rhythm is *Yes* and a new disease is found in this refinement.

---

*inv*1 : $Disease\_step4 \in Disease\_Codes\_Step4$
*inv*2 : $ST\_seg\_ele \in LEADS \rightarrow \mathbb{N}$
*inv*3 : $ST\_depression \in LEADS \rightarrow \mathbb{N}$
*inv*4 : $Sinus = Yes \wedge Disease\_step4 \in \{Acute\_inferior\_MI,$
      $Acute\_anterior\_MI \Rightarrow$
      $Heart\_State = KO$
*inv*5 : $Sinus = Yes \wedge Disease\_step4 = STEMI$
      $\Rightarrow$
      $Heart\_State = KO$
*inv*6 : $Sinus = Yes \wedge Disease\_step4 \in \{Troponin, CK\_MB\}$
      $\Rightarrow$
      $Heart\_State = KO$
*inv*7 : $Sinus = Yes \wedge Disease\_step4 = Non\_STEMI$
      $\Rightarrow$
      $Heart\_State = KO$
*inv*8 : $Sinus = Yes \wedge Disease\_step4 = Ischemia$
      $\Rightarrow$
      $Heart\_State = KO$

Four new events *ST_seg_elevation_YES*, *ST_seg_elevation_NOTCKMB_Yes*, *ST_seg_elevation_NO_TCKMB_No* and *Acute_IA_MI* are defined to cover *diagnosis* related to the ECG signals. All these events are used to interpret about the

ECG signal using ST-segment elevation or depression features [16]. To assess the ST-segments elevation or depression; we have formalised the following the textual criteria:

- Focus on the ST-segment for elevation or depression. ST-elevation ≥ 1000 μm (0.1 mV) in two or more contiguous ECG leads in a patient with chest pain indicates ST elevation MI (STEMI). The diagnosis is strengthened if there is reciprocal depression.
- ST-elevation in leads II, III, and aVF, with marked reciprocal depression in leads I and aVL, diagnostic of acute inferior MI.
- ST-segment elevation in V1 through V5, caused by extensive acute anterior MI.
- The ECG of a patient with a subtotal occlusion of the left main coronary artery. Note the ST elevation in aVR is greater than the ST elevation in V1, a recently identified marker of left main coronary disease.
- Features of non-ST-elevation MI (non-Q-wave MI).
- Elevation of the ST-segment may occur as a normal variant and ST-segment abnormalities and MI.

These textual sentences are formulated in the incremental development of our ECG protocol. This refinement advises scrutiny of the ST-segment before assessment of the T-waves, electrical axis, QT interval, and hypertrophy because the diagnosis of acute MI or ischemia is vital and depends on careful assessment of the ST-segment. Above given criteria are more complex and too ambiguous to represent. Therefore, we have formalised this part through careful cross reading of many reliable sources such as literature and encounter suggestions of the medical experts.

The event *ST_seg_elevation_YES* presents a diagnoses process for the ST Elevation Myocardial Infarction (STMEI). A set of guard predicates characterised the heart state and shows that the sinus rhythm is *Yes*, the ST elevation is TRUE and the length of ST segment elevation is greater than or equal to 1000 μm in two or more leads (II, III, aVF), or the ST elevation is TRUE and the length of ST segment elevation is greater than or equal to 1000 μm in two or more contiguous precordial leads V1 to V6, and disease must be Acute anterior MI or Acute inferior MI.

EVENT ST_seg_elevation_YES
  WHEN
    grd1 : $Sinus = Yes$
    grd2 : $(\exists l, k \cdot l \in \{II, III, aVF\} \wedge k \in \{II, III, aVF\} \wedge$
        $(ST\_elevation(l) = TRUE \wedge ST\_elevation(k) = TRUE)$
        $\wedge$
        $(ST\_seg\_ele(l) \geq 1000 \wedge ST\_seg\_ele(k) \geq 1000)$
        $\wedge l \neq k)$

```
        ∨
        ((∃l1, k1 · l1 ∈ {V1, V2, V3, V4, V5, V6} ∧ k1 ∈ {V1, V2, V3, V4, V5, V6}∧
        (ST_elevation(l1) = TRUE ∧ ST_elevation(k1) = TRUE)
        ∧
        (ST_seg_ele(l1) ≥ 1000 ∧ ST_seg_ele(k1) ≥ 1000)
        ∧l1 ≠ k1
        ∧
        (
        (l1 = V1 ∧ k1 = V2)∨
        (l1 = V2 ∧ k1 = V3)∨
        (l1 = V3 ∧ k1 = V4)∨
        (l1 = V4 ∧ k1 = V5)∨
        (l1 = V5 ∧ k1 = V6)
        )
        ))
    grd3 : Disease_step4 ∈ {Acute_inferior_MI, Acute_anterior_MI}
 THEN
    act1 : Disease_step4 := STEMI
END
```

The event $ST\_seg\_elevation\_NOTCKMB\_Yes$ is used to trace the symptoms of the Non-ST Elevation Myocardial Infarction (Non-STMEI). A set of guard predicates characterised the heart state and shows that the sinus rhythm is *Yes*, ST elevation is TRUE and the length of ST segment elevation is greater than or equal to 1000 μm in anyone lead (II, III, aVF), or the ST elevation is FALSE and the length of ST segment elevation is less than 1000 μm in all leads (II, III, aVF), the ST depression is greater than or equal to 1000 μm in two or more leads (LEADS), and disease must be Troponin, CK-MB.

```
EVENT ST_seg_elevation_NOTCKMB_Yes Refines ST_seg_elevation_NO
   WHEN
      grd1 : Sinus = Yes
      grd2 : (∃l, k · l ∈ {II, III, aVF} ∧ k ∈ {II, III, aVF}∧
               (ST_elevation(l) = TRUE ∧ ST_elevation(k) = TRUE)
               ∧
               (ST_seg_ele(l) ≥ 1000 ∧ ST_seg_ele(k) ≥ 1000)
               ∧l = k)
               ∨
               (∀l1 · l1 ∈ {II, III, aVF}⇒
               (ST_elevation(l1) = FALSE ∧ ST_seg_ele(l1) < 1000))
      grd3 : ∃l, k · l ∈ LEADS ∧ k ∈ LEADS∧
               (ST_depression(l) ≥ 1000 ∧ ST_depression(k) ≥ 1000)
               ∧l ≠ k
      grd4 : Disease_step4 ∈ {Troponin, CK_MB}
   THEN
      act1 : Disease_step4 := Non_STEMI
END
```

The event $ST\_seg\_elevation\_NO\_TCKMB\_No$ captures the essential conditions to determine the ischemia. A set of guards of this event describes that the sinus rhythm is *Yes*, the ST elevation is TRUE and the length of ST segment elevation is greater than or equal to 1000 μm in anyone lead (II, III, aVF), or the ST elevation is FALSE and the length of ST segment elevation is less than 1000 μm in all leads (II, III, aVF), ST depression is greater than or equal to 1000 μm in two or more leads (LEADS), and disease must be Troponin, CK-MB.

EVENT ST_seg_elevation_NO_TCKMB_No Refines ST_seg_elevation_NO
  WHEN
     $grd1 : Sinus = Yes$
     $grd2 : (\exists l, k \cdot l \in \{II, III, aVF\} \wedge k \in \{II, III, aVF\} \wedge$
             $(ST\_elevation(l) = TRUE \wedge ST\_elevation(k) = TRUE)$
             $\wedge$
             $(ST\_seg\_ele(l) \geq 1000 \wedge ST\_seg\_ele(k) \geq 1000)$
             $\wedge l = k)$
             $\vee$
             $(\forall l1 \cdot l1 \in \{II, III, aVF\} \Rightarrow$
             $(ST\_elevation(l1) = FALSE \wedge ST\_seg\_ele(l1) < 1000))$
     $grd3 : \exists l, k \cdot l \in LEADS \wedge k \in LEADS \wedge$
             $(ST\_depression(l) \geq 1000 \wedge ST\_depression(k) \geq 1000)$
             $\wedge l \neq k$
     $grd4 : Disease\_step4 \notin \{Troponin, CK\_MB\}$
  THEN
     $act1 : Disease\_step4 := Ischemia$
  END

The event *Acute_IA_MI* presents a diagnoses process for the Acute inferior MI and Acute anterior MI. A set of guard predicates characterised the heart state and shows that the sinus rhythm is *Yes*, the ST elevation is TRUE and the length of ST segment elevation is greater than or equal to 1000 μm in two or more leads (II, III, aVF), or the ST elevation is TRUE and the length of ST segment elevation is greater than or equal to 1000 μm in two or more contiguous pre-cordial leads V1 to V6.

EVENT Acute_IA_MI
  WHEN
     $grd1 : Sinus = Yes$
     $grd2 : (\exists l, k \cdot l \in \{II, III, aVF\} \wedge k \in \{II, III, aVF\} \wedge$
             $(ST\_elevation(l) = TRUE \wedge ST\_elevation(k) = TRUE)$
             $\wedge$
             $(ST\_seg\_ele(l) \geq 1000 \wedge ST\_seg\_ele(k) \geq 1000)$
             $\wedge l \neq k)$
             $\vee$
             $((\exists l1, k1 \cdot l1 \in \{V1, V2, V3, V4, V5, V6\} \wedge k1 \in \{V1, V2, V3, V4, V5, V6\} \wedge$
             $(ST\_elevation(l1) = TRUE \wedge ST\_elevation(k1) = TRUE)$
             $\wedge$
             $(ST\_seg\_ele(l1) \geq 1000 \wedge ST\_seg\_ele(k1) \geq 1000)$
             $\wedge l1 \neq k1$
             $\wedge$

$$($$
$$(l1 = V1 \wedge k1 = V2) \vee$$
$$(l1 = V2 \wedge k1 = V3) \vee$$
$$(l1 = V3 \wedge k1 = V4) \vee$$
$$(l1 = V4 \wedge k1 = V5) \vee$$
$$(l1 = V5 \wedge k1 = V6)$$
$$)$$
$$))$$

THEN

act1 : $Disease\_step4 :\in \{Acute\_inferior\_MI, Acute\_anterior\_MI\}$

END

10.5.5 Fourth Refinement: Assess for Pathologic Q-wave

This refinement only introduces new guidelines to interpret Q-wave feature of the ECG signal and assessment-related diseases to the Q-wave and R-wave [16]. Some new variables are represented by a set of invariants ($inv1$–$inv2$) to handle the required features of the Q-wave and R-wave to diagnose the ECG signal. The functions Q_Normal_Status and R_Normal_Status represent the normal state of the Q and R-waves in a boolean type. The next three invariants ($inv3$–$inv5$) are used to declare new variables in form of total functions mapping leads (LEADS) to $\mathbb{N}$, and an invariant ($inv6$) is also total function mapping leads (LEAD) to $BOOL$. The functions Q_Width, Q_Depth and R_Depth calculate the Q-wave width, Q-wave depth and R-wave depth, respectively. The last function Q_Wave_State represents the boolean state of the Q-wave for all leads. Two other new variables Age_of_Inf and $Mice\_State$ represent infarction age and miscellaneous states. An enumerated set of infarction age and miscellaneous states define as $Age\_of\_Infarct = \{recent,$ $indeterminate, old\}$ and $Mice\_State5 = \{Exclude\_Mimics\_MI, late\_transition, normal\_variant, borderline\_Qs, NMS\}$, respectively in the context. The variable $Disease\_step5$ represents a group of diseases of this refinement level as analysis of the Q-wave from the ECG signals. Some invariants ($inv10$–$inv13$) are introduced as representing the safety properties to confirm an abnormal state of the heart (KO). All invariants have similar form for checking the heart state under the various disease conditions. These invariants state that if the sinus rhythm is Yes and a new disease is found, then the heart must be in the abnormal (KO) state.

$inv1 : Q\_Normal\_Status \in BOOL$
$inv2 : R\_Normal\_Status \in BOOL$
$inv3 : Q\_Width \in LEADS \rightarrow \mathbb{N}$
$inv4 : Q\_Depth \in LEADS \rightarrow \mathbb{N}$
$inv5 : R\_Depth \in LEADS \rightarrow \mathbb{N}$
$inv6 : Q\_Wave\_State \in LEADS \rightarrow BOOL$
$inv7 : Age\_of\_Inf \in Age\_of\_Infarct$
$inv8 : Mice\_State \in Mice\_State5$
$inv9 : Disease\_step5 \in Disease\_Codes\_Step5$

$inv10 : Sinus = Yes \land Disease\_step4 = Acute\_anterior\_MI$
$\Rightarrow$
$Heart\_State = KO$
$inv11 : Sinus = Yes \land Disease\_step4 = Acute\_inferior\_MI$
$\Rightarrow$
$Heart\_State = KO$
$inv12 : Sinus = Yes \land Disease\_step5 = Hypertrophic\_cardiomyopathy$
$\Rightarrow$
$Heart\_State = KO$
$inv13 : Sinus = Yes \land Disease\_step5 \in$
$\{anterior\_MI, LVH, emphysema, lateral\_MI\}$
$\Rightarrow$
$Heart\_State = KO$

In this level of refinement, we have introduced nine events (*Q_Assessment_ Normal*, *Q_Assessment_Abnormal_AMI*, *Q_Assessment_Abnormal_IMI*, *Determine_Age_of_Infarct*, *Exclude_Mimics*, *R_Assessment_Normal*, *R_Assessment_ Abnormal*, *R_Q_Assessment_R_Abnormal_V1234* and *R_Q_Assessment_R_Abnormal_V56*) for assessing the Q-wave and R-wave in all leads of the ECG signals. We have represented the formal notation of following guidelines, which are used to assess the Q-wave and the R-wave:

- Assess for the loss of R-waves-pathologic Q-waves in leads I, II, III, aVL, and aVF.
- Assess for R-wave progression in V2 through V4. The variation in the normal QRS configuration that occurs with rotation. The R-wave amplitude should measure from 1000 μm to at least 20000 μm in V3 and V4. Loss of R-waves in V1 through V4 with ST-segment elevation indicates acute anterior MI.
- Loss of R-wave in leads V1 through V3 with the ST-segment isoelectric and the T-wave inverted may be interpreted as anteroseptal MI age indeterminate (i.e., infarction in the recent or distant past). Features are given of old anterior MI and lateral infarction in this refinement.

Sometimes, R-wave progression in leads V2 through V4 are very poor, may be caused by the following reasons: improper lead placement, late transition, anteroseptal or anteroapical MI, LVH Severe chronic obstructive pulmonary disease, particularly emphysema may cause QS complexes in leads V1 through V4, which may mimic MI; a repeat ECG with recording electrodes placed one intercostal space below the routine locations should cause R-waves to be observed in leads V2 through V4, Hypertrophic cardiomyopathy, LBBB [16].

The event *Q_Assessment_Normal* presents a diagnoses process to test the normal state of the Q-wave. A set of guard predicates of this event shows that the width of Q-wave is less than 40 ms and the depth of Q-wave is less than or equal to 3000 μm in leads II and aVF, the width of Q-wave is less than 40 ms in lead aVL, the width of Q-wave is less than 40 ms and the depth of Q-wave is less than or equal to 7000 μm in lead III and the width of Q-wave is less than or equal to 7000 μm in lead aVL, and the depth of Q-wave is less than 40 ms and less than or equal to 1500 μm in lead I.

EVENT Q_Assessment_Normal
   WHEN
      grd1 : $Q\_Width(II) < 40 \land Q\_Depth(II) \leq 3000 \land$
               $Q\_Width(aVF) < 40 \land Q\_Depth(aVF) \leq 3000 \land$
               $Q\_Width(aVL) < 40$
      grd2 : $Q\_Width(III) \leq 40 \land Q\_Depth(III) \leq 7000 \land Q\_Depth(aVL) \leq 7000$
      grd3 : $Q\_Depth(I) < 40 \land Q\_Depth(I) \leq 1500$
   THEN
      act1 : $Q\_Normal\_Status := TRUE$
END

The event *Q_Assessment_Abnormal_AMI* is used to identify the Acute_anterior_ MI symptoms of the heart using ECG signal. A list of guards are defined to cover the conditions of the diagnosis process. These guards express that the sinus rhythm is *Yes*, ST elevation is TRUE and the length of ST segment elevation is greater than or equal to 1000 µm in two or more leads (II, III, aVF), or the ST elevation is TRUE and the length of ST segment elevation is greater than or equal to 1000 µm in two or more contiguous pre-cordial leads V1 to V6, the width of Q-wave is greater than or equal to 40 ms and the depth of Q-wave is greater than or equal to 3000 µm in leads V5 and V6, the width of Q-wave is greater than or equal to 40 ms and depth of Q-wave is greater to 7000 µm in lead aVL, the width of Q-wave is greater than or equal to 40 ms and the depth of Q-wave is greater to 1500 µm in lead I, and the normal state of the Q-wave is FALSE.

EVENT Q_Assessment_Abnormal_AMI
   WHEN
      grd1 : $Sinus = Yes$
      grd2 : $(\exists l, k \cdot l \in \{II, III, aVF\} \land k \in \{II, III, aVF\} \land$
               $(ST\_elevation(l) = TRUE \land ST\_elevation(k) = TRUE)$
               $\land$
               $(ST\_seg\_ele(l) \geq 1000 \land ST\_seg\_ele(k) \geq 1000)$
               $\land l \neq k)$
               $\lor$
               $((\exists l1, k1 \cdot l1 \in \{V1, V2, V3, V4, V5, V6\} \land k1 \in \{V1, V2, V3, V4, V5, V6\} \land$
               $(ST\_elevation(l1) = TRUE \land ST\_elevation(k1) = TRUE)$
               $\land$
               $(ST\_seg\_ele(l1) \geq 1000 \land ST\_seg\_ele(k1) \geq 1000)$
               $\land l1 \neq k1$
               $\land$
               $($
               $(l1 = V1 \land k1 = V2) \lor$
               $(l1 = V2 \land k1 = V3) \lor$
               $(l1 = V3 \land k1 = V4) \lor$
               $(l1 = V4 \land k1 = V5) \lor$
               $(l1 = V5 \land k1 = V6)$
               $)$
               $))$

```
        grd3 : Q_Width(V5) ≥ 40 ∧ Q_Depth(V5) > 3000∧
                Q_Width(V6) ≥ 40 ∧ Q_Depth(V6) > 3000
        grd4 : Q_Width(aVL) ≥ 40 ∧ Q_Depth(aVL) > 7000
        grd5 : Q_Width(I) ≥ 40 ∧ Q_Depth(I) > 1500
        grd6 : Q_Normal_Status = FALSE
    THEN
        act1 : Disease_step4 := Acute_anterior_MI
END
```

The event *Q_Assessment_Abnormal_IMI* is used to characterised the symptoms of Acute_inferior_MI symptoms. A set of guards are used to satisfy the required condition for the symptoms of Acute_inferior_MI. A list of guards state that the sinus rhythm is *Yes*, the ST elevation is TRUE and the length of ST segment elevation is greater than or equal to 1000 μm in two or more leads (II, III, aVF), or the ST elevation is TRUE and the length of ST segment elevation is greater than or equal to 1000 μm in two or more contiguous pre-cordial leads V1 to V6, the width of Q-wave is greater than or equal to 40 ms and the depth of Q-wave is greater than or equal to 3000 μm in lead II, the width of Q-wave is greater than 40 ms and the depth of Q-wave is greater than or equal to 7000 μm in lead III, the width of Q-wave is greater than or equal to 40 ms and the depth of Q-wave is greater to 3000 μm in lead aVL, and the normal state of the Q-wave is FALSE.

```
EVENT Q_Assessment_Abnormal_IMI
    WHEN
        grd1 : Sinus = Yes
        grd2 : (∃l, k · l ∈ {II, III, aVF} ∧ k ∈ {II, III, aVF}∧
                (ST_elevation(l) = TRUE ∧ ST_elevation(k) = TRUE)
                ∧
                (ST_seg_ele(l) ≥ 1000 ∧ ST_seg_ele(k) ≥ 1000)
                ∧l ≠ k)
                ∨
                ((∃l1, k1 · l1 ∈ {V1, V2, V3, V4, V5, V6} ∧ k1 ∈ {V1, V2, V3, V4, V5, V6}∧
                (ST_elevation(l1) = TRUE ∧ ST_elevation(k1) = TRUE)
                ∧
                (ST_seg_ele(l1) ≥ 1000 ∧ ST_seg_ele(k1) ≥ 1000)
                ∧l1 ≠ k1
                ∧
                (
                (l1 = V1 ∧ k1 = V2)∨
                (l1 = V2 ∧ k1 = V3)∨
                (l1 = V3 ∧ k1 = V4)∨
                (l1 = V4 ∧ k1 = V5)∨
                (l1 = V5 ∧ k1 = V6)
                )
                ))
        grd3 : Q_Width(II) ≥ 40 ∧ Q_Depth(II) > 3000∧
                Q_Width(III) > 40 ∧ Q_Depth(III) > 7000∧
```

$$Q\_Width(aVF) \geq 40 \wedge Q\_Depth(aVF) > 3000$$

> grd4 : $Q\_Normal\_Status = FALSE$
> **THEN**
>> act1 : $Disease\_step4 := Acute\_inferior\_MI$
> **END**

The event *Determine_Age_of_Infarct* is used to determine the age of Infarct during diagnosis process. The age of Infarct can be in different states as *recent*, *old*, and *indeterminate*. These states can be determined if the heart disease can be classified using anyone disease that is given in the guards of the event.

> **EVENT Determine_Age_of_Infarct**
>> **WHEN**
>>> grd1 : $Disease\_step4 = Acute\_inferior\_MI$
>>>
>>> $\vee$
>>>
>>> $Disease\_step5 \in \{anterior\_MI, LVH, emphysema\}$
>>>
>>> $\vee$
>>>
>>> $Mice\_State = Exclude\_Mimics\_MI$
>>>
>>> $\vee$
>>>
>>> $Disease\_step2 = LBBB$
>> **THEN**
>>> act1 : $Age\_of\_Inf :\in \{recent, old, indeterminate\}$
> **END**

The event *Exclude_Mimics* is used to identify the Hypertrophic cardiomyopathy. The guards of this event state that the heart has the condition of Acute inferior MI, and the miscellaneous state of the heart confirms the Exclude Mimics MI.

> **EVENT Exclude_Mimics**
>> **ANY** *exmi*
>> **WHERE**
>>> grd1 : $Disease\_step4 = Acute\_inferior\_MI$
>>> grd2 : $exmi \in Mice\_State5 \wedge exmi = Exclude\_Mimics\_MI$
>> **THEN**
>>> act1 : $Disease\_step5 := Hypertrophic\_cardiomyopathy$
>>> act2 : $Mice\_State := borderline\_Qs$
> **END**

The event *R_Assessment_Normal* presents a diagnoses process to test the normal state of the R-wave. A set of guard predicates of this event shows that the depth of R-wave is greater than or equal to 0 μm and less than or equal to 6000 μm in lead V1 and age is greater than 30 years, the depth of R-wave is greater than 200 μm and less than or equal to 12000 μm in lead V2 and age is less than 30, and the depth of R-wave is greater than or equal to 1000 μm and less than or equal to 24000 μm in lead V3 and age is greater than 30. Here, the age is relevant to the diagnosis of myocardial infarction.

```
EVENT R_Assessment_Normal
    ANY age
    WHERE
        grd1 : R_Depth(V1) ≥ 0 ∧ R_Depth(V1) ≤ 6000 ∧ age > 30
        grd2 : R_Depth(V2) > 200 ∧ R_Depth(V2) ≤ 12000 ∧ age < 30
        grd3 : R_Depth(V3) ≥ 1000 ∧ R_Depth(V3) ≤ 24000 ∧ age > 30
    THEN
        act1 : R_Normal_Status := TRUE
END
```

The event *R_Assessment_Abnormal* is used to identify the miscellaneous states of the heart, when the R-wave of the ECG signal is abnormal.

```
EVENT R_Assessment_Abnormal
    WHEN
        grd1 : R_Normal_Status = FALSE
    THEN
        act1 : Mice_State :∈ {late_transition, normal_variant}
END
```

The event *R_Q_Assessment_R_Abnormal_V1234* is used to determine the anterior MI, LVH and emphysema with miscellaneous state Exclude Mimics MI. A set guards shows that the normal state of the R-wave is FALSE, the state of Q-wave is TRUE in leads V1 to V4.

```
EVENT R_Q_Assessment_R_Abnormal_V1234
    WHEN
        grd1 : R_Normal_Status = FALSE
        grd2 : Q_Wave_State(V1) = TRUE∧
               Q_Wave_State(V2) = TRUE∧
               Q_Wave_State(V3) = TRUE∧
               Q_Wave_State(V4) = TRUE
    THEN
        act1 : Disease_step5 :∈ {anterior_MI, LVH, emphysema}
        act1 : Mice_State := Exclude_Mimics_MI
END
```

The event *R_Q_Assessment_R_Abnormal_V56* diagnose the lateral MI and Hypertrophic cardiomyopathy. The guards of this event state that the state of Q-wave is TRUE in leads V5 and V6, and the heart state is in abnormal state (*KO*).

```
EVENT R_Q_Assessment_R_Abnormal_V56
  WHEN
      grd1 : Q_Wave_State(V5) = TRUE∧
                Q_Wave_State(V6) = TRUE
      grd3 : Heart_State = KO
  THEN
      act1 : Disease_step5 :∈ {lateral_MI, Hypertrophic_cardiomyopathy}
END
```

10.5.6 Fifth Refinement: P-wave

This refinement level introduces a criterion to assess the P-wave for abnormalities, including the atrial hypertrophy in the ECG signal [16]. A new variable *Disease_step6* is introduced in this refinement to introduce a set of diseases related to the P-wave. Some new variables are also introduced to assess the P-wave from 12-leads ECG signals, which are represented by *inv2–inv4*. The first two invariants introduce new variables in form of total functions mapping from leads (LEADS) to $\mathbb{N}$. These functions return height and broadness of the P-waves. The next invariant (*inv4*) represents total function mapping leads (LEADS) to *BOOL*. It returns diphasic state in a boolean type. A set of invariants (*inv5–inv7*) are representing the confirmation of an abnormal state of the heart (*KO*). These invariants state that if the sinus rhythm is *Yes* and a new disease is found, then the heart will be in an abnormal state. The invariant (*inv5*) is checking for existence of multiple diseases during the P-wave diagnosis. Five new events *P_Wave_assessment_Peaked_Broad_No*, *P_Wave_assessment_Peaked_Yes*, *P_Wave_assessment_Peaked_Yes_Check_RAE*, *P_Wave_assessment_Broad_Yes* and *P_Wave_assessment_Broad_Yes_Check_LAE* are introduced to assess the P-wave.

```
inv1 : Disease_step6 ∈ Disease_Codes_Step6
inv2 : P_Wave_Peak ∈ LEADS → ℕ
inv3 : P_Wave_Broad ∈ LEADS → ℕ
inv4 : Diphasic ∈ LEADS → BOOL
inv5 : Sinus = Yes ∧ Disease_step6 ∈
            {RVH, RV_strain, pulmonary_embolism,
            RAE, mitral_stenosis, mitral_regurgitation, LV_failure,
            LAE, dilated_cardiomyopathy, LVH_cause}
            ⇒
            Heart_State = KO
inv6 : Sinus = Yes ∧ Disease_step6 = LAE ⇒ Heart_State = KO
inv7 : Sinus = Yes ∧ Disease_step6 = RAE ⇒ Heart_State = KO
```

The textual representation of formal notation of the P-wave assessment is given in [16]. We have formalised all the textual guidelines.

The event *P_Wave_assessment_Peaked_Broad_No* shows that there is not any particular condition related to the heart disease under the specified guards. The guard of this event state that the peak of P-wave is less than 3000 μm in leads II and VI, or the broad of P-wave is less than 110 ms in leads II and VI, or the diphasic is FALSE in lead (II or VI).

```
EVENT P_Wave_assessment_Peaked_Broad_No
  WHEN
    grd1 : (P_Wave_Peak(II) < 3000∧
            P_Wave_Peak(V1) < 3000)
          ∨
          (P_Wave_Broad(II) < 110 ∧ P_Wave_Broad(V1) < 110)∨
          Diphasic(II) = FALSE∨
          Diphasic(V1) = FALSE
  THEN
    act1 : Disease_step6 := NDS6
END
```

The event *P_Wave_assessment_Peaked_Yes* is used to assess the heart condition using ECG signal. The guards of this events state that the peak of P-wave is greater than or equal to 3000 μm in lead II and VI and the heart is in abnormal state.

```
EVENT P_Wave_assessment_Peaked_Yes
  WHEN
    grd1 : P_Wave_Peak(II) ≥ 3000
    grd2 : P_Wave_Peak(V1) ≥ 3000
    grd3 : Heart_State = KO
  THEN
    act1 : Disease_step6 := RAE
END
```

The event *P_Wave_assessment_Peaked_Yes_Check_RAE* is used to identify several diseases related to the RVH, RV strain, and pulmonary. The guards of this event are very simple that formalise basic assessment process to discover the disease from the ECG signal. The guards of this event state that the peak of P-wave is greater than or equal to 3000 μm in lead II and VI, the heart is in abnormal state and the heart condition must be equivalent by RAE.

```
EVENT P_Wave_assessment_Peaked_Yes_Check_RAE
Refines P_Wave_assessment_Peaked_Yes
  WHEN
    grd1 : P_Wave_Peak(II) ≥ 3000
    grd2 : P_Wave_Peak(V1) ≥ 3000
    grd3 : Heart_State = KO
    grd4 : Disease_step6 = RAE
  THEN
    act1 : Disease_step6 :∈ {RVH, RV_strain, pulmonary_embolism}
END
```

The event *P_Wave_assessment_Broad_Yes* is used to trace the heart condition for the left atrial enlargement (LAE). The guards of this event formalise to assess the disease from the ECG signal. The guards of this event state that the broad of P-wave is greater than or equal to 110 ms in leads II and VI, or the diphasic is TRUE in lead (II or VI), and the heart state is in abnormal state.

EVENT P_Wave_assessment_Broad_Yes
 WHEN
  grd1 : $(P\_Wave\_Broad(II) \geq 110 \wedge P\_Wave\_Broad(V1) \geq 110) \vee$
    $Diphasic(II) = TRUE \vee$
    $Diphasic(V1) = TRUE$
  grd2 : $Heart\_State = KO$
 THEN
  act1 : $Disease\_step6 := LAE$
END

The event *P_Wave_assessment_Broad_Yes_Check_LAE* is refinement of *P_Wave_assessment_Broad_Yes* and it is used to identify the several diseases (mitral stenosis, mitral regurgitation, LV failure, dilated cardiomyopathy, LVH cause). The guards of this event state that the broad of P-wave is greater than or equal to 110 ms in leads II and VI, or the diphasic is TRUE in lead (II or VI), the heart state is in abnormal state, and the traced disease be equivalent to LAE.

EVENT P_Wave_assessment_Broad_Yes_Check_LAE
Refines P_Wave_assessment_Broad_Yes
 WHEN
  grd1 : $(P\_Wave\_Broad(II) \geq 110 \wedge P\_Wave\_Broad(V1) \geq 110) \vee$
    $Diphasic(II) = TRUE \vee$
    $Diphasic(V1) = TRUE$
  grd2 : $Heart\_State = KO$
  grd3 : $Disease\_step6 = LAE$
 THEN
  act1 : $Disease\_step6 :\in \{mitral\_stenosis, mitral\_regurgitation, LV\_failure,$
    $dilated\_cardiomyopathy, LVH\_cause\}$
END

10.5.7 Sixth Refinement: Assess for Left and Right Ventricular Hypertrophy

The Left Ventricular Hypertrophy (LVH) and Right Ventricular Hypertrophy (RVH) are assessed by this refinement. The criteria for LVH and RVH are not applicable if the bundle branch block is present [16]. Thus, it is essential to exclude the

LBBB and RBBB early in the interpretive sequences as delineated previously in refinement 2 and refinement 3. This refinement introduces two new variables *S_Depth* and *R_S_Ratio* in form of total functions mapping leads (LEADS) to $\mathbb{N}$. These functions are used to calculate the S-wave depth and ratio of R-wave and S-wave from the 12-leads ECG signal.

Invariants (*inv3–inv4*) are used to verify an abnormal state (*KO*) of the heart in case of detecting any disease. Two new events (*LVH_Assessment* and *RVH_Assessment*) are introduced to assess the LVH and RVH from the 12-leads ECG. Detailed textual representation of assessment of the LVH and RVH is given in [16].

$inv1 : S\_Depth \in LEADS \rightarrow \mathbb{N}$
$inv2 : R\_S\_Ratio \in LEADS \rightarrow \mathbb{N}$
$inv3 : Sinus = Yes \land Disease\_step6 = RVH \Rightarrow Heart\_State = KO$
$inv4 : Sinus = Yes \land Disease\_step6 = LVH\_cause \Rightarrow Heart\_State = KO$

The event *LVH_Assessment* refines *P_Wave_assessment_Broad_Yes_Check_LAE*. This event is used to assess the Left Ventricular Hypertrophy (LVH) causes. A set of guards is used to satisfy the required condition for the symptoms of LVH. The guards of this event state that the broad of P-wave is greater than or equal to 110 ms in leads II and V1, or the diphasic is TRUE in lead II or V1, through the previous assessment of the disease indicates that the symptoms of LAE, sex is 0 or 1, where 0 denotes for man and 1 denotes for woman, an addition of the depth of S-wave in lead V1 and R-wave in lead V5 is greater than 35000 µm or an addition of depth of S-wave in lead V1 and R-wave in lead V6 is greater than 35000 µm, an addition of the depth of S-wave in lead aVL and R-wave in lead V1 is greater than or equal to 24000 µm for a man or 18000 µm for woman, LVH specificity is equal to 90 and sensitivity is less than 40, if the previous assessment of the disease indicates the symptoms of LAE then LVH specificity should be less than 98, and heart state is in abnormal state.

EVENT LVH_Assessment Refines P_Wave_assessment_Broad_Yes_Check_LAE
  ANY *LVH_specificity, sensitivity, sex*
  WHERE
    grd1 : $(P\_Wave\_Broad(II) \geq 110 \land P\_Wave\_Broad(V1) \geq 110)\lor$
        $Diphasic(II) = TRUE\lor$
        $Diphasic(V1) = TRUE$
    grd2 : $Disease\_step6 = LAE$
    grd5 : $sex \in \{0, 1\}$
    grd3 : $((S\_Depth(V1) + R\_Depth(V5)) > 35000$
        $\lor$
        $(S\_Depth(V1) + R\_Depth(V6)) > 35000)$
    grd4 : $((R\_Depth(aVL) + S\_Depth(V1) \geq 24000) \land sex = 0)$
        $\lor$
        $((R\_Depth(aVL) + S\_Depth(V1) \geq 18000) \land sex = 1)$

```
        grd6 : LVH_specificity = 90
                    ∧
                sensitivity < 40
        grd7 : Disease_step6 = LAE ⇒ LVH_specificity < 98
        grd8 : Heart_State = KO
    THEN
        act1 : Disease_step6 := LVH_cause
    END
```

The event *RVH_Assessment* refines *P_Wave_assessment_Broad_Yes_Check_RAE*. This event is used to identify the Right Ventricular Hypertrophy RVH. A list of guards presents the required conditions for the symptoms of RVH. The guards of this event state that the peak of P-wave is greater than or equal to 3000 μm in leads II and V1, using previous assessment of the disease indicates the symptoms of RAE, the depth of R-wave is greater than or equal to 7000 μm and age is greater than 30 years, the depth of S-wave is greater than or equal to 7000 μm in leads V5 or V6, the ratio of R- and S-wave is greater than or equal to 1 in lead V1, the ratio of R-wave and S-wave is less than or equal to 1 in lead V5 or V6, angular axis is greater than or equal to 110 degree, the previous assessment of the disease does not indicate the symptoms of LBBB or RBBB, QRS interval is less than 120 ms, and heart state is in abnormal state.

```
    EVENT RVH_Assessment Refines P_Wave_assessment_Peaked_Yes_Check_RAE
        ANY age, aixs
        WHERE
            grd1 : P_Wave_Peak(II) ≥ 3000
            grd2 : P_Wave_Peak(V1) ≥ 3000
            grd3 : Disease_step6 = RAE
            grd4 : R_Depth(V1) ≥ 7000 ∧ age > 30
            grd5 : S_Depth(V5) ≥ 7000∨
                    S_Depth(V6) ≥ 7000
            grd6 : R_S_Ratio(V1) ≥ 1
            grd7 : R_S_Ratio(V5) ≤ 1
                    ∨
                    R_S_Ratio(V6) ≤ 1
            grd8 : aixs ∈ 0 .. 360 ∧ aixs ≥ 110
            grd9 : Disease_step2 ∉ {LBBB, RBBB}
            grd10 : QRS_Int < 120
            grd11 : Heart_State = KO
        THEN
            act1 : Disease_step6 := RVH
    END
```

10.5.8 Seventh Refinement: Assess T-wave

This refinement is used to assess the pattern of T-wave changes in the 12-leads ECG signals. The T-wave changes are usually nonspecific [16]. The T-wave inversion associated with the ST-segment depression or elevation indicates myocardial ischemia. A new variable *T_Normal_Status* represents as a boolean state like *TRUE* is for normal state, and *FALSE* is for abnormal state. A variable *Disease_step8* is introduced in this refinement to assess a set of diseases related to T-wave from the ECG signals. Invariants (*inv3–inv8*) represent variables in form of total functions mapping leads (LEADS) to possible other attributes (*T_State*, *T_State_B*, *BOOL*, $\mathbb{N}$ and *T_State_l_d*).

The function *T_Wave_State* represents the T-wave states like peaked or flat, or inverted. Similarly, the function *T_Wave_State_B* also represents the T-wave states like upright or inverted, or variable using second method of diagnosis of the T-wave. The function *Abnormal_Shaped_ST* and *Asy_T_Inversion_strain* returns boolean state of the abnormal ST-shape and asymmetric T-wave inversion strain pattern, respectively. The Function *T_inversion* calculates deep the T-wave inversion and the last function *T_inversion_l_d* represents the localised and diffuse T-inversion.

From *inv9* to *inv15* represent an abnormal state of the heart due to finding some diseases. All these invariants are similar to the previous level of refinements. This refinement is very complex, and we have formalised two alternate diagnosis for the ECG signal. We have introduced many events to assess the T-wave from the ECG signals and to predict the various diseases related to the T-wave. Events are *T_Wave_Assessment_Peaked_V123456*, *T_Wave_Assessment_Peaked_V12*, *T_Wave_Assessment_Peaked_V12_MI*, *T_Wave_Assessment_Flat*, *T_Wave_Assessment_Inverted_Yes*, *T_Wave_Assessment_Inverted_No*, *T_Wave_Assessment_Inverted_Yes_PM*, *T_Wave_Assessment_B*, *T_Wave_Assessment_B_DI*, *T_Inversion_Likely_Ischemia*, *T_Inversion_Diffuse_B*. All these events estimate a different kinds of properties from the T-wave signal for obtaining the correct heart disease. A long textual representation for analysing the T-wave is given in [16].

$inv1 : T\_Normal\_Status \in BOOL$
$inv2 : Disease\_step8 \in Disease\_Codes\_Step8$
$inv3 : T\_Wave\_State \in LEADS \rightarrow T\_State$
$inv4 : T\_Wave\_State\_B \in LEADS \rightarrow T\_State\_B$
$inv5 : Abnormal\_Shaped\_ST \in LEADS \rightarrow BOOL$
$inv6 : Asy\_T\_Inversion\_strain \in LEADS \rightarrow BOOL$
$inv7 : T\_inversion \in LEADS \rightarrow \mathbb{N}$
$inv8 : T\_inversion\_l\_d \in LEADS \rightarrow T\_State\_l\_d$
$inv9 : Sinus = Yes \wedge Disease\_step8 = Nonspecific \Rightarrow Heart\_State = KO$
$inv10 : Sinus = Yes \wedge Disease\_step8 = Nonspecific\_ST\_T\_changes$
$\qquad \Rightarrow$
$\qquad Heart\_State = KO$

$inv11 : Sinus = Yes \land Disease\_step8 = posterior\_MI \Rightarrow Heart\_State = KO$
$inv12 : Sinus = Yes \land Disease\_step8 \in \{Definite\_ischemia,$
$\qquad\qquad Probable\_ischemia, Digitalis\_effect\}$
$\qquad\qquad \Rightarrow$
$\qquad\qquad Heart\_State = KO$
$inv13 : Sinus = Yes \land Disease\_step8 = Definite\_ischemia \Rightarrow Heart\_State = KO$
$inv14 : Sinus = Yes \land Disease\_step8 = Probable\_ischemia \Rightarrow Heart\_State = KO$
$inv15 : Sinus = Yes \land Disease\_step8\_B \in \{Cardiomyopathy, other\_nonspecific\}$
$\qquad\qquad \Rightarrow$
$\qquad\qquad Heart\_State = KO$

The event *T_Wave_Assessment_Peaked_V123456* presents basic symptoms for assessing the hyperkalaemia. The guards of this event state that the heart is in abnormal state, and the state of T-wave is peaked in leads from V1 to V6.

EVENT T_Wave_Assessment_Peaked_V123456
  WHEN
    $grd1 : Heart\_State = KO$
    $grd2 : \forall l \cdot l \in \{V1, V2, V3, V4, V5, V6\} \Rightarrow T\_Wave\_State(l) = Peaked$
  THEN
    $act1 : Disease\_step8 := Hyperkalemia$
END

The event *T_Wave_Assessment_Peaked_V12* is used to assess normal variant in the ECG signal. A list of conditions for assessing the normal variant is given in the guards. The guards of this event state that the normal status of the R-wave is FALSE, the state of T-wave is peaked in leads V1 and V2, the ST elevation is TRUE and the ST segment elevation is greater than or equal to 1000 μm, or the abnormal shape of ST segment is TRUE in anyone lead, or the ST elevation is FALSE or the ST segment elevation is less than 1000 μm, and the abnormal shape of ST segment is FALSE in any two leads, inversion in T-wave is less than 5000 μm in all leads, and the status of T-wave is FALSE.

EVENT T_Wave_Assessment_Peaked_V12
  WHEN
    $grd1 : R\_Normal\_Status = FALSE$
    $grd2 : T\_Wave\_State(V1) = Peaked \land$
    $\qquad\quad T\_Wave\_State(V2) = Peaked$
    $grd3 : ((\exists l, k \cdot l \in LEADS \land k \in LEADS \land$
    $\qquad\quad (ST\_elevation(l) = TRUE \land ST\_elevation(k) = TRUE)$
    $\qquad\quad \land$
    $\qquad\quad ((ST\_seg\_ele(l) \geq 1000 \land ST\_seg\_ele(k) \geq 1000)$
    $\qquad\quad \lor$
    $\qquad\quad (Abnormal\_Shaped\_ST(l) = TRUE \land Abnormal\_Shaped\_ST(k) = TRUE))$
    $\qquad\quad \land l = k)$
    $\qquad\quad \lor$

$(\forall l1, k1 \cdot l1 \in LEADS \wedge k1 \in LEADS \wedge$
$((ST\_elevation(l1) = FALSE \vee ST\_elevation(k1) = FALSE)$
$\vee$
$((ST\_seg\_ele(l1) < 1000 \vee ST\_seg\_ele(k1) < 1000)$
$\wedge$
$(Abnormal\_Shaped\_ST(l1) = FALSE \vee$
$Abnormal\_Shaped\_ST(k1) = FALSE)))$
$\Rightarrow l1 \neq k1))$

grd4 : $\forall l \cdot l \in LEADS \Rightarrow T\_inversion(l) < 5000$
grd5 : $T\_Normal\_Status = FALSE$

THEN

act1 : $Mice\_State := normal\_variant$

END

The event *T_Wave_Assessment_Peaked_V12_MI* is used to discover the posterior MI from the ECG signal. A list of guards has characterised the conditions for assessing the posterior MI. These guards state that the state of T-wave is peaked in V1 and V2, the ST elevation is TRUE and the ST segment elevation is greater than or equal to 1000 µm, or the abnormal shape of ST segment is TRUE in anyone lead, or the ST elevation is FALSE or the ST segment elevation is less than 1000 µm, and the abnormal shape of ST segment is FALSE in any two leads, inversion in T-wave is greater than 5000 µm in all leads, and the deep inversion in T-wave is localised in leads from V2 to V5 and II, III, aVF.

EVENT T_Wave_Assessment_Peaked_V12_MI

WHEN

grd1 : $T\_Wave\_State(V1) = Peaked \wedge$
$T\_Wave\_State(V2) = Peaked$

grd2 : $((\exists l, k \cdot l \in LEADS \wedge k \in LEADS \wedge$
$(ST\_elevation(l) = TRUE \wedge ST\_elevation(k) = TRUE)$
$\wedge$
$((ST\_seg\_ele(l) \geq 1000 \wedge ST\_seg\_ele(k) \geq 1000)$
$\vee$
$(Abnormal\_Shaped\_ST(l) = TRUE \wedge Abnormal\_Shaped\_ST(k) = TRUE))$
$\wedge l = k)$
$\vee$
$(\forall l1, k1 \cdot l1 \in LEADS \wedge k1 \in LEADS \wedge$
$((ST\_elevation(l1) = FALSE \vee ST\_elevation(k1) = FALSE)$
$\vee$
$((ST\_seg\_ele(l1) < 1000 \vee ST\_seg\_ele(k1) < 1000)$
$\wedge$
$(Abnormal\_Shaped\_ST(l1) = FALSE \vee$
$Abnormal\_Shaped\_ST(k1) = FALSE)))$
$\Rightarrow l1 \neq k1))$

grd3 : $\forall l \cdot l \in LEADS \Rightarrow T\_inversion(l) > 5000$

grd4 : $T\_inversion\_l\_d(V2) = Localized \wedge$
$T\_inversion\_l\_d(V3) = Localized \wedge$
$T\_inversion\_l\_d(V4) = Localized \wedge$

$T\_inversion\_l\_d(V5) = Localized$

grd5 : $T\_inversion\_l\_d(II) = Localized \land$
$T\_inversion\_l\_d(III) = Localized \land$
$T\_inversion\_l\_d(aVF) = Localized$

grd7 : $T\_Normal\_Status = FALSE$

THEN

act1 : $Disease\_step8 := posterior\_MI$

END

The event *T_Wave_Assessment_Flat* is used to trace Nonspecific ST-T changes including other several diseases. To identify these diseases, a set of guards is given that represents the required conditions. These guards state that the state of T-wave is flat in all leads, the ST elevation is TRUE and the ST segment elevation is greater than or equal to 1000 μm, or the abnormal shape of ST segment is TRUE in anyone lead, or the ST elevation is FALSE or the ST segment elevation is less than 1000 μm, and the abnormal shape of ST segment is FALSE in any two leads, inversion in T-wave is less than 5000 μm in all leads, and the normal state of T-wave is FALSE.

EVENT T_Wave_Assessment_Flat
  WHEN
    grd1 : $\forall l \cdot l \in LEADS \Rightarrow T\_Wave\_State(l) = Flat$
    grd2 : $((\exists l, k \cdot l \in LEADS \land k \in LEADS \land$
        $(ST\_elevation(l) = TRUE \land ST\_elevation(k) = TRUE)$
        $\land$
        $((ST\_seg\_ele(l) \geq 1000 \land ST\_seg\_ele(k) \geq 1000)$
        $\lor$
        $(Abnormal\_Shaped\_ST(l) = TRUE \land Abnormal\_Shaped\_ST(k) = TRUE))$
        $\land l = k)$
        $\lor$
        $(\forall l1, k1 \cdot l1 \in LEADS \land k1 \in LEADS \land$
        $((ST\_elevation(l1) = FALSE \lor ST\_elevation(k1) = FALSE)$
        $\lor$
        $((ST\_seg\_ele(l1) < 1000 \lor ST\_seg\_ele(k1) < 1000)$
        $\land$
        $(Abnormal\_Shaped\_ST(l1) = FALSE \lor$
        $Abnormal\_Shaped\_ST(k1) = FALSE)))$
        $\Rightarrow l1 \neq k1))$
    grd3 : $\forall l \cdot l \in LEADS \Rightarrow T\_inversion(l) < 5000$
    grd5 : $T\_Normal\_Status = FALSE$
  THEN
    act1 : $Disease\_step8 := Nonspecific\_ST\_T\_changes$
    act1 : $Disease\_step8\_B :\in \{Cardiomyopathy, Electrolyte\_depletion,$
        $Alcohol, Myocarditis, Other\}$
  END

The event *T_Wave_Assessment_Inverted_Yes* presents basic symptoms for assessing the definite ischemia, probable ischemia, and digitalis effect. The guards of this event state that the state of T-wave is inverted and the ST elevation is TRUE in all leads, or the normal state of Q-wave is FALSE, and the heart is in abnormal state.

EVENT T_Wave_Assessment_Inverted_Yes
  WHEN
    grd1 : $\forall l \cdot l \in LEADS \Rightarrow T\_Wave\_State(l) = Inverted$
    grd2 : $\forall l \cdot l \in LEADS \Rightarrow ST\_elevation(l) = TRUE$
                $\vee$
            $Q\_Normal\_Status = FALSE$
    grd3 : $Heart\_State = KO$
  THEN
    act1 : $Disease\_step8 :\in \{Definite\_ischemia, Probable\_ischemia, Digitalis\_effect\}$
  END

The event *T_Wave_Assessment_Inverted_No* is used to trace the condition of nonspecific of the heart using ECG signal. The guards of this event specify that the state of T-wave is inverted and the ST elevation is FALSE in all leads, or the normal state of Q-wave is TRUE, and the heart is in abnormal state.

EVENT T_Wave_Assessment_Inverted_No
  WHEN
    grd1 : $\forall l \cdot l \in LEADS \Rightarrow T\_Wave\_State(l) = Inverted$
    grd2 : $\forall l \cdot l \in LEADS \Rightarrow ST\_elevation(l) = FALSE$
                $\vee$
            $Q\_Normal\_Status = TRUE$
    grd3 : $Heart\_State = KO$
  THEN
    act1 : $Disease\_step8 := Nonspecific$
  END

The event *T_Wave_Assessment_Inverted_Yes_PM* is used to find the symptoms for pulmonary embolism from the ECG signal. A set of guards is used that specifies underlined conditions for the pulmonary embolism. The guards of this event state that the peak of P-wave is greater than or equal to 3000 μm in leads II and VI, through the previous assessment RAE has been identified, the state of T-wave is inverted and the ST elevation is TRUE in all leads or the normal state of Q-wave is FALSE, the ST elevation is TRUE and the ST segment elevation is greater than or equal to 1000 μm, or the abnormal shape of ST segment is FALSE in anyone lead, or the ST elevation is FALSE and the ST segment elevation is less than 1000 μm, or the abnormal shape of ST segment is FALSE in any two leads, the Asymmetric T inversion strain is TRUE in leads V1 to V3, and the normal state of T-wave is FALSE.

EVENT T_Wave_Assessment_Inverted_Yes_PM
  WHEN
    grd1 : $P\_Wave\_Peak(II) \geq 3000$
    grd2 : $P\_Wave\_Peak(V1) \geq 3000$
    grd3 : $Disease\_step6 = RAE$
    grd4 : $((\forall p \cdot p \in LEADS \Rightarrow T\_Wave\_State(p) = Inverted) \wedge$
          $(\forall t \cdot t \in LEADS \Rightarrow ST\_elevation(t) = TRUE$
          $\vee$
          $Q\_Normal\_Status = FALSE))$
    grd5 : $((\exists l, k \cdot l \in LEADS \wedge k \in LEADS \wedge$
        $(ST\_elevation(l) = TRUE \wedge ST\_elevation(k) = TRUE)$
        $\wedge$
        $((ST\_seg\_ele(l) \geq 1000 \wedge ST\_seg\_ele(k) \geq 1000)$
        $\vee$
        $(Abnormal\_Shaped\_ST(l) = FALSE \wedge$
        $Abnormal\_Shaped\_ST(k) = FALSE))$
        $\Rightarrow l = k)$
        $\vee$
        $(\forall l1, k1 \cdot l1 \in LEADS \wedge k1 \in LEADS \wedge$
        $(ST\_elevation(l1) = FALSE \wedge ST\_elevation(k1) = FALSE)$
        $\wedge$
        $((ST\_seg\_ele(l1) < 1000 \wedge ST\_seg\_ele(k1) < 1000)$
        $\vee$
        $(Abnormal\_Shaped\_ST(l1) = FALSE \wedge$
        $Abnormal\_Shaped\_ST(k1) = FALSE))$
        $\Rightarrow l1 \neq k1))$
    grd6 : $Asy\_T\_Inversion\_strain(V1) = TRUE \wedge$
        $Asy\_T\_Inversion\_strain(V2) = TRUE \wedge$
        $Asy\_T\_Inversion\_strain(V3) = TRUE$
    grd8 : $T\_Normal\_Status = FALSE$
  THEN
    act1 : $Disease\_step6 := pulmonary\_embolism$
END

The event *T_Wave_Assessment_B* is used to identify the status of the T-wave. Moreover, this event assess the pattern of T-wave changes. The guards of this event state that the state of T-wave is upright in leads I, II, and V3 to V6, the state of T-wave is inverted in lead aVL, and the state of T-wave is variable in leads III, aVL, aVF, V1 and V2.

EVENT T_Wave_Assessment_B
  WHEN
    grd1 : $\forall l \cdot l \in \{I, II, V3, V4, V5, V6\} \Rightarrow T\_Wave\_State\_B(l) = Upright$
    grd2 : $T\_Wave\_State\_B(aVL) = Inverted\_B$
    grd3 : $\forall l \cdot l \in \{III, aVL, aVF, V1, V2\} \Rightarrow T\_Wave\_State\_B(l) = Variable$
  THEN
    act1 : $T\_Normal\_Status := TRUE$
END

The event *T_Wave_Assessment_B_DI* refines *T_Wave_Assessment_Inverted_Yes*. This event is used to discover the symptoms for definite ischemia from the ECG signal. A set of guards is used that specifies underlined conditions for definite ischemia. The guards of this event state that the ST elevation is TRUE in all leads or the normal status of Q-wave is FALSE, the normal status of T-wave is FALSE, the ST elevation is TRUE and the ST segment elevation is greater than or equal to 1000 μm, or the abnormal shape of ST segment is TRUE in any two leads.

EVENT T_Wave_Assessment_B_DI Refines T_Wave_Assessment_Inverted_Yes
WHEN
  $grd2 : \forall l \cdot l \in LEADS \Rightarrow ST\_elevation(l) = TRUE$
              $\lor$
      $Q\_Normal\_Status = FALSE$
  $grd3 : T\_Normal\_Status = FALSE$
  $grd4 : \exists l, k \cdot l \in LEADS \land k \in LEADS \land$
        $((ST\_seg\_ele(l) \geq 1000 \land ST\_seg\_ele(k) \geq 1000) \lor$
        $(ST\_elevation(l) = TRUE \land ST\_elevation(k) = TRUE)$
        $\lor$
        $(Abnormal\_Shaped\_ST(l) = TRUE \land Abnormal\_Shaped\_ST(k) = TRUE))$
        $\land$
        $l \neq k$
THEN
  $act1 : Disease\_step8 := Definite\_ischemia$
END

The event *T_Inversion_Likely_Ischemia* refines *T_Wave_Assessment_Inverted_Yes*. This event is used to trace the symptoms for probable ischemia from the ECG signal. A set of guards is used that specifies the required conditions for the probable ischemia. The guards of this event state that the state of T-wave is inverted in all leads, the ST elevation is TRUE in all leads or the normal status of Q-wave is FALSE, the inversion in T-wave is greater than 5000 μm in all leads, the ST elevation is TRUE and the ST segment elevation is greater than or equal to 1000 μm, or the abnormal shape of ST segment is TRUE in anyone lead, or the ST elevation is FALSE or the ST segment elevation is less than 1000 μm, and the abnormal shape of ST segment is FALSE in any two leads, the inversion in T-wave is localised in leads II, III, aVF, and V2 to V5, and the normal state of T-wave is FALSE.

EVENT T_Inversion_Likely_Ischemia Refines T_Wave_Assessment_Inverted_Yes
WHEN
  $grd1 : \forall l \cdot l \in LEADS \Rightarrow T\_Wave\_State(l) = Inverted$
  $grd2 : \forall l \cdot l \in LEADS \Rightarrow ST\_elevation(l) = TRUE$
              $\lor$
      $Q\_Normal\_Status = FALSE$
  $grd3 : \forall l \cdot l \in LEADS \Rightarrow T\_inversion(l) > 5000$

$grd4 : ((\exists l, k \cdot l \in LEADS \land k \in LEADS \land$
    $(ST\_elevation(l) = TRUE \land ST\_elevation(k) = TRUE)$
    $\land$
    $((ST\_seg\_ele(l) \geq 1000 \land ST\_seg\_ele(k) \geq 1000)$
    $\lor$
    $(Abnormal\_Shaped\_ST(l) = TRUE \land Abnormal\_Shaped\_ST(k) = TRUE))$
    $\land l = k)$
    $\lor$
    $(\forall l1, k1 \cdot l1 \in LEADS \land k1 \in LEADS \land$
    $((ST\_elevation(l1) = FALSE \lor ST\_elevation(k1) = FALSE)$
    $\lor$
    $((ST\_seg\_ele(l1) < 1000 \lor ST\_seg\_ele(k1) < 1000)$
    $\land$
    $(Abnormal\_Shaped\_ST(l1) = FALSE \lor$
    $Abnormal\_Shaped\_ST(k1) = FALSE)))$
    $\Rightarrow l1 \neq k1))$

$grd5 : T\_inversion\_l\_d(V2) = Localized \land$
    $T\_inversion\_l\_d(V3) = Localized \land$
    $T\_inversion\_l\_d(V4) = Localized \land$
    $T\_inversion\_l\_d(V5) = Localized$

$grd6 : T\_inversion\_l\_d(II) = Localized \land$
    $T\_inversion\_l\_d(III) = Localized \land$
    $T\_inversion\_l\_d(aVF) = Localized$

$grd7 : T\_Normal\_Status = FALSE$

THEN

    $act1 : Disease\_step8 := Probable\_ischemia$

END

The event *T_Inversion_Diffuse_B* is used to diagnose the symptoms for cardiomyopathy, other nonspecific from the ECG signal. A set of guards is used that specifies the required conditions that state that the ST elevation is TRUE and the ST segment elevation is greater than or equal to 1000 μm, or the abnormal shape of ST segment is TRUE in anyone lead, or the ST elevation is FALSE or the ST segment elevation is less than 1000 μm, and the abnormal shape of ST segment is FALSE in any two leads, the inversion in T-wave is greater than 5000 μm in all leads, the T inversion is diffuse, and the normal state of T-wave is FALSE.

T_Inversion_Diffuse_B
  WHEN
    $grd1 : ((\exists l, k \cdot l \in LEADS \land k \in LEADS \land$
      $(ST\_elevation(l) = TRUE \land ST\_elevation(k) = TRUE)$
      $\land$
      $((ST\_seg\_ele(l) \geq 1000 \land ST\_seg\_ele(k) \geq 1000)$
      $\lor$
      $(Abnormal\_Shaped\_ST(l) = TRUE \land$
      $Abnormal\_Shaped\_ST(k) = TRUE))$
      $\land l = k)$

$$\lor$$
$$(\forall l1, k1 \cdot l1 \in LEADS \land k1 \in LEADS \land$$
$$((ST\_elevation(l1) = FALSE \lor ST\_elevation(k1) = FALSE)$$
$$\lor$$
$$((ST\_seg\_ele(l1) < 1000 \lor ST\_seg\_ele(k1) < 1000)$$
$$\land$$
$$(Abnormal\_Shaped\_ST(l1) = FALSE \lor$$
$$Abnormal\_Shaped\_ST(k1) = FALSE)))$$
$$\Rightarrow l1 \neq k1))$$

$grd2 : \forall l \cdot l \in LEADS \Rightarrow T\_inversion(l) > 5000$

$grd3 : \forall l \cdot l \in LEADS \Rightarrow T\_inversion\_l\_d(l) = Diffuse$

$grd4 : T\_Normal\_Status = FALSE$

THEN

$act1 : Disease\_step8\_B :\in \{Cardiomyopathy, other\_nonspecific\}$

END

10.5.9 Eighth Refinement: Assess Electrical Axis

After finding all kinds of information about abnormal ECG, it is also essential to check the electrical axis (see Table 10.1) using two simple clues:

- If leads I and aVF are upright; the axis is normal.
- The axis is perpendicular to the lead with the most equiphasic or smallest QRS deflection. Left-axis deviation and the commonly associated left anterior fascicular block are visible in ECG signal.

This refinement is very essential refinement for the ECG interpretation because of the different angle of the ECG signal gives different output and angle based prediction can be changed [16]. So, for accuracy of the ECG interpretation electrical axis must be included. New variables *minAngle*, *maxAngle*, *Axis_Devi* and *Dis-*

Table 10.1 Electrical axis

Most equiphasic lead	Lead perpendicular	Axis
		Lead I and aVF positive = normal axis
III	aVR	Normal = +30 degrees
aVL	II	Normal = +60 degrees
		Lead I positive and aVF negative = Left axis
II	aVL (QRS positive)	Left = −30 degrees
aVR	III (QRS negative)	Left = −60 degrees
I	aVF (QRS negative)	Left = −90 degrees
		Lead I negative and aVF positive = right axis
aVR	III (QRS positive)	Right = +120 degrees
II	aVL (QRS negative)	Right = +150 degrees

ease_step9 have been defined here for assessment of the electrical axis. A new variable *QRS_Axis_State* is defined as a total function mapping from leads (LEADS) to *QRS_directions*. This function represents the QRS-axis direction of the leads. Two invariants (*inv6–inv7*) represent the safety properties in assessment of the correct axis. These invariants are verifying an abnormal state of the heart (*KO*) using axis position.

$$
\begin{aligned}
&inv1 : minAngle \in -90 \ldots 180 \\
&inv2 : maxAngle \in -90 \ldots 180 \\
&inv3 : Axis\_Devi \in Axis\_deviation \\
&inv4 : Disease\_step9 \in Disease\_Codes\_Step9 \\
&inv5 : QRS\_Axis\_State \in LEADS \rightarrow QRS\_directions \\
&inv6 : Disease\_step9 \in \{LPFB, Dextrocardia, NV\_MSEC\} \;\wedge \\
&\qquad\quad maxAngle = 180 \wedge minAngle = 110 \\
&\qquad\quad \Rightarrow \\
&\qquad\quad Heart\_State = KO \\
&inv7 : Disease\_step9 \in \{LAFB, MSCHD, Some\_Form\_VT, ED\_OC\} \\
&\qquad\quad \wedge maxAngle = -90 \wedge minAngle = -30 \\
&\qquad\quad \Rightarrow \\
&\qquad\quad Heart\_State = KO
\end{aligned}
$$

In this refinement level, we introduce various events for assessing different kinds of features from 12 leads ECG signal corresponding to the angle. Following events are introduced in this refinement: *Axis_Assessment_QRS_upright_Yes_Age_less_40*, *Axis_Assessment_QRS_upright_Yes_Age_gre_40*, *Axis_Assessment_QRS_upright_No_QRS_positive*, *Axis_Assessment_QRS_upright_No_QRS_negative*, *Misc_Disease_Step9_LAD*, *Misc_Disease_Step9_RAD*, *R_Q_Assessment_R_Abnormal_V56_axis_deviation*.

The event *Axis_Assessment_QRS_upright_Yes_Age_less_40* refines *Axis_Assessment_QRS_upright_Yes*. This event is used to find the electrical axis. A set of guards is used that specifies that the QRS axis state is upright in leads I and aVF, and age is less than 40 years.

```
EVENT Axis_Assessment_QRS_upright_Yes_Age_less_40
Refines Axis_Assessment_QRS_upright_Yes
    ANY age
    WHERE
        grd1 : QRS_Axis_State(I) = D_Upright∧
                QRS_Axis_State(aVF) = D_Upright
        grd2 : age ∈ ℕ ∧ age < 40
    THEN
        act1 : minAngle := 0
        act2 : maxAngle := 110
END
```

The event *Axis_Assessment_QRS_upright_Yes_Age_gre_40* refines *Axis_Assessment_QRS_upright_Yes*. This event is similar to the last event that is also used to assess the electrical axis. The minimum angle is −30 and maximum angle is 90. A set of guards is used that defines that the QRS axis state is upright in leads I and aVF, and age is greater than 40 years.

```
EVENT Axis_Assessment_QRS_upright_Yes_Age_gre_40
Refines Axis_Assessment_QRS_upright_Yes
    ANY age
    WHERE
        grd1 : QRS_Axis_State(I) = D_Upright∧
                QRS_Axis_State(aVF) = D_Upright
        grd2 : age ∈ ℕ ∧ age > 40
    THEN
        act1 : minAngle := −30
        act2 : maxAngle := 90
END
```

The event *Axis_Assessment_QRS_upright_No_QRS_positive* refines *Axis_Assessment_QRS_upright_No*. This event is used to determine the electrical axis and left axis deviation (LAD) in leads. A set of guards is used that defines that the QRS axis state is not upright in leads I and aVF, the QRS axis state is positive in leads I and aVF, and the heart is in abnormal state.

```
EVENT Axis_Assessment_QRS_upright_No_QRS_positive
Refines Axis_Assessment_QRS_upright_No
    WHEN
        grd1 : ¬(QRS_Axis_State(I) = D_Upright∧
                QRS_Axis_State(aVF) = D_Upright)
        grd2 : QRS_Axis_State(I) = D_Positive∧
                QRS_Axis_State(aVF) = D_Positive
        grd3 : Heart_State = KO
    THEN
        act1 : minAngle := −30
        act2 : maxAngle := −90
        act3 : Axis_Devi := LAD
END
```

The event *Axis_Assessment_QRS_upright_No_QRS_negative* refines *Axis_Assessment_QRS_upright_No*. This event is used to identify the electrical axis and right axis deviation (RAD) in leads. A set of guards is used that defines that the QRS axis state is not upright in leads I and aVF, the QRS axis state is negative in leads I and aVF, and the heart is in abnormal state.

```
EVENT Axis_Assessment_QRS_upright_No_QRS_negative
Refines Axis_Assessment_QRS_upright_No
    WHEN
        grd1 : ¬(QRS_Axis_State(I) = D_Upright∧
                  QRS_Axis_State(aVF) = D_Upright)
        grd2 : QRS_Axis_State(I) = D_Negative∧
                  QRS_Axis_State(aVF) = D_Negative
        grd3 : Heart_State = KO
    THEN
        act1 : minAngle := 110
        act2 : maxAngle := 180
        act3 : Axis_Devi := RAD
END
```

The event *Misc_Disease_Step9_LAD* assess miscellaneous diseases like LAFB, MSCHD, etc. A set of guards is used that defines that the axis deviation is left axis deviation (LAD) in leads, negative minimum angle is −30, negative maximum angle is −90 and the heart is in abnormal state.

```
Misc_Disease_Step9_LAD
    WHEN
        grd1 : Axis_Devi = LAD∧
                  minAngle = −30∧
                  maxAngle = −90
        grd2 : Heart_State = KO
    THEN
        act1 : Disease_step9 :∈ {LAFB, MSCHD, Some_Form_VT, ED_OC}
END
```

The event *Misc_Disease_Step9_LAD* assess several diseases like LPFB, Dextrocardia, NV MS-EC. A set of guards is used that defines that the axis deviation is right axis deviation (RAD) in leads, positive minimum angle is 110, positive maximum angle is 180 and the heart is in abnormal state.

```
Misc_Disease_Step9_RAD
    WHEN
        grd1 : Axis_Devi = RAD∧
                  minAngle = 110∧
                  maxAngle = 180
        grd2 : Heart_State = KO
    THEN
        act1 : Disease_step9 :∈ {LPFB, Dextrocardia, NV_MSEC}
END
```

The event *R_Q_Assessment_R_Abnormal_V56_axis_deviation* refines *R_Q_Assessment_R_Abnormal_V56*. This event is used to identify the lateral MI. A set of guards is used that formalises that the state of Q-wave is TRUE in leads V5 and V6, the axis deviation is right axis deviation (RAD) in leads, positive minimum angle is 110, positive maximum angle is 180 and the heart is in abnormal state.

```
EVENT R_Q_Assessment_R_Abnormal_V56_axis_deviation
Refines R_Q_Assessment_R_Abnormal_V56
   WHEN
      grd1 : Q_Wave_State(V5) = TRUE∧
             Q_Wave_State(V6) = TRUE
      grd2 : Axis_Devi = RAD∧
             minAngle = 110∧
             maxAngle = 180
      grd3 : Heart_State = KO
   THEN
      act1 : Disease_step5 := lateral_MI
END
```

10.5.10 Ninth Refinement: Assess for Miscellaneous Conditions

There are lots of heart diseases, and it is very difficult to predict everything. A lot of conditions make it more and more ambiguous. This refinement level keeps multiple miscellaneous conditions about the ECG interpretation [16]. Following conditions are given for miscellaneous conditions as follows:

- Artificial pacemakers: If electronic pacing is confirmed, usually no other diagnosis can be made from the ECG.
- Prolonged QT syndrome: See normal QT parameters listed in Table 10.2. No complicated formula is required for assessment of the QT intervals.

A variable $MC\_Step10\_Test\_Needed$ is declared to represent miscellaneous condition tests as a boolean type $TRUE$ or $FALSE$. Variable $Disease\_step10$ is introduced in this refinement to assess a set of diseases of miscellaneous conditions from the ECG signal. The next two invariants ($inv2$–$inv3$) represent the abnormality of the heart state (KO) in case of discovery of new miscellaneous diseases. In this refinement, we introduce only two events ($Miscellaneous\_Conditions\_Step10$ and $Misc\_Disease\_Step10\_Dextrocardia\_Test$) to discover miscellaneous conditions from the ECG signal.

	Heart rate (bpm)	Male	Female
Table 10.2 Clinically useful approximation of upper limit of QT interval (ms)			
	45–65	<470	<480
	66–100	<410	<430
	>100	<360	<370

$inv1 : MC\_Step10\_Test\_Needed \in BOOL$
$inv2 : Disease\_step10 \in Misc_{Disease}\_Codes\_Step10$
$inv3 : Sinus = Yes \land Disease\_step10 \in \{Incomplete\_RBBB,$
           $Long\_QT, Hypokalemia, Digitalis\_toxicity, Hypothermia,$
           $Electronic\_pacing, Pericarditis, Hypercalcemia\}$
           $Electrical\_alternans$
           $\Rightarrow$
           $Heart\_State = KO$
$inv4 : Sinus = Yes \land Disease\_step9 = Dextrocardia$
           $\Rightarrow$
           $Heart\_State = KO$

The event *Miscellaneous_Conditions_Step10* is used to assess miscellaneous disease. It is very difficult to identify all the possible diseases using ECG signal, therefore a set of disease is classified under the miscellaneous conditions. This event is used to find the several diseases. A set of guards is used that specifies that the further test is needed that is presented as a boolean type, and the heart is in abnormal state.

EVENT Miscellaneous_Conditions_Step10
  WHEN
    $grd1 : MC\_Step10\_Test\_Needed = TRUE$
    $grd2 : Heart\_State = KO$
  THEN
    $act1 : Disease\_step10 :\in \{Incomplete\_RBBB, Pericarditis, Long\_QT, Hypokalemia,$
         $Digitalis\_toxicity, Electrical\_alternans, Electronic\_pacing, Hypothermia,$
         $Hypercalcemia\}$
  END

The event *Misc_Disease_Step10_Dextrocardia_Test* refines *Misc_Disease_Step9_RAD* and this event is modelled to assess the Dextrocardia. A list of required conditions is formalised in form of guards. These guards present that the axis deviation is right axis deviation (RAD) in leads, minimum angle is 110, maximum angle is 180, boolean state for further testing is TRUE, and the heart is in abnormal state.

EVENT Misc_Disease_Step10_Dextrcardia_Test Refines Misc_Disease_Step9_RAD
  WHEN
    $grd1 : Axis\_Devi = RAD \land$
         $minAngle = 110 \land$
         $maxAngle = 180$
    $grd2 : MC\_Step10\_Test\_Needed = TRUE$
    $grd3 : Heart\_State = KO$
  THEN
    $act1 : Disease\_step9 := Dextrocardia$
  END

10.5.11 Tenth Refinement: Assess Arrhythmias

This is the final refinement of the ECG interpretation of the system. In this refinement, we introduce different kinds of tachyarrhythmias and give the protocols for assessment as follows:

- Narrow complex tachycardia: Gives the differential diagnosis of narrow QRS complex tachycardia.
- Wide complex tachycardia: Gives the differential diagnosis of wide QRS complex tachycardia.

$inv1 : NW\_QRS\_Tachycardia\_RT\_State \in$
  $NW\_QRS\_Tachycardia\_RI$
$inv2 : Disease\_step11 \in Misc\_Disease\_Codes\_Step11$
$inv3 : Sinus = Yes \wedge Disease\_step11 \in$
  $\{Ventricular\_Premature\_Beats, Nodal\_Premature\_Beats,$
  $Bradyarrhythmias, Narrow\_QRS\_Tachycardias,$
  $Wide\_QRS\_Tachycardias, Atrial\_Premature\_Beats\}$
  $\Rightarrow Heart\_State = KO$

$inv4 : Sinus = Yes \wedge Distease\_step11\_NW\_QRST \in$
  $\{Sinus\_Tachycardia, Supraventricular\_Tachycardia,$
  $WPW\_Syndrome\_Orthodromic, Torsades\_de\_pointes,$
  $Atrial\_Tachycardia, AF\_Fixed\_AV\_Conduction, AVNRT,$
  $Ventricular\_Tachycardia, WPW\_Syndrome\_Antidromic,$
  $AF\_Variable\_AV\_Conduction\_BBB\_WPW\_Synd\_Anti,$
  $AF\_BBB\_WPW\_Synd\_Antidromic\}$
  $\Rightarrow Heart\_State = KO$

$inv5 : Sinus = Yes \wedge Distease\_step11\_NW\_QRST \in$
  $\{AF\_Variable\_AV\_Conduction, AVNRT,$
  $AT\_Paroxysmal\_NParoxysmal, AT\_Variable\_AV\_Block,$
  $AF\_Fixed\_AV\_Conduction, WPW\_Syndrome\_OCMT,$
  $Sinus\_Tachycardia, Multifocal\_Atrial\_Tachycardia,$
  $Atrail\_Fibrillation\}$
  $\Rightarrow Heart\_State = KO$

$inv6 : NW\_QRS\_Tachycardia\_RT\_State = Regular \wedge$
  $Distease\_step11\_NW\_QRST \in \{Sinus\_Tachycardia,$
  $WPW\_Syndrome\_OCMT, AF\_Fixed\_AV\_Conduction,$
  $AVNRT, AT\_Paroxysmal\_NParoxysmal\}$
  $\Rightarrow Heart\_State = KO$

$inv7 : NW\_QRS\_Tachycardia\_RT\_State = Irregular \wedge$
  $Distease\_step11\_NW\_QRST \in \{Atrail\_Fibrillation,$
  $AT\_Variable\_AV\_Block, AF\_Variable\_AV\_Conduction,$
  $Multifocal\_Atrial\_Tachycardia\}$
  $\Rightarrow Heart\_State = KO$

$inv8 : NW\_QRS\_Tachycardia\_RT\_State = Regular \wedge$
$\qquad Disease\_step11\_NW\_QRST \in \{Ventricular\_Tachycardia,$
$\qquad Sinus\_Tachycardia, AF\_Fixed\_AV\_Conduction,$
$\qquad Supraventricular\_Tachycardia, Atrial\_Tachycardia,$
$\qquad AVNRT, WPW\_Syndrome\_Antidromic,$
$\qquad WPW\_Syndrome\_Orthodromic\}$
$\qquad \Rightarrow Heart\_State = KO$

$inv9 : NW\_QRS\_Tachycardia\_RT\_State = Irregular \wedge$
$\qquad Disteavse\_step11\_NW\_QRST \in$
$\qquad \{AF\_Variable\_AV\_Conduction\_BBB\_WPW\_Synd\_Anti,$
$\qquad Torsades\_de\_pointes, AF\_BBB\_WPW\_Synd\_Antidromic\}$
$\qquad \Rightarrow Heart\_State = KO$

A new variable *NW_QRS_Tachycardia_RT_State* is defined to express the QRS tachycardia regular or irregular state using *inv*1. A variable *Disease_step11* is introduced in this refinement to assess arrhythmias from the ECG signals. All rest of the invariants (*inv*3–*inv*9) represents an abnormal state (*KO*) of the heart after analysing the arrhythmia and related disease. All invariants have similar kinds of properties. We introduce five new events to assess tachyarrhythmias from the 12-leads ECG signals in case of abnormal rhythm. Five events are *Rhythm_test_FALSE_Step11, Step11_N_QRS_Tachycardia_Regular, Step11_N_QRS_Tachycardia_Irregular, Step11_W_QRS_Tachycardia_Regular* and *Step11_W_QRS_Tachycardia_Irregular.*

The event *Rhythm_test_FALSE_Step11* is used to identify the heart state, sinus rhythm, heart rate and several diseases that are not identified through the last assessment process. The guards of this event shows that the equidistant of PP interval is FALSE or the equidistant of RR interval is FALSE, the RR interval is not equal to the PP interval in leads II, V1, V2, or the positive state of P-wave is FALSE, and the heart rate is within the range of 1 to 300 bps.

Rhythm_test_FALSE_Step11
  ANY *rate*
  WHERE
    $grd1 : (\forall l \cdot l \in \{II, V1, V2\} \Rightarrow PP\_Int\_equidistant(l) = FALSE \vee$
        $RR\_Int\_equidistant(l) = FALSE \vee$
        $RR\_Interval(l) \neq PP\_Interval(l))$
        $\vee$
        $P\_Positive(II) = FALSE$
    $grd2 : rate \in 1 .. 300$
  THEN
    $act1 : Sinus := No$
    $act2 : Heart\_Rate := rate$
    $act3 : Heart\_State := KO$
    $act4 : Disease\_step11 :\in \{Atrial\_Premature\_Beats, Ventricular\_Premature\_Beats,$
        $Bradyarrhythmias, Narrow\_QRS\_Tachycardias, Wide\_QRS\_Tachycardias,$
        $Nodal\_Premature\_Beats\}$
  END

The event *Step11_N_QRS_Tachycardia_Regular* refines Step11_N_QRS_Ta-chycardia. This event assesses the different kinds of diseases like sinus tachycardia, AVNRT, etc. A set of guards of this event is used to formalise the required conditions. These conditions present that the heart has no sinus rhythm, the heart is in abnormal state, the heart rate is within 1 to 60 or 100 to 300 range, through previous assessment the heart has the conditions of narrow QRS tachycardia, and the state of narrow QRS tachycardia is regular.

EVENT Step11_N_QRS_Tachycardia_Regular Refines Step11_N_QRS_Tachycardia
  WHEN
   grd1 : $Sinus = No$
   grd2 : $Heart\_State = KO$
   grd3 : $Heart\_Rate \in 1 .. 300 \setminus 60 .. 100$
   grd4 : $Disease\_step11 = Narrow\_QRS\_Tachycardias$
   grd5 : $NW\_QRS\_Tachycardia\_RT\_State = Regular$
  THEN
   act1 : $Disease\_step11\_NW\_QRST :\in \{Sinus\_Tachycardia, AVNRT,$
       $AF\_Fixed\_AV\_Conduction, AT\_Paroxysmal\_NParoxysmal,$
       $WPW\_Syndrome\_OCMT\}$
  END

The event *Step11_N_QRS_Tachycardia_Irregular* refines Step11_N_QRS_Ta-chycardia. The action of this event specifies to identify several diseases using ECG signal. The guards of this event state that the heart has no sinus rhythm, heart is in abnormal state, the heart rate is within 1 to 60 or 100 to 300 range, through previous assessment the heart has the conditions of narrow QRS tachycardia, and the state of narrow QRS tachycardia is irregular.

EVENT Step11_N_QRS_Tachycardia_Irregular Refines Step11_N_QRS_Tachycardia
  WHEN
   grd1 : $Sinus = No$
   grd2 : $Heart\_State = KO$
   grd3 : $Heart\_Rate \in 1 .. 300 \setminus 60 .. 100$
   grd4 : $Disease\_step11 = Narrow\_QRS\_Tachycardias$
   grd5 : $NW\_QRS\_Tachycardia\_RT\_State = Irregular$
  THEN
   act1 : $Disease\_step11\_NW\_QRST :\in \{AF\_Variable\_AV\_Conduction,$
       $Atrail\_Fibrillation, AT\_Variable\_AV\_Block, Multifocal\_Atrial\_Tachycardia\}$
  END

The event *Step11_W_QRS_Tachycardia_Regular* refines Step11_W_QRS_Ta-chycardia. As similar to the last event, the action of this event also specifies to identify several diseases from the ECG signal. A set of guards presents required conditions. These required conditions show that the heart has no sinus rhythm, heart is in abnormal state, the heart rate is within 1 to 60 or 100 to 300 range, through previous assessment the heart has the conditions of wide QRS tachycardia, and the state of narrow QRS tachycardia is regular.

EVENT Step11_W_QRS_Tachycardia_Regular Refines Step11_W_QRS_Tachycardia
   WHEN
      grd1 : $Sinus = No$
      grd2 : $Heart\_State = KO$
      grd3 : $Heart\_Rate \in 1 .. 300 \setminus 60 .. 100$
      grd4 : $Disease\_step11 = Wide\_QRS\_Tachycardias$
      grd5 : $NW\_QRS\_Tachycardia\_RT\_State = Regular$
   THEN
      act1 : $Distease\_step11\_NW\_QRST :\in \{Ventricular\_Tachycardia,$
            $Supraventricular\_Tachycardia, AVNRT, WPW\_Syndrome\_Orthodromic,$
            $Sinus\_Tachycardia, Atrial\_Tachycardia, AF\_Fixed\_AV\_Conduction,$
            $WPW\_Syndrome\_Antidromic\}$
  END

The event *Step11_W_QRS_Tachycardia_Irregular* refines Step11_W_QRS_Tachycardia. A list of guards presents that the heart has no sinus rhythm, heart is in abnormal state, the heart rate is within 1 to 60 or 100 to 300 range, through previous assessment of the heart has the conditions of wide QRS tachycardia, and the state of narrow QRS tachycardia is irregular. The action of this event is used to identify several diseases from the ECG signal that are given in the action.

EVENT Step11_W_QRS_Tachycardia_Irregular Refines Step11_W_QRS_Tachycardia
   WHEN
      grd1 : $Sinus = No$
      grd2 : $Heart\_State = KO$
      grd3 : $Heart\_Rate \in 1 .. 300 \setminus 60 .. 100$
      grd4 : $Disease\_step11 = Wide\_QRS\_Tachycardias$
      grd5 : $NW\_QRS\_Tachycardia\_RT\_State = Irregular$
   THEN
      act1 : $Distease\_step11\_NW\_QRST :\in \{AF\_BBB\_WPW\_Synd\_Antidromic,$
            $AF\_Variable\_AV\_Conduction\_BBB\_WPW\_Synd\_Anti, Torsades\_de\_pointes\}$
  END

Here, we have given required safety properties in form invariants in all refinements. All these properties are derived from the original protocol to verify the correctness and consistency of the system. These properties are formulated through logic experts as well as cardiologist experts according to the original protocol. The main advantage of this technique is that if any property is not holding by the model, then it helps to find anomalies or to find missing parts of the model such as required conditions and parameters. A technical report [21] contains the complete formal representation of the ECG interpretation protocol.

10.5.12 Proof Statistics

All the proof obligations for all ten refinements are generated and proved using the Rodin prover [29]. Table 10.3 shows statistics of the ECG interpretation protocol us-

Table 10.3 Proof statistics

Model	Total number of POs	Automatic proof	Interactive proof
Abstract model	41	33 (80 %)	8 (20 %)
First refinement	61	54 (88 %)	7 (12 %)
Second refinement	41	38 (92 %)	3 (8 %)
Third refinement	51	36 (70 %)	15 (30 %)
Fourth refinement	60	35 (58 %)	25 (42 %)
Fifth refinement	43	22 (51 %)	21 (49 %)
Sixth refinement	38	14 (36 %)	24 (64 %)
Seventh refinement	124	29 (23 %)	95 (77 %)
Eighth refinement	52	30 (57 %)	22 (43 %)
Ninth refinement	21	9 (42 %)	12 (52 %)
Tenth refinement	67	43 (64 %)	24 (36 %)
Total	599	343 (58 %)	256 (42 %)

ing refinement approach. In the table, the POs column represents the total number of proof obligations generated for each level. The interactive POs column represents the number of those proof obligations that have to be proved interactively. Those proof obligations that are not proved interactively are proved completely automatically by the prover. The complete development of the ECG interpretation protocol system results in 599 (100 %) proof obligations, in which 343 (58 %) are proved automatically by the Rodin tool. The remaining 256 (42 %) proof obligations are proved interactively using Rodin tool. In seventh refinement, numbers of POs are higher than other refinements because significantly in this level; number of variables and events are higher than another level of refinements. All the proofs are discharged completely automatic as well as interactive for all refinement levels. All these proofs are involved either by the complexity of the formal expression that proved by *do case* or finiteness constraints on a set of leads. The main interactive steps involved instantiating for total function of the different features of the ECG interpretation in every level of refinement. In order to guarantee the correctness of the system, we have established various invariants in the stepwise refinement. All these invariants are derived from the original protocol to verify the correctness and consistency of the system under the guidance of the cardiologist expert. Most of the invariants are introduced for checking the abnormality of the features of the ECG signal. Detection of an abnormal criteria, the heart shows surety of a particular disease or a set of diseases. A set of diseases are distinguished in next level of refinements.

10.6 Lesson Learnt

The task of modelling of the ECG interpretation protocol in the Event-B has required a significant effort. It is a typical knowledge engineering task, where the knowledge is the original document, is transformed into the Event-B formal notation, which provides a significant hierarchical structure for analysing the ECG interpretation protocol and to diagnose different kinds of heart diseases. As the result, the Event-B ECG interpretation protocol specification is much more lengthy than the original text: the original ECG interpretation protocol. The complete formal specification of the ECG interpretation protocol in the Event-B is more than 200 pages.

We consider that logic-based modelling approach is very difficult to model a complex medical protocol. This approach has required a good understanding of logic as well as knowledge of the medical protocol. We have spent lots of time with medical experts to understand the structure of the medical protocols for formalising purpose. For modelling the ECG protocol, we have consulted with cardiologist and medical experts. The formal model of ECG protocol is based on original protocol and checked by medical experts [21, 22].

We cannot strictly say that the formal representation of the ECG interpretation protocol in the Event-B modelling language has contributed to the improvement of the original protocol. Most important contribution is refinements-based formal development of the ECG interpretation protocol and to generate a new optimal way of the ECG interpretation protocol for diagnosing the ECG signal. The developed formal model is proved and verified according to the given protocol properties as discussed in the formal development. Furthermore, the Event-B formalisation has served to disambiguate unclarities in the original document that resulted from the modelling stage: a number of ambiguity and repetition diagnosis problems with original document are uncovered and resolved by refining the formal specification of the ECG interpretation protocol in the Event-B. The formal model can help to restructure the original document of guidelines and protocols.

The verification attempts have served to clarify any remaining problems in the original ECG interpretation protocol document. More importantly, we have shown that it is possible in practice to systematically analyse whether a protocol formalised in the Event-B complies with certain medically relevant properties. Various properties of the ECG interpretation protocol have been the object of formal verification using the Event-B system, with different type of results. Mostly, the given properties of the ECG interpretation protocol have been confirmed by the formal representation of the ECG interpretation protocol. However, in other cases, verification is not simple and lots of ambiguous informations, i.e. it is not possible to complete the proof or further development of the model due to ambiguity. We have introduced some additional assumptions with the help of cardiologist experts for describing the conditions needed to make the property true and added more conditions to remove the ambiguity. These assumptions are missing piece of information in the medical protocol, which helps to improve the medical protocol. We have applied a pragmatic approach to collect lots of information through literature survey and medical experts advises for finding the exact facts to introduce new assumptions and conditions for discharging all the generated proof obligations.

For example, pieces of informations missing from the original ECG interpretation protocol like it is not given that how many leads should hold particular property during diagnosis. As per our solution, we have applied test for particular properties in all leads. This results in a characterisation of the circumstances under which the property holds. The obtained characterisation is analysed by the medical experts under all the possible conditions, and it can be used either to redefine the property or to improve the original ECG interpretation protocol text by documenting the cases under which the property does (or does not) hold.

More importantly, numerous anomalies became apparent during the Event-B modelling of the ECG interpretation protocol. Here, we have used term anomaly to refer to any issues that are not able to represent satisfactory of the original ECG interpretation protocol. Some set of anomalies, which have found during the development of the system are described below. We have grouped all anomalies in three well known general categories: ambiguity, inconsistency and incompleteness.

10.6.1 Ambiguous

Ambiguous is a well-known anomaly in the area of formal representation, and it is very hard to interpret. For instance, a problem we encountered while modelling the ECG interpretation protocol is determining whether the terms "ST-depression" and "ST-elevation" had the same meaning or not. These are terms that are used in the ECG interpretation original protocol, but not defined elsewhere. Similarly, what is the difference between "ischemia", "definite ischemia", "probable ischemia" and "likely ischemia".

In the ECG interpretation, there are 12 leads ECG signals, which are used for interpretation, but a lot of places in the original document not clarify in which lead the particular property should hold. Such kinds of information are very ambiguous and give lots of confusions to model the system.

10.6.2 Inconsistencies

Inconsistencies are other kinds of anomalies which are always given conflicting results or different decisions on same patient data. The problems derived from inconsistent elements are very serious and as such must be avoided during development. The ECG interpretation protocol presents several inconsistencies. For instance, we found an inconsistency in form of applicable conditions in the ECG protocol. It expresses that the conditions are applicable to both "male" and "female" under some certain circumstances. However, elsewhere in the protocol an action is advised that these conditions of the protocol are not applicable to "female".

10.6.3 Incompleteness

Either missing pieces of information or insufficient information in the original document are always related to the incompleteness anomaly. In either case, incompleteness hinders a correct interpretation of the guidelines and protocols. For example, the original protocol contains "normal variant" factors to be considered when assessing the T-wave. However, what "normal variant" exactly means is missing in the protocol. As an example of insufficient information for "normal variant", we provide the class of diseases for further analysis the system.

10.7 Summary

Refinement is a key concept for developing the complex systems, since it starts with a very abstract model and incrementally adds new details to the set of requirements. We have outlined an incremental refinement-based approach for formalising medical protocols using the Rodin tool. The approach we have taken is not specific to the Event-B. We believe a similar approach could be taken using others state-based notations such as ASM, TLA$^+$, Z, etc. The Rodin proof tool is used to generate the hundreds of proof obligations and to discharge those obligations automatically and interactively. Another key role of the tool is in helping us to discover appropriate gluing invariants to prove the refinements. In summary, some key lessons are that incremental development with small refinement steps; appropriate abstractions at each level and powerful tool support are all invaluable in such a kind of formal development.

In this chapter, we have shown the formal representation of medical protocol. The formal model of medical protocol is verified, and this verified model is not only feasible but also useful for improving the existing medical protocol. We have fully formalised a real-world medical protocols (ECG interpretation) in an incremental refinement-based formalisation process, and we have used proof tools to systematically analyse whether the formalisation complies with certain medically relevant protocol properties [21, 22]. The formal verification process has discovered a number of anomalies which all are discussed in the previous section. Throughout this process, we have obtained the following concrete results:

- A formal specification language like Event-B is used for modelling a complex system, is used to model the medical practice protocols. The Event-B is a general modelling language tool. The Event-B is used to present a formal specification for a real-life medical protocols; ECG interpretation.
- The ECG interpretation protocol is formalised in the Event-B modelling language. The medical protocol ECG interpretation is used in our study has been developed in incremental way and finally transformed into a concrete formal representation. Each proved refinement level of the formal model of the protocol represents feasibility and correctness.

- In our formal verification process of the ECG interpretation, we have obtained a list of anomalies.
- Verification proofs for the ECG interpretation protocol, and properties have proved using the Rodin proof tool. Generated proof obligations and proofs show that formal verification of the ECG interpretation protocols is feasible.
- Original protocol of the ECG is also based on some hierarchy, but in that hierarchy, some diagnosis is repeating in multiple branches (see in [16]). We have also discovered an optimised hierarchical structure for the ECG interpretation efficiently using incremental refinement approach, which can help to diagnose more efficiently then old techniques, and this obtained hierarchical structure is verified through medical experts.

The ECG interpretation protocol [21, 22] is very complex, and it interprets various kinds of heart diseases. Improving quality of medical protocol using the formal verification tools like highly mathematical based modelling languages; Event-B, is the main contribution of our work. We have also discovered a hierarchical structure for the ECG interpretation efficiently that helps to discover a set of conditions that can be very helpful to diagnose particular disease an early stage of the diagnosis without using multiple diagnosis. Our hierarchical tree structure provides more concrete solutions for the ECG interpretation protocol and helps to improve the original ECG interpretation protocol. Our objective behind this work is that if any medical protocol is developed under particular circumstances to handle a set of specific properties according to the medical experts, formal verification can also meet whether the protocol actually complies with them. This has been the first attempt ever in verifying medical protocols with mathematical rigour with the generalised formal modelling tool Event-B. The main objective of this approach to test correctness and consistency of the medical protocol using refinement based incremental development. This approach is not only for diagnosis purpose, but it may be applicable to covering a large group of other categories (i.e. treatment, management, prevention, counselling, evaluation, etc.)[3] related to the medical protocols.

References

1. Abrial, J.-R. (2010). *Modeling in Event-B: System and software engineering* (1st ed.). New York: Cambridge University Press.
2. Advani, A., Goldstein, M., Shahar, Y., & Musen, M. A. (2003). Developing quality indicators and auditing protocols from formal guideline models: Knowledge representation and transformations. In *AMIA annual symposium proceedings* (pp. 11–15).
3. Balser, M., Reif, W., Schellhorn, G., & Stenzel, K. (1999). KIV 3.0 for provably correct systems. In D. Hutter, W. Stephan, P. Traverso, & M. Ullmann (Eds.), *Lecture notes in computer science: Vol. 1641. Applied formal methods—FM-trends 98* (pp. 330–337). Berlin: Springer.
4. Barold, S. S., Stroobandt, R. X., & Sinnaeve, A. F. (2004). *Cardiac pacemakers step by step*. London: Futura. ISBN 1-4051-1647-1.

---

[3]http://www.guideline.gov/.

5. Bäumler, S., Balser, M., Dunets, A., Reif, W., & Schmitt, J. (2006). Verification of medical guidelines by model checking—a case study. In A. Valmari (Ed.), *Lecture notes in computer science: Vol. 3925. Model checking software* (pp. 219–233). Berlin: Springer. doi: 10.1007/11691617_13.

6. Bottrighi, A., Giordano, L., Molino, G., Montani, S., Terenziani, P., & Torchio, M. (2010). Adopting model checking techniques for clinical guidelines verification. *Artificial Intelligence in Medicine, 48*, 1–19.

7. Cansell, D., & Méry, D. (2008). The Event-B modelling method: Concepts and case studies. In D. Bjørner & M. C. Henson (Eds.), *Monographs in theoretical computer science. Logics of specification languages* (pp. 47–152). Berlin: Springer.

8. Clarke, E. M., Grumberg, O., & Peled, D. (2001). *Model checking.* Cambridge: MIT Press.

9. Ellenbogen, K. A., & Wood, M. A. (2005). *Cardiac pacing and ICDs* (4th ed.). Oxford: Blackwell. ISBN 1-4051-0447-3.

10. Epstein, A. E., DiMarco, J. P., Ellenbogen, K. A., Estes, N. A. M., III, Freedman, R. A., Gettes, L. S., et al. (2008). ACC/AHA/HRS 2008 guidelines for device-based therapy of cardiac rhythm abnormalities: A report of the American College of Cardiology/American Heart Association task force on practice guidelines (writing committee to revise the ACC/AHA/NASPE 2002 guideline update for implantation of cardiac pacemakers and antiarrhythmia devices) developed in collaboration with the American Association for Thoracic Surgery and Society of Thoracic Surgeons. *Journal of the American College of Cardiology, 51*(21), e1–e62.

11. Field, M. J., & Lohr, K. N. (1990) *Clinical practice guidelines: Directions for a new program.* Washington: National Academy Press.

12. Fox, J., Johns, N., & Rahmanzadeh, A. (1998). Disseminating medical knowledge: The proforma approach. *Artificial Intelligence in Medicine, 14*(1–2), 157–182.

13. Hesselson, A. (2003). *Simplified interpretations of pacemaker ECGs.* Oxford: Blackwell. ISBN 978-1-4051-0372-5.

14. Holzmann, G. J. (1997). The model checker SPIN. *IEEE Transactions on Software Engineering, 23*, 279–295.

15. Isern, D., & Moreno, A. (2008). Computer-based execution of clinical guidelines: A review. *International Journal of Medical Informatics, 77*(12), 787–808.

16. Khan, M. G. (2008). *Rapid ECG interpretation.* Clifton: Humana Press.

17. Kosara, R., Miksch, S., Seyfang, A., & Votruba, P. (2002). *Tools for acquiring clinical guidelines in Asbru.*

18. Love, C. J. (2006). *Cardiac pacemakers and defibrillators.* Georgetown: Landes Bioscience. ISBN 1-57059-691-3.

19. Malmivuo, J. (1995). *Bioelectromagnetism.* Oxford: Oxford University Press. ISBN 0-19-505823-2.

20. Marcos, M., Berger, G., van Harmelen, F., ten Teije, A., Roomans, H., & Miksch, S. (2001). Using critiquing for improving medical protocols: Harder than it seems. In *Proceedings of the 8th conference on AI in medicine in Europe: Artificial intelligence medicine*, AIME'01 (pp. 431–441). London: Springer.

21. Méry, D., & Singh, N. K. (2011). Technical report on interpretation of the electrocardiogram (ECG) signal using formal methods. MOSEL-LORIA-INRIA-CNRS: UMR7503-Université Henri Poincaré-Nancy I-Université Nancy II-Institut National Polytechnique de Lorraine. http://hal.inria.fr/inria-00584177/en/.

22. Méry, D., & Singh, N. K. (2012). Medical protocol diagnosis using formal methods. In Z. Liu & A. Wassyng (Eds.), *Lecture notes in computer science: Vol. 7151. Foundations of health informatics engineering and systems* (pp. 1–20). Berlin: Springer.

23. Miksch, S., Hunter, J., & Keravnou, E. T. (Eds.) (2005). In *Lecture notes in computer science: Vol. 3581. Proceedings, 10th conference on artificial intelligence in medicine*, AIME'05, Aberdeen (pp. 23–27). Berlin: Springer.

24. Miller, P. L. (1985). *A critiquing approach to expert computer advice: Attending.* Marshfield: Pitman.

25. Miller, D. W., Frawley, S. J., & Miller, P. L. (1999). Using semantic constraints to help verify the completeness of a computer-based clinical guideline for childhood immunization. *Computer Methods and Programs in Biomedicine, 58*(3), 267–280.

26. Musen, M. A., Tu, S. W., Das, A. K., & Shahar, Y. (1995). A component-based architecture for automation of protocol-directed therapy. In *AIME* (pp. 3–13).

27. Peleg, M., Tu, S., Bury, J., Ciccarese, P., Fox, J., Greenes, R. A., et al. (2003). Comparing computer-interpretable guideline models: A case-study approach. *Journal of the American Medical Informatics Association, 10*, 52–68.

28. Pérez, B., & Porres, I. (2010). Authoring and verification of clinical guidelines: A model driven approach. *Journal of Biomedical Informatics, 43*(4), 520–536.

29. RODIN (2004). Rigorous open development environment for complex systems. http://rodin-b-sharp.sourceforge.net.

30. Rumbaugh, J., Jacobson, I., & Booch, G. (Eds.) (1999). *The unified modeling language reference manual*. Essex: Addison-Wesley Longman.

31. Schmitt, J., Hoffmann, A., Balser, M., Reif, W., & Marcos, M. (2006). Interactive verification of medical guidelines. In J. Misra, T. Nipkow, & E. Sekerinski (Eds.), *Lecture notes in computer science: Vol. 4085. FM 2006: Formal methods* (pp. 32–47). Berlin: Springer. doi:10.1007/11813040_3.

32. Seyfang, A., Miksch, S., Marcos, M., Wittenberg, J., Polo-Conde, C., & Rosenbrand, K. (2006). Bridging the gap between informal and formal guideline representations. In *Proceedings of the 2006 conference on ECAI 2006: 17th European conference on artificial intelligence*, Riva del Garda, August 29–September 1, 2006 (pp. 447–451). Amsterdam: IOS Press.

33. Shahar, Y., Miksch, S., & Johnson, P. (1998). The Asgaard project: A task-specific framework for the application and critiquing of time-oriented clinical guidelines. In *Artificial intelligence in medicine* (pp. 29–51).

34. Shiffman, R. N. (1997). Representation of clinical practice guidelines in conventional and augmented decision tables. *Journal of the American Medical Informatics Association, 4*(5), 382–393.

35. Shiffman, R. N., & Greenes, R. A. (1994). Improving clinical guidelines with logic and decision-table techniques: Application to hepatitis immunization recommendations. *Medical Decision Making, 14*(3), 245–254.

36. Ten Teije, A., Marcos, M., Balser, M., van Croonenborg, J., Duelli, C., van Harmelen, F., et al. (2006). Improving medical protocols by formal methods. *Artificial Intelligence in Medicine, 36*(3), 193–209.

37. van Croonenborg, J., Duelli, C., van Harmelen, F., Jovell, A., Lucas, P., Marcos, M., et al. (2004). Protocure: Supporting the development of medical protocols through formal methods. In *Lecture notes in artificial intelligence. Proceedings of the symposium of computerised protocols and guidelines*, SCPG-04, Prague. Berlin: Springer.

38. Wang, D., Peleg, M., Tu, S. W., Boxwala, A. A., Greenes, R. A., Patel, V. L., et al. (2002). Representation primitives, process models and patient data in computer-interpretable clinical practice guidelines: A literature review of guideline representation models. *International Journal of Medical Informatics, 68*(1–3), 59–70.

39. Warmer, J., & Kleppe, A. (2003). *The object constraint language: Getting your models ready for MDA* (2nd ed.). Boston: Addison-Wesley Longman.

Chapter 11
Conclusion

Abstract This chapter concludes the book through summarising important points of each chapter. The main contribution of this book is to propose the formal methods based development life-cycle and associated techniques and tools, that are exemplified by the grand challenge related to the cardiac pacemaker. Additionally, this book provides a technique for identifying anomalies in the standard ECG protocol through incremental formalisation in Event-B.

11.1 Introduction

Highly critical systems, such as medical, avionic, and automotive systems require high integrity, software reliability, and proof based development for complying with certification standards [2, 5, 8, 9], which evaluate the systems before their usage. In this framework, adaptation of the formal method has become the state-of the-art tech to meet the high demands on safety and reliability by certification bodies [6]. However, adaptation of formal methods significantly complicates the development process of a system due to complexity of the modelling as well as a system itself. Refinement based modelling techniques reduce verification effort significantly by designing the whole system using the stepwise development process. The complete system is verified with the help of theorem prover, model checker and animation tools. Moreover, critical systems can be analysed already at the early stages of their development, which allow to explore conceptual errors, ambiguities, requirement correctness and design flaws before implementation of the actual system, and this approach helps to correct errors more easily and with less cost.

This book presents a new development life-cycle methodology, which is an extension of the waterfall model for developing the critical systems, where each phase has used different kinds of techniques based on formal techniques. In current system development process, formal methods are used only at the early stage of the system development for verifying the requirements. We have proposed new development methodology, which supports formal methods at every stage of the system development process. We have not only used existing development life-cycle steps, but also introduced some new steps in the life-cycle methodology. The proposed new recursive approach is based on refinement techniques to build the whole system from requirement analysis to code generation. New introduced techniques and tools

N.K. Singh, *Using Event-B for Critical Device Software Systems*,
DOI 10.1007/978-1-4471-5260-6_11, © Springer-Verlag London 2013

based on formal methods support refinement based formal development, essential verification, and validation steps and automatic code generation in the process of critical system development. The proposed techniques and tools are the development methodology, framework for real-time animator [15], refinement chart [24], automatic code generation tools [3, 14, 16, 17], and formal logic based heart model for closed-loop modelling [19, 21, 22].

In Chap. 1, we have given a list of objectives, which all are covered in this book through giving a new development life-cycle methodology and a set of associated techniques and tools for developing the critical systems. Assessment of the development methodology and a set of techniques and tools are given through well known case study related to the medical domain. This work has established a unified theory for the critical system development, and proposed techniques and tools fulfil the other objectives. We have given a rigorous approach for the system development rather than the traditional development of critical systems. In traditional development, formal methods are used to provide safety assurances and to meet the requirements of the standard of the certification bodies. Our new approach based completely on formal techniques, develops the whole system rigorously from requirement analysis to code implementation, satisfying all requirements of the standard certification bodies. In addition, the methodology provides a safety assessment approach to analyse the whole development life cycle of the critical system, which meets requirements of the certification standard bodies.

Complexity of the critical system makes, it is hard to understand and to verify. Several approaches exist for the verification of critical systems, including model checking, theorem proving, or simulation based validation. There exists a vast variety of problems related to the critical systems and several solutions for each problem. Rigorous reasoning about the system behaviour is required to ensure that a desired behaviour is achieved. Event-B is a modelling language, which describes a system abstractly, and introduces system details through refinement steps to obtain the final concrete system. The Rodin [1, 25] tools provide significant automated proof support for generating the proof obligations and discharging them. Generated proof obligations help to understand the complexity of the problem and to ensure the correctness of the system. In the following sections, we have made several contributions towards an integration of refinement based development using Event-B with formal specification, verification and code implementation for the critical systems.

11.2 Life-Cycle Methodology

A major step forward is the new life-cycle methodology, exploits the mathematical base to carry out a complete rigorous proof based system development using formal techniques in every step from requirement analysis to automatic code generation. This life-cycle methodology is used for developing the critical systems for obtaining the certificate standards, such as IEC-62304 [7] and the Common Criteria [2, 4, 12]. This development methodology combines the refinement approach with verification tool, model checker tool, real-time animator, and finally generates the source code using the automatic tools. System development process is concurrently assessed by safety assessment approach [11] to comply with certification standards. Applying these new approaches for highly critical systems have many benefits, i.e. the exposure of errors, which might not have been detected without formal methods. The guidance of NITRD [6] allows adoption of formal methods into an established set of processes for development and verification of a high confidence medical device to be an evolutionary refinement rather than an abrupt change of methodology.

11.3 Techniques and Tools

The book work also advances the development of new techniques and tools for supporting the new life-cycle methodology, and is explained in subsequent phases:

Real time animator is used to validate the formal model with real-time data set at an early stage of system development without generating the source code [15], and to bridge the gap between software engineers and stakeholders to build quality system and discover all ambiguous informations from the requirements. The combined approach of formal verification and real-time animation allows the systematic development of a clear, concise, precise and unambiguous specification of a software system and enables software engineers to animate the formal specification at an early stage of the development. Moreover, there are scientific and legal applications as well, where the formal model based animation can be used to simulate (or emulate) certain scenarios to glean more information or better understandings of the system to improve the final given system.

Another significant contribution towards improving techniques and tools section is the "refinement chart", which is used to present the whole system using layering approach in graphical block diagrams, where functional blocks are divided into multiple simpler blocks in a new refinement level, without changing the original behaviour of the system. The refinement chart offers a clear view of assistance in "system" integration. This approach also gives a clear view about the system assembling based on operating modes and different kinds of features. This is an important issue not only for being able to derive system-level performance and correctness guarantees, but also for being able to assemble components in a cost-effective manner. The complexity of design is reduced by structuring systems using modes and by detailing this design using refinement.

Automatic code generation from a proved formal model to the target programming language is an essential step for system implementation, which is an equally important contribution. We have developed the main principles, rules, and implementation solutions for the translation tool, and also code verification techniques for generating target programming language (C, C++, Java and C#) code satisfying Event-B specifications [3, 14, 16, 17]. The syntax adopted is restrictive, but with many salient and essential characteristics for the most numeric applications, supports powerful static-analysis methods and generates fast and safe source code in the target programming languages. The benefits of developing and enhancing the translation tool [3, 14, 16, 17] presented stem primarily from their increased support for automated translation between the two components of a formal model and target programming language. The adaptations of the translation rules require more complete experiments, especially with large formal models for checking the impact on the execution time for some specific platforms. The gains rely then on the guarantees provided using a formal method and on the certification level which can be obtained by this way. As far as we know, only few formal methods support code generation, which is as time and space efficient as handwritten code.

Development of an environment for closed-loop modelling using formal techniques [21] is our another remarkable contribution of this book. We have presented a methodology for modelling a mathematical heart model based on logico-mathematical theory. The most important goal is that this formal model helps to obtain a certification for the medical devices related to the heart system such as cardiac pacemaker and ICDs. It can be also used as a diagnostic tool to identify a critical state of the patient using a patient environment model. The heart model is based on electrocardiography analysis, which models the heart circulatory system at the cellular level. This has been one of the most challenging problems to validate and verify the correct behaviour of the developed system model (a cardiac pacemaker or ICDs) under biological environment (i.e. heart). This approach for formalising and reasoning about impulse propagation into the heart system through the conduction network. The heart model suggests that such an approach can yield a viable model that can be subjected to useful validation against medical device software at an early stage in the development process (i.e. cardiac pacemaker). The heart model is verified with the help of physiologist and cardiologist experts.

11.4 Applications

Assessment of proposed development life-cycle methodology and a set of associated techniques and tools are made through the development of the industrial-scale case study, which cover medical domains. The well-known case study is the cardiac pacemaker [13, 15, 18]. We have applied development methodology and associated techniques and tools for system implementation. The combined approaches of the formal verification, and validation, refinement chart, real-time animator, and automatic code generation, cover enumerated claims like certifiable assurance and safety, error-free system development and system integration. Refinement chart specially covers component-based design frameworks and decomposition, integration of critical infrastructure and device integration. Our case study on cardiac pacemaker illustrates the potential value of a formal specification, and its subsequent animation can bring to the comprehension and clarification of the informal requirements. The case study has shown that requirement specifications could be used directly in real-time environment without modifications for automatic test result evaluation using our approach. We can see from our pacemaker case study that all these claims help to design an error-free system and different phases of the system have been shown by refinements in form of formal development as well as refinement charts. We have presented evidence that such an analysis is fruitful for both formal and non-formal group of people. The second observation from our experiments is that development of multiple models helped us not only find errors in the requirements documents but also gave us an opportunity to better understand intricate requirements such as the control algorithm of a critical system. Moreover, we believe that the effort needed is commensurate with the benefits we derive from developing the multiple models.

In order to assess the overall utility of our approach, a selection of the results of the formalisation and verification steps have been presented to a group of pacemaker developers (French-Italian based pacemaker company). The developers are satisfied by the result of pacemaker development using this methodology in sense of incremental development as well as integration of hardware and software. They really agreed on the refinement charts for showing operating mode relation and their mode transitions. Throughout our case study, we have shown formal specification and verification of the cardiac pacemaker system and the models must be validated to ensure that they meet requirements. Hence, validation must be carried out by both formal modelling and domain experts. Based on the experiment described above and our conclusions we are convinced of the usefulness on certain areas, and therefore, we are considering to use this methodology for designing the highly critical systems. The proposed framework and developed techniques and tools offer system development from formal verification to code generation, which offer to obtain that challenge of complying with FDA's QSR, ISO/IEC and IEEE standards quality system directives [2, 5, 8–10] and help to get certification for the highly complex critical systems.

11.5 Medical Protocol

This book also contributes in the area of formal representation of the medical protocol. The formal model of medical protocol is verified, and this verified model is not only feasible but also useful for improving the existing medical protocol. We have fully formalised a real-world medical protocol (ECG interpretation) in an incremental refinement-based formalisation process, and we have used proof tools to systematically analyse whether the formalisation complies with certain medically relevant protocol properties [20, 23]. The formal verification process has discovered a number of anomalies. We have also discovered a hierarchical structure for the ECG interpretation efficiently that helps to discover a set of conditions that can be very helpful to diagnose particular disease at early stage of the diagnosis without using multiple diagnosis. Our hierarchical tree structure provides more concrete solutions for the ECG interpretation protocol and helps to improve the original ECG interpretation protocol. The main objective of this approach is to test correctness and consistency of the medical protocol. This approach is not only for diagnosis purpose, but it may be applicable to covering a large group of other categories (i.e. treatment, management, prevention, counselling, evaluation, etc.)[1] related to the medical protocols.

References

1. Abrial, J.-R. (2010). *Modeling in Event-B: System and software engineering* (1st ed.). New York: Cambridge University Press.
2. CC. Common criteria. http://www.commoncriteriaportal.org/.
3. EB2ALL (2011). Automatic code generation from Event-B to many programming languages. http://eb2all.loria.fr/.
4. Farn, K.-J., Lin, S.-K., & Fung, A. R.-W. (2004). A study on information security management system evaluation—assets, threat and vulnerability. *Computer Standards & Interfaces, 26*(6), 501–513.
5. FDA. Food and Drug Administration. http://www.fda.gov/.
6. High Confidence Software and Systems Coordinating Group (2009). *High-confidence medical devices: Cyber-physical systems for 21st century health care* (Technical report). NITRD. http://www.nitrd.gov/About/MedDevice-FINAL1-web.pdf.
7. IEC62304 (2006). International Electrotechnical Commission: Medical device software—software life-cycle processes. http://www.iec.ch/.
8. IEEE-SA. IEEE Standards Association. http://standards.ieee.org/.
9. ISO. International Organization for Standardization. http://www.iso.org/.
10. Keatley, K. L. (1999). A review of the FDA draft guidance document for software validation: Guidance for industry. *Quality Assurance, 7*(1), 49–55.
11. Leveson, N. G. (1991). Software safety in embedded computer systems. *Communications of the ACM, 34*, 34–46.
12. Mead, N. R., Mead, N. R., & Scondras, C. (2003). *International liability issues for software quality.*
13. Méry, D., & Singh, N. K. (2009). *Pacemaker's functional behaviors in Event-B* (Research report). MOSEL-LORIA-INRIA-CNRS: UMR7503-Université Henri Poincaré-Nancy I-Université Nancy II-Institut National Polytechnique de Lorraine. http://hal.inria.fr/inria-00419973/en/.
14. Méry, D., & Singh, N. K. (2010). *EB2C: A tool for Event-B to C conversion support.* Poster and tool demo submission, published in a CNR technical report in SEFM.
15. Méry, D., & Singh, N. K. (2010). Real-time animation for formal specification. In M. Aiguier, F. Bretaudeau, & D. Krob (Eds.), *Complex systems design & management* (pp. 49–60). Berlin: Springer.
16. Méry, D., & Singh, N. K. (2011). Automatic code generation from Event-B models. In *Proceedings of the second symposium on information and communication technology*, SoICT'11 (pp. 179–188). New York: ACM.
17. Méry, D., & Singh, N. K. (2011). *EB2J: Code generation from Event-B to Java.* Short paper presented at the 14th Brazilian symposium on formal methods, SBMF'11.
18. Méry, D., & Singh, N. K. (2011). Functional behavior of a cardiac pacing system. *International Journal of Discrete Event Control Systems, 1*(2), 129–149.
19. Méry, D., & Singh, N. K. (2011). Technical report on formalisation of the heart using analysis of conduction time and velocity of the electrocardiography and cellular-automata. MOSEL-LORIA-INRIA-CNRS: UMR7503-Université Henri Poincaré-Nancy I-Université Nancy II-Institut National Polytechnique de Lorraine. http://hal.inria.fr/inria-00600339/en/.

---

[1] http://www.guideline.gov/.

20. Méry, D., & Singh, N. K. (2011). Technical report on interpretation of the electrocardiogram (ECG) signal using formal methods. MOSEL-LORIA-INRIA-CNRS: UMR7503-Université Henri Poincaré-Nancy I-Université Nancy II-Institut National Polytechnique de Lorraine. http://hal.inria.fr/inria-00584177/en/.
21. Méry, D., & Singh, N. K. (2012). Closed-loop modeling of cardiac pacemaker and heart. In *Foundations of health informatics engineering and systems.*
22. Méry, D., & Singh, N. K. (2012). Formalization of heart models based on the conduction of electrical impulses and cellular automata. In Z. Liu & A. Wassyng (Eds.), *Lecture notes in computer science: Vol. 7151. Foundations of health informatics engineering and systems* (pp. 140–159). Berlin: Springer.
23. Méry, D., & Singh, N. K. (2012). Medical protocol diagnosis using formal methods. In Z. Liu & A. Wassyng (Eds.), *Lecture notes in computer science: Vol. 7151. Foundations of health informatics engineering and systems* (pp. 1–20). Berlin: Springer.
24. Méry, D., & Singh, N. K. (2013). Formal specification of medical systems by proof-based refinement. *ACM Transactions on Embedded Computing Systems, 12*(1), 15:1–15:25.
25. RODIN (2004). Rigorous open development environment for complex systems. http://rodin-b-sharp.sourceforge.net.

Appendix
Certification Standards

A.1 What Are Standards?

Standards are documented agreements containing technical specifications, which produce precise criteria, consistent rules, procedures to ensure reliability, software processes, methods, products, services and use of products are fit for their purpose in this world. Standards include a set of issues corresponding to the product functionality and compatibility, facilitate interoperability, including designing, developing, enhancing, and maintaining. A set of protocols and guidelines, which are produced by the standards, are consistent and universally acceptable for product development. Standards allow to understand the quality of different products for competing with them and provides a way to verify the credibility of new products [13, 18]. A basic definition of standards is defined by ISO [18] as follows:

Standards are documented agreements containing technical specifications or other precise criteria to be used consistently as rules, guidelines, or definitions of characteristics, to ensure that materials, products, processes and services are fit for their purpose.

Different nations tend to have different views of what a standard is and what standardisation is for. Standards are varied from nation to nation. For instance, UK and Europe standards define a product. Implementation dependencies should be reduced, and rigorous testing of products should satisfy the standards. The standard is a description of an artifact that is to be built precisely according to the provisions of the standard.

Since software plays an increasingly important role in software-based products related to medical, automotive and avionic systems. Because of the uncertainty of the reliability and compatibility of these software-based products, different kinds of national and international standards related to certification bodies (FDA's QSR and ISO's 13485, etc.) need effective means for ensuring that the developed software-based system is safe and reliable.

There is a wide variety of standards bodies. More than 300 software standards and 50 organisations are developing software standards [8]. Standards come in many different flavours, for example, de-facto standards, local, national and international

N.K. Singh, *Using Event-B for Critical Device Software Systems*,
DOI 10.1007/978-1-4471-5260-6, © Springer-Verlag London 2013

Table A.1 Standards organisations

AIAA	American Institute of Aeronautics and Astronauts
ANS	American Nuclear Society
ANSI	American National Standards Institute
ASTM	American Society for Testing and Materials
BSI	British Standards Institution
CCITT	Telecommunication Standardization Bureau
CEN	European Committee for Standardization
CSA	Canadian Standards Association
CSE	Communications Security Establishment
DEF	British Defence Standards
DIN	Drug Information Association
DIN	Deutsches Institute für Normung
DoD	U.S. Department of Defense
ISO	International Organization for Standardization
IEC	International Electrotechnical Committee
IEEE	Institute of Electronic and Electrical Engineers
CC	Common Criteria
FDA	The Food & Drug Administration

standards. Some of the standards are more specific related to the defence, financial, medical, nuclear, transportation, etc. Some of the major software standards are given in Table A.1 [8].

In the next sections, we describe here only international standards related to the information technology by ISO/IEC (the International Organization for Standardization/International Electrotechnical Commission), IEEE (Institute of Electronic and Electrical Engineers), FDA (Food and Drug Administration) and CC (Common Criteria).

A.2 ISO/IEC Standards

IEC (International Electrotechnical Commission) is established in 1906 and ISO (International Organization for Standardization) is a non-governmental organisation is established in 1947 [6, 8, 18]. The ISO is a worldwide federation of national standards bodies from more than 140 countries, one from each country, which facilitate the international coordination and unification of the industrial standards [18]. The primary preoccupation of international standards is to eliminate *technical barriers to trade*; the view is that world-wide standards help rationalise the international trading process [6, 10].

There are number of standards addressing safety and security of a system related to the software development. For example, avionics RTCA-Do-178B [22] or the

IEC 61508 [9, 12] as the fundamental standard for functional safety of the E/E/EP systems [9, 12]. The IEC 62304 [11] standard is for software life-cycles of medical device development, which addresses to achieve more specific goals through standard process activity. The process standard IEC 62304 [11] is a collection of two other standards ISO 14791 and ISO 13485, where ISO 14791 standards are for quality, and ISO 13485 is for risk management. Here, we have presented a brief introduction about IEC 61508 and IEC 62304 standards, which may be achieved using our proposed methodologies.

A.2.1 IEC 61508—Software Safety in E/E/EP Systems

Systems constitute of electrical and/or electronic elements, which can be used to perform safety functions in many application sectors. ISO/IEC 61508 [9, 12] constitutes a generic approach for all safety life cycle activities of the electrical and/or electronic and/or programmable electronic (E/E/PE) systems to perform safety functions. It provides a generic development approach for achieving a rational and consistent technical policy for all kinds of electrical systems to the safety-related system. This standard provides some frameworks to consider safe and reliable for the safety-related systems that are developed in other technologies. It covers a wide variety of complexity, hazard and risk potentials related to the E/E/PE systems. Main objective of this standard is to define a life-cycle for safety-critical software considering best practices and recommendations from early phases of requirements and development to operation, maintenance and disposal. A complete detail description about *Software Architecture Design* related to the properties for systematic integrity, software design and development are given in a tabular form [9, 10, 12]. The main objective of the IEC 61508 is to provide software architecture design, including design activity of the system, which are defined as follows:

- Selection of techniques and verify the satisfiable level according to the safety requirements
- Partitioning of the system
- Software/hardware interaction
- Unambiguous representation of the architecture
- Treatment of safety integrity of data
- Specification of architecture integration tests

Besides generic quality goals, the IEC 61508 also covers process dependencies and concrete characteristics of the architecture related to the completeness and correctness according to the requirements, no design faults, simple modular and structure-able, satisfiable desired behaviour, verifiable and testable design, and fault tolerance against system failure due to common cause [10, 12].

A.2.2 IEC 62304—Process Requirements for Medical Device Software

The IEC 62304 [11] standard specifies a framework of the life cycle processes for medical devices, which helps to design a safe system. All necessary requirements for each life cycle process are provided by the IEC 62304. Life cycle process is divided into a subset of activities and is controlled by the risk management and quality management. The risk-management process is defined by the ISO 14971 standard and quality management is defined by the ISO 13485 standards.

The ISO 14971 and ISO 13485 standards [18] provide risk-based quality management that determines the required rigour of software quality assurance from the risk, which appears from a medical device in form of undesired behaviour of the system. Software can be an important part of a medical device providing safety and effectiveness of the software-based a medical device requires to fulfil requirements and to use of software without any risk. When a software is contributing to a hazard, which is determined by hazard identification activity of the risk-management process. Hazards could be indirectly caused by software, which can be considered that software is a contributing factor. The use of software to control risk is made during the risk control activity and risk management process under consideration of the ISO 14971 and ISO 13485 standards, respectively. The software-development process consists of a number of activities related to the service or maintenance of a medical device system, including software updates. All these activities are also considered as an important task of the software-development process. The IEC 62304 mentions six sub-activities for the architectural design step, which are as follows:

- Realisation of the requirements
- Interface design
- Specification of functional and non-functional software components
- Specification of the environment of software components
- Partitioning due to the risk mitigation strategy
- Verification of the architecture

The software safety classification ranges from A—no harm or injury—to C—death or severe injury is possible. The classification defines the principle level of rigour, and consequently, the efforts to be undertaken, is required for all software development and maintenance activities [10]. The IEC 62304 standards provide assurance for medical software system and guarantees that the software does not contribute to hazardous failure of the system due to its systematic safety-oriented process and implementation of the functional requirements are performed carefully for the required activities. The requirement analysis, architecture, design, implementation and integration are main phases of the development process for handling the complexity of a system. Each phase of the development process is controlled by the IEC 62304, which recommends activities to plan, track, control and communicate possible problems to prevent the risk of systematic errors. The complete process development with risk management for a medical device is described in [8, 11].

A.3 IEEE Standards Association

The Institute of Electrical and Electronics Engineers (IEEE) standard [13] provides the safety assurance level for industries, including: power and energy, biomedical and health care, information technology, transportation, nanotechnology, telecommunication, information assurance, and many more. The IEEE standard is internationally recognised and technical experts from all over the world participate in the development of it [13, 17]. The IEEE standards documents are prepared within the IEEE societies. The IEEE standards are developed by both groups of experts related to the subject within the IEEE societies and outside from the IEEE societies. The IEEE societies built a group from the broad range of individuals and organisations from worldwide with different kinds of expert to assist in standards development and standards-related collaboration. This group helps for innovation and expansion of technologies on the criteria of international market demand related to the safety systems. The IEEE standard is approved by authority and considers the users recommendations before apply into the development process. All these standards are reviewed at least every five years to qualify the new amendments in the systems. IEEE societies provide standards for almost every area of engineering, which are enumerated as follows:

- Aerospace Electronics
- Antennas & Propagation
- Batteries
- Communications
- Computer Technology
- Consumer Electronics
- Electromagnetic Compatibility
- Green & Clean Technology
- Healthcare IT
- Industry Applications
- Instrumentation & Measurement
- National Electrical Safety Code
- Nuclear Power
- Power & Energy
- Power Electronics
- Smart Grid
- Software & Systems Engineering
- Transportation
- Wired & Wireless

We have given some basic details about related to the Software & Systems Engineering, which are defined as follows:

Fig. A.1 The standards
development life-cycle of
IEEE

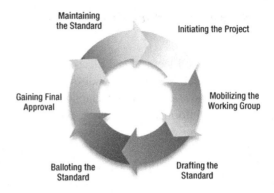

A.3.1 IEEE Standard 1012

The IEEE Standard 1012 is particularly used for both critical and non-critical software related to the Software Verification and Validation Plans (SVVP). Critical software is *software in which a failure could have an impact on safety or could cause large, financial or social losses* [14]. The SVVP mainly used for first, verification of the software product according to the previously defined life-cycle phases, and second validation of the final product according to the existing software and system requirements [16].

A.3.2 IEEE Standard 730

The IEEE Standard 730 [15] is related to the Software Quality Assurance Plans (SQAP), which provides minimum acceptable requirements for the software. This standard helps specially for development and maintenance of the critical software. A subset of requirements of this standard is applicable to non-critical and already developed software.

A.3.3 IEEE Standard 1074

The IEEE Standard 1074 is used for developing a process of a software project life cycle. This standard mainly controls the architecture of the process, which is particularly useful for organisation that is responsible to complete development process of the software projects [17]. The development life cycle of the IEEE standards is depicted in Fig. A.1, which describes a process for developing the IEEE standards using six stages life cycle under the fixed time frame along with the effective and trusted process. A detailed description about each level of the development life cycle of the IEEE standards is available in [13].

A.4 FDA

The Food and Drug Administration (FDA) [20] is established by US Department of Health and Human Services (HHS) in 1930 for regulating the various kinds of product like food, cosmetics, medical devices, etc. The FDA is now using standards in the regulatory review process to provide safety to the public before using any product. The FDA allows manufacturers to submit the declaration of conformity to satisfy premarket review requirements. The FDA provides some guidelines on the recognition use of and consensus standards. The FDA is interested in standards because they can help to serve as a common yardstick to assist with mutual recognition, based on the signed Mutual Recognition Agreement between the European Union and United States. More than ever before, standards will have the more prominent role for the review of medical devices. The FDA also recognises ISO/IEC and IEEE standards [13, 14]. Basic goals of the FDA standard are:

- To promote health by reviewing research and approving new products.
- To ensure foods and drugs are safe and properly labelled.
- To work with other nations to "reduce the burden of regulation".
- To cooperate with scientific experts and consumers to effectively carry out these obligations.

The FDA standard classifies the medical devices based on risk and use of medical devices. The FDA provides some standard guidelines for medical devices, and medical devices have required to meet these standards. Time to time lots of amendments have been done in the FDA standards [7, 20] according to the use of medical devices to provide safety.

The Center for Devices and Radiological Health (CDRH) [5] is the branch of the FDA, which is responsible for ensuring the safety of medical devices and eliminating unnecessary radiation from the medical products [7, 19, 20]. It provides standards for medical products from the simple toothbrush to complex devices such as pacemakers. The CDRH [5] also checks the safety performance of non-medical devices, which emit certain types of electromagnetic radiation like cellular phones, screening equipment, microwave ovens, etc. The CDRH has some standards, which are used to describe many aspects of a medical device related to premarket and post-market issues. Here, we briefly mention some basic concepts [7, 20] involved in FDA regulation for medical devices:

- *Class I* devices are defined as non-life sustaining. These products are the least complicated and their failure poses little risk.
- *Class II* devices are more complicated and present more risk than Class I, though are also non-life sustaining. They are also subject to any specific performance standards.
- *Class III* devices sustain or support life, so that their failure is life threatening.

Table A.2 CC user groups (consumers, developers and evaluators)

	Consumers	Developers	Evaluators
Part 1: Introduction and General Model	For background information and reference purposes	For background information and reference for the development of requirements and formulating security specifications for TOEs	For background information and reference purposes. Guidance structure for PPs and STs
Part 2: Security Functional Requirements	For guidance and reference when formulating statements of requirements for security functions	For reference when interpreting statements of requirements and formulating functional specifications of TOEs	Mandatory statement of evaluation criteria when determining whether TOE effectively meets claimed security functions
Part 3: Security Assurance Requirements	For guidance when determining required levels of assurance	For reference when interpreting statements of assurance requirements and determining assurance approaches of TOEs	Mandatory statement of evaluation criteria when determining the assurance of TOEs and when evaluating PPs and STs

A.5 Common Criteria

The Common Criteria (CC) [1] is an international standard that allows evaluation of security for IT products and technology. The CC is an international standard (ISO/IEC 15408) [18] for computer security certification. The CC is a collection of existing criteria: European (Information Technology Security Evaluation Criteria (ITSEC)), US (Trusted Computer Security Evaluation Criteria (TCSEC)) and Canadian (Canadian Trusted Computer Product Evaluation Criteria (CTCPEC)) [2–4]. The CC [1] contributes for developing an international standard and provides a way to worldwide mutual recognition and evaluation results.

The Common Criteria enable an objective evaluation to validate that a particular product or system satisfies a defined set of security requirements. The CC provides a framework for computer users, vendors and testing organisations for fulfil their requirements and ensure that the process of specification, implementation and testing of the product has been conducted in a rigorous and standard manner. The CC has mainly three parts, which has been described in Table A.2 to show the interest of three different kinds of users (Consumers, Developers and Evaluators) [2].

CC objectives [2–4] are described as follows:

- To ensure that evaluations of Information Technology (IT) products and protection profiles are performed to high and consistent standards and are seen to contribute significantly to confidence in the security of those products and profiles.
- To improve the availability of evaluated, security-enhanced IT products and protection profiles.
- To eliminate the burden of duplicating evaluations of IT products and protection profiles.
- To continuously improve the efficiency and cost-effectiveness of the evaluation and certification/validation process for IT products and protection profiles.

A.5.1 CC Evaluation Assurance Level (EAL)

The Common Criteria (CC) certification provided insurance coverage by measuring the level of security based the likelihood of threats and their impact. The Common Criteria defines two classes of security requirements: functional and assurance. The objectives of these two classes vary depending upon the security classification level. There are seven levels of assurance that is known as Evaluation Assurance Levels (EALs). The numerical rating of the EAL [4] describes development and presentation of the product's evaluation. Each EAL corresponds to the Security Assurance Requirements (SARs), which cover the product development within the level of strictness. The assurance level from EAL1 to EAL7 represents an increasing order of evaluation assurance level. In the EALs, the first level being when the threat and impact are very low and the seventh is when the threat and impact are very strong, means the higher level provides more confidence and assurance safety. The last level of EAL involves verification of the developed software based on logical reasoning and theorem proving techniques. Higher level of EALs do not necessarily imply "better security", they only mean that the security claimed is extensively verified. All the Evaluation Assurance Levels (EALs) [21] of safety are described as follows:

EAL1: Functionally Tested. It applies when you require confidence in a product's correct operation, but do not view threats to security as serious. An evaluation at this level should provide evidence that the target of evaluation functions in a manner consistent with its documentation, and that it provides useful protection against identified threats.

EAL2: Structurally Tested. It applies when developers or users require low to moderate independently assured security, but the complete development record is not readily available. This situation may arise when there is limited developer access or when there is an effort to secure legacy systems.

EAL3: Methodically Tested and Checked. It applies when developers or users require a moderate level of independently assured security and require a thorough investigation of the target of evaluation and its development, without substantial re-engineering.

EAL4: Methodically Designed, Tested, and Reviewed. It applies when developers or users require moderate to high independently assured security in conventional commodity products and are prepared to incur additional security-specific engineering costs.

EAL5: Semi-formally Designed and Tested. It applies when developers or users require high, independently assured security in a planned development and require a rigorous development approach that does not incur unreasonable costs from specialist security engineering techniques.

EAL6: Semi-formally Verified Design and Tested. It applies when developing security targets of evaluation for application in high-risk situations where the value of the protected assets justifies the additional costs.

EAL7: Formally Verified Design and Tested. It applies to the development of security targets of evaluation for application in extremely high-risk situations, as well as when the high value of the assets justifies the higher costs.

References

1. CC. Common criteria. http://www.commoncriteriaportal.org/.
2. CC (2009). Common criteria for information technology evaluation, part 1: Introduction and general model. http://www.iec.ch/.
3. CC (2009). Common criteria for information technology security evaluation, part 2: Security functional requirements. http://www.iec.ch/.
4. CC (2009). Common criteria for information technology security evaluation, part 3: Security assurance components. http://www.iec.ch/.
5. CDRH (2006). Safety of marketed medical devices. Center for Devices and Radiological Health, US FDA.
6. Duce, D. A. (1997). Formal methods and standards: An idiosyncratic view. In *Proceedings of the 2nd BCS-FACS conference on northern formal methods*, 2FACS'97 (p. 5). Swinton: British Computer Society.
7. FDA. Food and Drug Administration. http://www.fda.gov/.
8. Fries, R. C. (2011). *Handbook of medical device design*. New York: Dekker.
9. Gall, H. (2008). Functional safety IEC 61508/IEC 61511 the impact to certification and the user. In *Proceedings of the 2008 IEEE/ACS international conference on computer systems and applications*, AICCSA'08 (pp. 1027–1031). Washington: IEEE Comput. Soc.
10. Huhn, M., & Zechner, A. (2010). Arguing for software quality in an IEC 62304 compliant development process. In T. Margaria & B. Steffen (Eds.), *Lecture notes in computer science: Vol. 6416. Leveraging applications of formal methods, verification, and validation* (pp. 296–311). Berlin: Springer.
11. IEC62304 (2006). International Electrotechnical Commission: Medical device software—software life-cycle processes. http://www.iec.ch/.
12. IEC61508 (2008). IEC functional safety and IEC 61508: Working draft on functional safety of electrical/electronic/programmable electronic safety-related systems. http://www.iec.ch/.
13. IEEE-SA. IEEE Standards Association. http://standards.ieee.org/.
14. IEEE Std. 610.12-1990 (1990). IEEE standard glossary of software engineering terminology (p. 1).
15. IEEE Std. 730-1998. IEEE standard for software quality assurance plans. http://standards.ieee.org/.
16. IEEE Std. 1012-1998. IEEE standard for software verification and validation. http://standards.ieee.org/.

17. IEEE Std. 1074-1997. IEEE standard for developing software life cycle processes. http://standards.ieee.org/.

18. ISO. International Organization for Standardization. http://www.iso.org/.

19. Jetley, R., Purushothaman Iyer, S., & Jones, P. (2006). A formal methods approach to medical device review. *Computer, 39*(4), 61–67.

20. Keatley, K. L. (1999). A review of the FDA draft guidance document for software validation: Guidance for industry. *Quality Assurance, 7*(1), 49–55.

21. Mead, N. R., Mead, N. R., & Scondras, C. (2003). *International liability issues for software quality.*

22. RTCA (1992). Do-178B, software considerations in airborne systems and equipment certification. Committee: SC-167. http://www.rtca.org/.

Index

Printed in the United States
By Bookmasters

Printed in the United States
By Bookmasters